Psychopathology of Rare and Unusual Syndromes

Psychopathology of Rare and Unusual Syndromes

Femi Oyebode
University of Birmingham

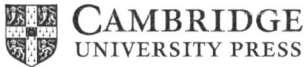

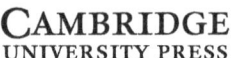

CAMBRIDGE
UNIVERSITY PRESS

University Printing House, Cambridge CB2 8BS, United Kingdom

One Liberty Plaza, 20th Floor, New York, NY 10006, USA

477 Williamstown Road, Port Melbourne, VIC 3207, Australia

314–321, 3rd Floor, Plot 3, Splendor Forum, Jasola District Centre, New Delhi – 110025, India

103 Penang Road, #05–06/07, Visioncrest Commercial, Singapore 238467

Cambridge University Press is part of the University of Cambridge.

It furthers the University's mission by disseminating knowledge in the pursuit of education, learning, and research at the highest international levels of excellence.

www.cambridge.org
Information on this title: www.cambridge.org/9781108716772
DOI: 10.1017/9781108591652

First published 2021

A catalogue record for this publication is available from the British Library.

Library of Congress Cataloging-in-Publication Data
Names: Oyebode, Femi, author.
Title: Psychopathology of rare and unusual syndromes / Femi Oyebode.
Description: Cambridge, United Kingdom ; New York, NY : Cambridge University Press, [2021] | Includes bibliographical references and index.
Identifiers: LCCN 2021024682 (print) | LCCN 2021024683 (ebook) | ISBN 9781108716772 (paperback) | ISBN 9781108591652 (ebook)
Subjects: MESH: Mental Disorders – physiopathology | Rare Diseases – physiopathology | BISAC: PSYCHOLOGY / Mental Health | PSYCHOLOGY / Mental Health
Classification: LCC RC454 (print) | LCC RC454 (ebook) | NLM WM 140 | DDC 616.89–dc23
LC record available at https://lccn.loc.gov/2021024682
LC ebook record available at https://lccn.loc.gov/2021024683

ISBN 978-1-108-71677-2 Paperback

....

Contents

'Rare and unusual is often precious. So is this book which contains colourful descriptions of psychiatric conditions and phenomena that are not common in everyday clinical practice but when encountered remind us why we chose psychiatry as a profession and why the study of the human mind is so interesting and challenging.'

Aleksandar Janca, Emeritus Professor, University of Western Australia

'In *Psychopathology of Uncommon Rare and Unusual Syndromes*, Professor Oyebode has produced a great masterpiece. Each of the conditions in this book has been comprehensively described and thoroughly researched, each syndrome replete with historical and contemporary case examples, thus enabling vivid impressions to be formed in the minds of the reader. While actual aetiologies are often unclear, the author has integrated philosophical, psychodynamic and biological theories to explain these conditions. What shines through is the author's immense literary talents, his love for writing, teaching, researching and his enthusiasm in sharing his keen observations of the phenomenology of psychiatric disorders with his readers.

This book is destined to become a classic. I highly recommend it as a "must read" for every student and practitioner of psychiatry. I cannot wait to get hold of a copy for myself.'

Leslie Lim, Associate Professor, Senior Consultant Psychiatrist, Singapore General Hospital

Preface

This book focuses on psychiatric phenomena that are typically regarded as rare and unusual. These phenomena include the delusional misidentification syndromes, various abnormalities of perception such as Charles Bonnet syndrome, multimodal perceptual experiences such as synaesthesia, abnormalities of the self such as autoscopy and abnormalities of experience of the body such as Côtard syndrome. These phenomena, sometimes termed syndromes, are of great theoretical and conceptual interest to psychiatrists precisely because they are often discrete abnormalities that transcend diagnostic categories but yet allow for the opportunity to carefully examine and elucidate fundamental aspects of abnormal phenomena.

The current preoccupation with nosology, with the categorization of disorders, has resulted in a premature assumption that the only underlying mechanisms worthy of study are those which relate to disease processes to the exclusion of the possibility of carefully studying elemental abnormal phenomena with a view to furthering our understanding of the underlying processes and mechanisms that make these phenomena possible.

In this book, these various and disparate conditions are explored in detail, examining their conceptual value, their relationship to other more common and mundane phenomena, while at the same time discussing what we know about their underlying neuropsychology, the neural mechanisms that are likely to be at play and the neuropsychiatric conditions that form the structural and, potentially, the functional bases of these phenomena.

To illustrate these points, take as an example the delusional misidentification syndromes (Capgras, Frègoli, delusion of intermetamorphosis and reduplicative paramnesia). The inter-relationships between the basic phenomena are described and their neuropsychiatric and functional psychiatric settings explored. The express purpose is to see how the structural and functional brain abnormalities relate to the apparent impairments of face processing and face recognition systems and how these jointly result in psychopathological abnormalities, namely various kinds of delusions.

The aim of this book is ambitious to the degree that the goal is to make the case that discrete phenomena merit our interest and concern – indeed, that a focus on these phenomena to the exclusion of preoccupation with nosology is likely to be fruitful. Underlying and covert brain mechanisms are made more overt and apparent. This model of theoretical psychiatry, built on the foundation of phenomenology and psychopathology, without the prejudices of arbitrary and moot boundaries between so-called disorders, is aimed at establishing and consolidating a different approach to clinical psychiatry.

In addition to the desire to heighten interest in psychopathology, there is also the goal of demonstrating the value of taking an approach that draws widely, introducing and emphasizing the absolute relevance of evolutionary theory to our understanding of jealousy, for example, indicating how fundamental social psychological findings in persuasive communication are to any understanding of folie à deux, and drawing on the immense contribution of social anthropology to the theory of possession trance and ultimately to possession states in psychiatry.

If there is a method to this approach, it is simply to restate the obvious: psychiatry is a subject that inescapably synthesizes knowledge, and it thrives when the fullness of the person is understood as a whole and when the perspectives of the humanities and the social sciences are conjoined with the undeniable incisiveness of the biological sciences in the project of understanding a person. In short, the method speaks to richness and plurality. And my hope is that my exploration of these disparate but nonetheless interconnected abnormal phenomena demonstrates what can be gained from an inquiry that analyzes and disaggregates while at the same time finding connections in the most unexpected places.

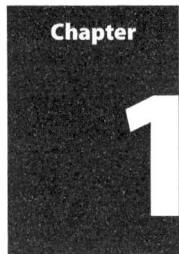

Chapter

Delusional Misidentification Syndromes

1.1 Introduction

The delusional misidentification syndromes include Capgras syndrome, Frégoli syndrome, syndrome of intermetamorphosis, syndrome of subjective doubles, delusion of inanimate doubles and reduplicative paramnesia (Capgras, 1923; Anderson & Williams, 1994; Ellis, Luauté & Retterstøl, 1994; Christodoulou et al., 2009). These conditions are of great and continuing interest to psychiatrists, neuropsychologists, neuroscientists and philosophers alike because of their intriguing clinical presentations and the fact of the possibility of linking discrete beliefs to neural and neuropsychological underpinnings.

Capgras syndrome is perhaps one of the best known and most discussed examples of the delusional misidentification syndromes. It is characterized by the firmly held but false belief that an impostor has replaced a familiar person (Silva & Leong, 1992; Ellis, Whitley & Luauté, 1994; Christodoulou et al., 2009; Abbate et al., 2012).

In Frégoli syndrome, the subject believes that an unfamiliar person is really a disguised familiar person, whereas in the syndrome of intermetamorphosis, the subject believes that the unfamiliar and familiar persons are identical because of shared physical characteristics such as hair colour or shape of nose. The syndrome of subjective doubles is characterized by the belief that a double of the self is abroad in the world acting in such a way as to damage the subject's reputation. The delusion of inanimate doubles refers to the belief that inanimate objects have been duplicated and replaced, whereas reduplicative paramnesia refers to the belief that places have been duplicated.

Central to these conditions is the concept of the 'double', a concept that was present in mythology in antiquity and has carried on into the fictional narrative in the present day. Plautus's *Amphitryon* is a Roman tragicomedy in which Jupiter takes on Amphitryon's appearance in order to sleep with Alcmena, Amphitryon's wife. Mercury takes on Sosia's (Amphitryon's servant) appearance in order to delay Amphitryon's return. The success of this comedy of errors turns on the concept of doubles – Jupiter acting as Amphitryon and Mercury as Sosia. This story was the source of the original name for Capgras syndrome, namely *illusion de Sosie*. This literary preoccupation with the concept of the double is present in Dostoyevsky's *The Double* and Shusaku Endo's *Shame*.

The concept of the double is important in popular culture and as a device in literature because of the implications regarding the fragility of identity by way of facial recognition and also because of the challenges it posits to our notion of the physical uniqueness of persons, a uniqueness that is only truly breached in the case of identical twins. The possibility that persons, objects, places and even time might not be unique is at the core of delusional misidentification syndromes. This idea that duplication is possible and even probable and that against better judgement it can be firmly held as self-evident and established even in the face of counterargument and factual impossibility raises a welter of queries – as much about normal processes as about abnormal phenomena. Among the many questions is how we come to recognize faces, people, objects, places and so on and how we come to mark them as unique examples of a class even in the context of marked changes over time. I mean by this the fact that we continue to identify an individual from cradle to grave as the same person despite significant changes in physical appearance over time. The urgent and continuing fascination with the delusional misidentification syndromes derives at least from the many theoretical, philosophical and empirical matters they raise. There is the added underlying assumption that these conditions may provide the basis for examining and investigating the neurological basis of delusions in general, as is argued later.

Delusional misidentification syndromes are commonly regarded as rare conditions. Estimates of the prevalence range from 0.001 to 4.1 per cent (Joseph, 1994; Kirov, Jones & Lewis, 1994; Moselhy & Oyebode, 1997; Tamam et al., 2003). However, the prevalence in neurodegenerative disorders may be as high as 16.6 per cent in Lewy body dementia, 15.7 per cent in Alzheimer's dementia and 8.3 per cent in semantic dementia (Harciarek & Kertesz, 2008). Early reports suggested that these disorders occur exclusively in females, but it is now clearly established that males are afflicted as well.

These conditions can occur in schizophrenia, affective disorders and organic brain diseases (Förstl et al., 1994; Joseph, O'Leary, Kurland & Ellis, 1999b; Feinberg & Roane, 2005; Sidoti & Lorusso, 2007; Oyebode, 2008; Christodoulou et al., 2009). There is evidence that the right hemisphere has a role in the pathogenesis of these disorders (Cutting, 1991; Ellis, 1994) and that impairment of face processing including impairment of face-recognition memory is an important underlying anomaly in subjects who present with delusional misidentification syndrome (Paillère-Martinot et al., 1994; Edelstyn et al., 1996; Edelstyn, Oyebode & Barrett, 1998; Breen, Caine & Coltheart, 2000). The fact that delusional misidentification syndromes are associated with neurological, neuropsychological and neurophysiological correlates makes them ideal subjects for further investigation as to the origin and genesis of delusions (Christodoulou & Malliara-Loulakaki, 1981; Förstl et al., 1994; Munro, 1994; Paillère-Martinot et al., 1994; Papageorgiou et al., 2005; Ismail et al., 2012). In other words, these conditions, being relatively discrete and susceptible to clear description, allow for the study of the neurological underpinnings of delusional beliefs and perhaps even underscoring the processes and functional impairments that determine the nature of delusions.

In the next section, I will focus on the original case descriptions, concentrating on the distinctive aspects of the respective syndromes and drawing attention to issues that are yet to be resolved. I will then turn to the classification and pathogenesis of delusional misidentification syndromes and the relevance of these to our understanding of the nature of delusions in general.

1.2 Classical Case Descriptions

1.2.1 Capgras Syndrome

Capgras syndrome was first formally described in 1923 by Capgras and Reboul-Lachaux (Capgras, 1923). The patient was a 53-year-old woman, Mme M, who had a 10-year history of presenting with the systematized belief that many people including her husband and daughter had been transformed into doubles. It is a complex case presenting with predominantly delusions of grandeur and persecution, but it is remembered for the fact that Mme M believed that numerous people had been transformed into doubles. The principal beliefs in this case that are of relevance to Capgras phenomenon are as follows:

1. Mme M believed that she was substituted at birth and that her father had acted criminally to abduct and hide her from her real parents, the Duke of Broglie and Mlle de Rio-Branco, the daughter of the Duke of Luynes. Mme M said, '[N]ever having divulged my birth, many people only know the name of the person who brought me up; it's these doubles who have given me the name of their children, that's why they have changed my personal details.' (Ellis, Whitley & Luaute, 1994, p. 125)

2. She believed that she had two or three doubles who were known to her and said, 'I was blond, they have made me chestnut, with eyes three times the size; they were rounded in front, now they are flat: they put drops in my meals to take away the features of my eyes, and the same with my hair; as for my chest, I no longer have one … and that's why no-one recognizes me anymore and why people are making use of my good previous history [delusion of subjective doubles and reverse Frégoli syndrome].' (Ellis, Whitley & Luaute, 1994, p. 122)

3. She believed that her children were objects of substitution. She said, '[T]hey always gave me some other girl, who in turn was taken away and then immediately replaced. … As soon as they took one child away they gave me another who looks just the same: I have had more than two thousand in five years: they are doubles.' (Ellis, Whitley & Luaute, 1994, p. 122)

4. She believed that her husband was a double. She said, '[I]f this person is my husband, he is more than unrecognizable, he is a completely transformed person. I can assure you that the imposter [sic] husband that they are trying to insinuate as my own husband, has not existed for ten years, is not the person who is keeping me here.' (Ellis, Whitley & Luaute, 1994, p. 122)

5. She believed that the concierges were doubles, as were the other tenants in the building. And in hospital at Maison-Blanche she believed that nearly everyone was a double. She said, '[T]he theatre that is played out by these doubles is unbelievable.' The doctors, nurses and patients were also involved. She said, '[T]he doctors that come here wearing capes, don't tell me there is only one of them, I know at least fifteen! … [T]he sister is sometimes kind, sometimes annoyed: these are doubles. For each sister there are fifty, they give their orders through doubles. The young daughter of this Sister also has doubles. The number of sisters who have disappeared is unbelievable [clonal pluralization].' (Ellis, Whitley & Luaute, 1994, p. 124–5)

6. She explained why she is convinced of there being doubles, saying, '[T]hat can be seen by certain details … a little mark in the ear … a thinner face … a longer moustache … different colour eyes … the way of speaking … the way of walking.' She explained what she meant by doubles: 'Doubles … are people who resemble each other.' (Ellis, Whitley & Luaute, 1994, p. 129)

These features of Capgras phenomenon remain the essential characteristic features, namely the belief in 'duplicates' or 'doubles' of persons, usually familiar persons. However, there are other autobiographical accounts of the same phenomenon that predate the description by Capgras and Reboul-Lachaux. For example, Daniel Schreber, in his *Memoirs of My Nervous Illness*, which was published in 1903 (Schreber & Macalphine, 1955, p. 104), wrote

I saw there several ladies, among them Mrs W., the wife of a Pastor in Fr., and my own mother, also several gentlemen, among them the Councillor of the County Court K., of

Dresden, with an ungainly enlarged head. Even if I wanted to try to convince myself now that I had only been deceived by fleeting similarities of external appearances, this would not suffice to explain to me the impressions I had at the time; I could understand such likeness occurring in two or three instances but not the fact that, as I will show, almost all the patients in the Asylum, that is to say at least several dozen human beings, looked like persons who had been more or less close to me in my life.

What is significant about Schreber's account is that it does not refer to the terms 'double' or 'duplicate', but nonetheless it is clear that his experience is grounded in the belief that he perceived identity between people who were well known to him and others that he saw in the asylum and that the identification was based on the identity of appearance. This allows us to grasp one of the fundamental and implicit aspects of delusional misidentification syndromes, namely that objects including human beings may not be unique and singular but also that they can be replicated as more or less accurate facsimiles. To extend this point, Capgras phenomenon does not merely relate to being in the presence of the supposed original but erroneously believing that the original is actually a copy but also to cases where in the presence of a novel object to believe that it is an exact replica of the original. The distinction between this and the following syndrome, Frégoli syndrome, is that in Frégoli syndrome it is accepted by the patient that the physical appearances are different, but this discrepancy merely covers the true facts that the real individual is hiding behind a mask, so to say.

Once this subtle variation in the form of Capgras phenomenon is recognized, then the account by John Perceval (1840/1962, p. 266) becomes understandable.

> During the same year, I also saw the faces of persons who approached me, clothed in the features of my nearest relations, and earliest acquaintances, so that I called out their names, and could have sworn, but for the immediate change of countenance, that my friends had been there.

Here we see the patient recognizing in disparate individuals familiar and distinct facial features of his close relatives such that he mistook these unfamiliar people as relations or acquaintances. What is notable is that the recognition is based on identity of distinct characterizing features. This description anticipates the delusion of intermetamorphosis that follows later.

It is less well recognized that Capgras phenomenon is not restricted to faces or persons. Indeed, this is a condition that can affect all the principal sensory modalities. It is not solely a phenomenon of visual perception, nor of facial recognition only. It is well accepted that visual objects other than the face can be affected (Oyebode & Sargeant, 1996), hence the description of delusions of inanimate doubles (Anderson & Williams, 1994), but the involvement of audition and gustation is less well recognized. But this is perhaps not surprising given the relative rarity of these presentations. Examples include

1. A young man who believed that his younger brother had switched his vinyl records for poor copies because the music sounded different when he played the records, and this difference was indefinable and not attributed to scratches. Superficially, this case pointed at duplicated vinyl records, but in fact the originating phenomenon was altered musical audition.

2. A female patient who claimed that her meals tasted differently including strawberries and concluded either that the meals had been tampered with in some manner or altered, with the purpose of poisoning her. Here her gustatory experience of the taste of strawberries did not match her expectation of what strawberries tasted like, and she then had the erroneous belief that her meals had been tampered with.

There is no reason to suppose that Capgras phenomenon does not affect olfaction or other sensory modalities except that examples of these are yet to be described.

What the above-mentioned cases demonstrate is that the underlying anomaly, at least in some cases, involves discrepancy between prior expectations of the nature and identity of a sensory object and the actuality of the experienced object. The beliefs expressed by the patients, on the face of it, seem merely to be attempts to reconcile these discrepancies. Hence beliefs about doubles are explanations given for the perceived but minute differences between the expected sensory object and the actually perceived object. By definition, the sensory object could be a visual, aural, gustatory, or other sensory object.

1.2.2 Frégoli Syndrome

In 1927, Courbon and Fail (1927) described the case of a 27-year-old woman who claimed that her 'persecutors are capable of all types of transformation and can impose such transformations on others: they are Frégoli who can frégolify any and everybody' (Ellis, Whitley & Luaute, 1994, p. 134). This syndrome was named after Léopoldo Frégoli, an Italian actor who was reputed to be able to transform himself into various people while on stage.

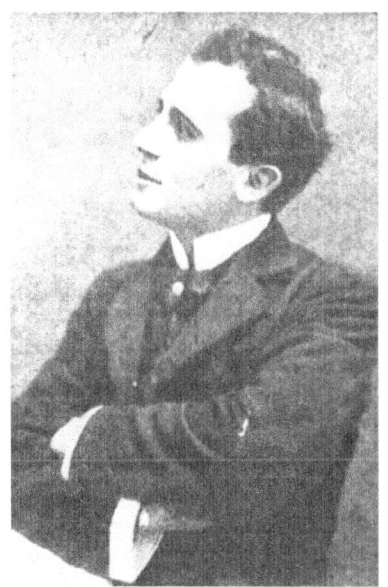

Leopoldo Fregoli 1857–1936

The patient believed that she was 'the victim of enemies, of whom the main culprits [were] the actresses Robine and Sarah Bernhardt, whom she often went to see in the theatre' (Ellis, Whitley & Luaute, 1994, p. 134). She believed that 'for years they [had] pursued her closely, taking the form of people she knows or meets, taking over her thoughts, preventing her from doing this or that, then forcing her to do things, stroking her and forcing her to masturbate'. She 'recognized members of her own family among the other actors. A female employer who had attempted to caress her three years earlier was Robine. The woman she met and attacked in the street because of the annoying sensation she felt coming from her was also Robine. . . . The hospital doctor who has never been to Choisy nor bears any resemblance to anyone she has ever known, becomes her dead father or even Dr Leroux, a doctor who saved her when she was three months old, whom she has never seen since and whose features she cannot recall. In the same way, the intern becomes her cousin' (Ellis, Whitley & Luaute, 1994, p. 135).

Courbon and Fail concluded that the defining features of their newly described syndrome were that (1) in Capgras syndrome, the doubles were distinct beings who could be confused with one another because of their perfect resemblance, but their personalities were distinct even if appearances were the same, and (2) in Frégoli syndrome, there was a single personality but numerous and varied appearances. In other words, there were several individuals who bore no resemblance to one another but who were incarnations of another person whom they did not resemble. To emphasize the point, in Frégoli syndrome, there is no physical similarity between the individual who is the target of recognition and the person to whom that individual is identified.

1.3 Syndrome of Intermetamorphosis

The syndrome of **intermetamorphosis** was first described by Courbon and Tusque in 1932 (Ellis & Young, 1990). The patient, Sylvanie G, was 49 years of age at the time of her presentation. She had been previously admitted to hospital in February 1924. The salient feature of her presentation was that 'people around her [were] transformed physically and psychologically into other people' (Ellis, Whitley & Luaute, 1994, p. 139). She said

> They have changed my hens, they've put two old ones in the place of two young ones, they had large combs instead of small ones. . . . I have seen women change into men, young women into old men. . . . In the street in Paris a quarter of an hour apart, I saw three boys like my son. They were dressed in the same way, with the same nose, the same rosy face, the same small mouth. But not one of them was my son, because they were teasing me, laughing happily, and young girls with them. . . . My aunt I saw in two different places at the same time, as if split in two. (p. 139)

In relation to her husband, she said

> In a second my husband is taller, smaller or younger. It's the individual into whom he is transformed who lives, who is in his skin, who moves. It's as if you put yourself into his skin, it was you and not him. It was not merely a *change*, but a true *transformation* [italics in the original]: I have changed with age, but have not transformed, I am still the same person. One day he changed into young M. Panier. He took on his mannerisms and face, spoke like him. (p. 140)

She concluded, 'They change as they wish. . . . [T]he whole of society is doing it, and with such great agility' (p. 140).

Courbon and Tusques (1932) make the point that their newly described syndrome is distinct from Frégoli syndrome in that in Frégoli syndrome there is false recognition without false physical semblance, whereas in intermetamorphosis there is both false recognition and false physical resemblance (Ellis, Whitley & Luaute, 1994). To restate this more clearly, in Frégoli syndrome, the patient recognizes a familiar person in someone who is demonstrably physically different from the familiar person. By contrast, intermetamorphosis involves the recognition of and identification of a familiar person in an unfamiliar person, but the recognition and identification are based on some shared characteristics. The degree to which the shared characteristics are in fact false physical resemblances is generally not appreciated.

1.4 Syndrome of Subjective Doubles

Christodoulou (1978a) described an 18-year-old female patient presenting with the belief that a

> female neighbour had succeeded, by means of elaborate transformations, in acquiring physical characteristics identical with her own ('same face, same build, same clothes, same everything'). She believed that this woman had special make-up, a wig, and a mask and characterized this transformation as a 'metamorphosis'. (p. 250)

On a subsequent admission,

> [s]he insisted that she had seen at least two female patients transformed into her own self. She attacked one of these patients and pulled her hair. When her hypothetical double

managed to escape from her Ms. A was agonized and begged her doctor to 'pull the mask' from the other patient's face to disclose her real identity.   (p. 250)

She wrote, in a letter, to her father:

> In here there is a girl as fat and as tall as I am. At night when everyone is asleep she puts on a wig and a mask and walks from the room stealing things in order to incriminate me. One night I woke and saw her with my own eyes. It is unfortunate that due to my confusion I failed to run to the window to shout to the people, 'Look here, this is me, and this is my double with a wig and a mask.'   (p. 250)

The original case of Capgras syndrome just described also presented with delusion of subjective doubles and anticipated the case described by Christodoulou. What is unclear in these cases is whether the belief is simply an abnormal belief or involves, as it seems to in this case, actual perception of the so-called doubles.

In addition, it is important, from the point of view of attempting to understand the origins of these experiences, that this patient had associated false memories of familiarity including *déjà vécu* and also depersonalizations and derealization. I will return to these issues later.

Christodoulou's case demonstrates very sharply one of the most tantalizing aspects of delusional misidentifications that is little remarked upon, namely that false physical resemblances take place. In other words, a patient can look at a physically distinct face and figure and come to the erroneous judgement that it is identical to her own face and body. The reverse is also true, that a patient can look at their own face and report significant physical changes (see the original case described by Capgras and Reboul-Lachaux discussed earlier). I emphasize this point in order to argue that these false physical resemblances or altered visual perceptions must be accounted for in any explanation of the underlying causal mechanisms.

1.5 Reduplicative Paramnesia

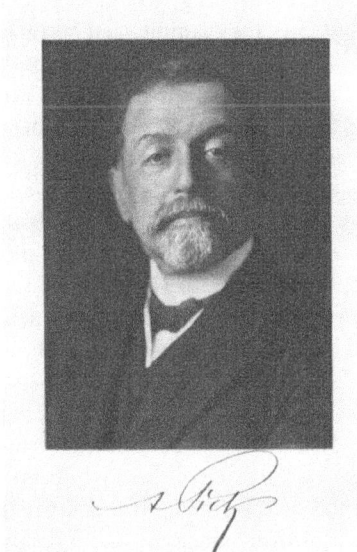

Arnold Pick 1851–1924

Pick (1903) described a new phenomenon that he termed reduplicative paramnesia. The case was a 67-year-old woman who was being treated in hospital in Prague. On the morning of May 24,

> she imagined she was in K., and in reply to the assistant's question how it was that he was in K. also, she said she was very pleased to see him *here too* [italics in the original]. On being questioned further how it was that the entire hospital, as well as the patients, came to be in K., she replied that the doctor had so arranged it. When examined later on, she recognized the author, but at first does not know where she is; had at first believed that she was in K., her birthplace. ... On being asked how it was that the professor had come to K., how had the entire surroundings come there, and to the objection how could the doctors have come there? 'Why, good God! Everything can go round about and back again.'   (p. 262)

In relation to additional inquiries, the patient said

> there had been a great swindle, and she had been dragged into it. . . . [S]he relate[d] that she had been in the clinic in Prague for five months; she had left there yesterday; this is a clinic, too, exactly like the one in Prague. . . . She . . . explains this is the same clinic as the former one, but at a different place. (p. 263)

In a previous case, Pick had described a man who had asserted that there were two independent clinics that were exactly alike and, in addition, that there were two professors of the same name at the head of these clinics.

Reduplicative paramnesia is treated as a subset of delusional misidentification syndromes because of the underlying notion of duplication. Generally, though, there is no associated misidentification of persons as such, except in a few cases (Patterson & Mack, 1985; Hudson & Grace, 2000b).

1.6 Classification of Delusional Misidentification Syndromes

Delusional misidentification syndromes are, strictly speaking, not syndromes at all but symptoms. As described earlier, these symptoms can occur in schizophrenia, mood disorder, delusional disorder or organic disorder such as Alzheimer's dementia (Oyebode & Sargeant, 1996). It is important to be aware of the range of other neurological and physical disorders that have been described in association with delusional misidentification syndromes such as multiple sclerosis (Sidoti & Lorusso, 2007), urinary tract infection (Salviati et al., 2013), parkinsonism (Roane et al., 1998), Parkinson's disease (Pagonabarraga et al., 2008), cortical atrophy (Joseph et al., 1999b), Alzheimer's dementia (Ismail et al., 2012; Jedidi et al., 2013), Lewy body dementia (Thaipisuttikul et al., 2013), subarachnoid haemorrhage (Bouckoms, Martuza, & Henderson, 1986) and cerebral infarction (de Pauw, Szulecka & Poltock, 1987; Jocic & Staton, 1993).

There have been repeated calls for consensus regarding terminology, definitions and classification of these conditions (de Pauw, 1994). Several authors have proposed differing classifications (Silva, Leong & Shaner, 1990; Weinstein, 1994; Roessner & Rössner, 2002). Silva et al. (1990) justify their proposed new nomenclature by arguing that the current classification is based upon the explanations given by the patients, for example, that familiar people have been replaced or are doubles. Their proposal attempts to classify at a more fundamental level based upon the notion that delusional misidentification syndromes are disorders of recognition of identities of the self and others and by structuring the classification on the degree to which the delusional belief involves beliefs about psychological or physical alterations in the target person or object of the delusional belief. This proposal fails to deal adequately with delusional beliefs involving objects or places and, in my view, ignores a more fundamental problem, which is that delusional misidentification syndromes can involve more than visual sensory objects. Perhaps more problematic, however, is the fact that in including 'subjective' Frégoli, 'reverse' intermetamorphosis and other new phenomena it is likely to unnecessarily widen the boundaries of delusional misidentifications syndromes. In any case, this radical alternative classification has not found wide usage.

Other authors have included misidentification of mirror images and television images and the so-called phantom boarder syndrome as part of the delusional misidentification syndromes (Förstl et al., 1991). Again, this approach seeks to widen the reach of these syndromes by including phenomena that do not have at their core notions of 'the double' or that are best construed in other ways. Misidentification of television and mirror images as real possibly points to loss of the capacity to distinguish between objects and their images. Some of the misidentification of mirror images of the self relates more to prosopagnosia for familiar faces than to delusional misidentification syndromes. This issue raises the distinction between misidentification and misrecognition. The idea here is that misidentification is a conscientious misidentification of a person as someone else despite evidence to the contrary, whereas misrecognition is a common place error, to do with mistaken recognition, and does not involve conviction and inflexibility in the face of counterargument. Roessner and Rössner (2002) make the case for their own classification system based upon the distinction between the target person or object being 'altered' or 'doubled'. On the face of it, this seems to be a simplified method, but in practice it is difficult to hold in mind and to apply with ease.

More recently, clonal pluralization of self, relatives or others has been proposed as a variant of delusional misidentification syndromes in which an individual believes that there are many physical and psychological copies of a given original (Ranjan et al., 2007). Weinstein has argued for a classification system that regards the delusional misidentification disorders as determined by a belief in duplicates and hence a classification according to whether the duplication is expressed in the modalities of person, place, time and event, objects, parts of the body or self. This approach might reduce complexity (Weinstein, 1994), but it is likely to lose sight of the commonalities between Capgras phenomenon for person, place, time and events, as these would all be classified differently, and the obvious conceptual links may ultimately be lost in the noise of multiple and unrelated categories.

There is little doubt that delusional misidentification syndromes occur as a continuum from a positive pole consisting of minor forms of déjà vu experience to reduplicative paramnesia and a negative pole from depersonalization to nihilistic delusions (Sno, 1994). What is significant is that there is at present no fully satisfactory classification of delusional misidentification syndromes. Derealization and depersonalization can occur in the prodromal phase of delusional misidentification syndromes, and hence there is some case for depersonalization having an intrinsic role in the process that produces delusional misidentification syndromes (Todd, Dewhurst & Wallis, 1981b). This at least means that the argument for regarding delusional misidentification syndromes as being part of a continuum as proposed by Sno (1994) is promising as a basis for further inquiry, but the central issue is the configuration of the continuum. In Sno's scheme, he envisages positive and negative poles, with the positive pole moving from déjà vu experiences to reduplicative paramnesia and the negative pole from depersonalization to Côtard syndrome. It is unstated where in the continuum Capgras syndrome, Frégoli syndrome, syndrome of subjective doubles, syndrome of intermetamorphosis and *jamais vu* phenomenon would reside. It is also unclear what role severity would play in determining the position of a syndrome along the continuum. Nonetheless, there is merit in regarding the negative and positive poles as potential ways of understanding the underlying mechanism of misidentification syndromes.

1.7 Explanatory Hypotheses

1.7.1 Psychodynamic Explanations

Coleman (1933) argued for ambivalence as an essential psychodynamic mechanism in delusional misidentification syndromes, namely that the misidentified individual is one with whom the patient has an ambivalent relationship. A clinical example might be the case of a young woman who is physically and emotionally abused by her parents and whose response is to say, 'They can't be my parents or they wouldn't treat me like this,' and to conclude that they must be impostors. These kinds of cases, where the erroneous belief is clearly understandable given the context, exist but are rare.

Coleman's view is shared by several other authors who also emphasize the fact that only a small number of specific individuals are misidentified, and this confirms that ambivalence is important and central to understanding why a particular individual is selected as the focus of the delusional belief (Enoch, Trethowan & Barker, 1967; Moskowitz, 1972; Vogel, 1974; Dally & Gomez, 1979). The problem with this approach is simply that it is not always obvious that the emotional relationship is marked either by ambivalence or by a negative attitude. And, in any case, delusional misidentification for objects and places for which ambivalence is far from obvious widely occurs (Moselhy & Oyebode, 1997).

Other authors have emphasized the role of splitting of internalized object representation (Berson, 1982) and regression to a phase in childhood before object constancy was established (Jackson et al., 1992) or regression to archaic forms of thinking that occurs in psychosis (Todd, Dewhurst & Wallis, 1981a) as the basic anomaly in delusional misidentification syndromes. What is clear is that these explanatory hypotheses cannot account for the range of cases seen, nor can they account for the associations with neurological lesions or impairments in face processing that have been demonstrated in delusional misidentification syndromes.

1.7.2 Neurological Explanations

Delusional misidentification syndromes have been associated with a number of neurological lesions (Moselhy & Oyebode, 1997). In a series of 29 cases, diffuse cortical atrophy and posterior fossa or subcortical abnormalities were demonstrated on computed tomographic scans, and cortical dysrhythmia and focal epileptiform discharges were reported on electroencephalogram (Joseph, 1985b). There is also substantial evidence for the role of the right (non-dominant) hemisphere in delusional misidentification syndromes (Cutting, 1991; Madoz-Gúrpide & Hillers-Rodríguez, 2010), including findings of a significantly enlarged right anterior horn region in patients with delusional misidentification syndrome in the context of Alzheimer's disease (Förstl et al., 1991) and the development of delusional misidentification syndromes following right temporoparietal infarction (de Pauw et al., 1987). In addition, in reduplicative paramnesia there is evidence of bilateral anterior cortical atrophy, subcortical atrophy and involvement of cerebellar vermis atrophy (Joseph et al., 1999b). But perhaps the most important findings are the reports of Capgras syndrome in association with interictal psychosis and infarction of the occipitotemporal junction, thereby drawing attention to the role of the occipital cortex in delusional misidentification syndromes (Lewis, 1987) and of direct involvement of the fusiform gyrus, therefore pointing to a role for the same brain areas in both delusional misidentification syndromes and prosopagnosia (Hudson & Grace, 2000a). Other investigators have shown that in Alzheimer's disease presenting with Capgras syndrome there is significant hypometabolism in orbitofrontal and cingulate regions bilaterally and in left median areas and relative hyper-metabolism in bilateral superior temporal and inferior parietal regions (Mentis et al., 1995). Indeed, Lewy body dementia, Capgras syndrome, phantom boarder syndrome and reduplication of person and place were all associated with hypoperfusion in the left hippocampus, insula, ventral striatum and bilateral inferior frontal gyri, whereas visual hallucinations of persons were associated with hypoperfusion in the left ventral occipital gyrus and bilateral parietal regions. It is probably true to say that an integrative model is required that relates the differing roles of the various cortical regions to the production of delusional beliefs, for example, identifying lesions in the right frontal regions as important in releasing left-sided hyper-inferential states that are liable to cause delusion formation (Ismail et al., 2012).

Christodoulou and Malliara-Loulakaki (1981) initially proposed psychophysiological changes and anomalies in delusional misidentification syndromes. More recently, there is emerging evidence of abnormal P300 in association with working memory in delusional misidentification syndromes, suggesting failure to allocate sufficient attentional resources to sensory stimuli (Papageorgiou et al., 2002, 2003, 2005).

1.7.3 Neuropsychological Explanations

There is growing evidence of impairment of face-recognition memory in the absence of impairment of verbal-recognition memory in delusional misidentification syndromes (Bidault, Luauté & Tzavaras, 1986; Ellis, 1994; Edelstyn et al., 1996; Edelstyn et al., 1998; Oyebode, 2008). These reported impairments are at least as severe as those in individuals with acquired right-sided brain injury (Edelstyn et al., 1998) and distinguish between patients with schizophrenia presenting with delusional misidentification syndromes and those without (Walther et al., 2010a). This is important and interesting precisely because it points to the same underlying mechanisms as in prosopagnosia. In prosopagnosia, it is now established that covert face recognition takes place via the intact ventral pathway linking the occipital cortex with medial temporal structures, thereby bypassing the damaged dorsal pathway that links the occipital cortex via longitudinal fasciculus with the parietal cortex (Bauer, 1984). This finding underscores the dual system underlying face recognition, namely (1) recognition of the face icon as being that of a specified individual and (2) the associated feeling of familiarity that is mediated by medial temporal structures. In normal situations, both systems work to determine accurate recognition of faces. In prosopagnosia, there is a failure to identify familiar faces, but covert recognition can be shown to be intact via skin conductance studies. It is hypothesized that in Capgras syndrome the dorsal pathway is impaired with a sparing of the ventral pathway (the opposite of what happens in prosopagnosia), with the result that face recognition is intact but the sense of familiarity is disrupted, thereby producing the belief that a familiar person is an impostor (Ellis et al., 1992). This is an elegant and testable hypothesis that has now been confirmed (Ellis et al., 1997; Hirstein & Ramachandran, 1997), with the proviso that the putative dorsal pathway is yet to be demonstrated (Breen et al., 2000) and that the dissociation between overt and covert recognition is not as clear-cut as once thought, thus making room for further elaborations and refinements to the original hypothesis. There is also evidence that in addition to the markedly reduced magnitude of skin conductance responses to familiar faces compared to normal samples, patients with Capgras syndrome also demonstrate impairment in judging gaze directions and conclude that models looking in different directions are different individuals (Hirstein & Ramachandran, 1997). It is also relevant that there may be differences in the demonstrable face processing impairments between Capgras and Frégoli syndromes (Walther et al., 2010b).

A recent study concluded that a single lesion can be responsible for delusional misidentification syndromes (Darby et al., 2017). These authors present findings on 2 patients of their own and 15 other patients drawn from the literature for whom imaging data existed. The patients from the literature were an assortment of patients with Capgras syndrome,

Frégoli syndrome and reduplicative paramnesia. The findings and propositions of this study must be read with this limitation in mind. In brief, these authors showed that the lesions shown to be involved in delusional misidentification syndromes were connected to the left retrospenial cortex and that this area is involved in recognition of familiarity. Secondly, they were also functionally connected to the right frontal cortex, an area thought to be involved in expectation violation, an aspect of belief evaluation. The conclusion was that delusional misidentification syndromes have a unique pattern of functional brain connectivity involving brain areas that deal with the sense of familiarity and that is distinct from the neurology of other kinds of delusions.

In a careful case study, Thiel et al. (2014) showed that in a patient presenting with a selective Capgras syndrome for his partner had a large right prefrontal lesion sparing the ventromedial and medial orbitofrontal cortex but showed paucity of activity on functional magnetic resonance imaging study in the left posterior cingulate cortex and left posterior temporal sulcus on presentation of his partner's face. There was also impaired functional connectivity of the left posterosuperior temporal sulcus with the left superior frontal gyrus. The authors concluded that Capgras syndrome is associated with impairment in the extended face processing system, including areas that deal with inference of mental state from face processing.

There are other proposals including the notion of disconnection between various cortico-visuo-limbic pathways that result in the lack of resolution of the differing representations of personal experience, including face representations (Joseph, 1985a), the role of preconscious perceptual processing (Fleminger, 1992; Fleminger, 1994), a form of agnosia of identification (Bidault et al., 1986), impairment of the attribution of uniqueness to self, others and objects (Margariti & Kontaxakis, 2006) and the place of 'mindreading' in delusional misidentification syndromes (Hirstein, 2010). These additional hypotheses have yet to be confirmed by further empirical study.

1.7.4 Reduplicative Paramnesia

The nature and pathogenesis of reduplicative paramnesia are often treated separately from the other delusional misidentification syndromes, with the emphasis on the neurological aspects of the condition. Benson, Gardner and Meadows (1976) reported on three cases following traumatic head injuries and argued that impairment of the right hemisphere and associated frontal lobe damage were responsible for the development of the syndrome. The suggestion that impairment of the right hemisphere is important has been subsequently confirmed (Staton, Brumback & Wilson, 1982; Patterson & Mack, 1985; Kapur, Turner & King, 1988; Murai et al., 1997; Moser et al., 1998). Staton et al. (1982) showed that a deep lesion in the temporoparietal-occipital junction and in the right posterior hippocampus was relevant in their case in which duplication of time, place and person occupied, and they postulated a disconnection between newly registered memory and long-term memory. A case reported by Filley and Jarvis (1987) demonstrated that not only is right hemisphere impairment important but reduplicative paramnesia can also occur as a delayed effect, three years after the original injury and despite apparent good recovery from the injury.

The proposed mechanism for reduplicative paramnesia is converging on the proposed mechanism for Capgras syndrome, namely that that there is disruption in the systems for recognition of familiarity in the absence of impairment of face-recognition (Capgras syndrome) or place-recognition reduplicative paramnesia (Lee et al., 2011). In a patient presenting with reduplicative paramnesia following a stroke affecting the right postero-inferior frontal region extending from the paraventricular and subventricular areas to the insular subcortical area, Lee et al. (2011) hypothesized that the longitudinal fasciculus and the fronto-occipital fasciculus, both of which are involved in visuospatial processing in common with involvement of both anterior thalamic radiation and uncinate fasciculus responsible for abnormal feelings of hyper-familiarity, were instrumental in causing reduplicative paramnesia in their patient. It is of interest that even though reduplicative paramnesia is founded on structural neurological change, it is at least temporarily amenable to improvement by exposure to distinct landmarks through perception of unequivocal topographic information (Pignat et al., 2013).

1.8 Violence and Delusional Misidentification Syndromes

Violence in patients with delusional misidentification syndromes, particularly Capgras syndrome, has been reported in the literature (Crane, 1976; Woytassek & Atwal, 1985; Silva et al., 1993, 1994; Thompson & Swan, 1993). It is now clear that violence occurs not only in Capgras syndrome but also in the syndrome of subjective doubles (Christodoulou, 1978a) and the syndrome of intermetamorphosis (Barton & Barton, 1986). The original case of Fregoli syndrome reported by Courbon and Fail (Courbon, 1927) involved a female patient who was admitted following an assault on a former employer whom the patient accused of being in disguise, and there are other more recent reports too (Ashraf et al., 2011; Carabellese et al., 2014). It is also worth noting that Capgras syndrome appears to be selectively associated with parricide, especially where the patient lives with elderly parents, particularly mothers (Ahn et al., 2012). But patients presenting with delusional misidentification syndrome can themselves be victims of violence as well as being perpetrators of violence (De Pauw & Szulecka, 1988). There is some evidence that individuals with delusional misidentification who are violent are less likely to use weapons than other patients who express delusional beliefs and that grandiose beliefs, thought disorder, generalized hostility and a previous history of violence are predictors of violence in individuals who present with delusional misidentification syndromes (Silva et al., 1995).

1.9 Conclusion

Delusional misidentification syndromes are exemplary conditions in that they are characterized by delusional beliefs that are discrete and circumscribed and that hence are relatively easy to investigate. Their similarity to prosopagnosia, a neurological condition that has relatively clear neural underpinnings, has stimulated neuropsychiatric and neuropsychological investigations that have yielded fruit. It is now clear that these conditions, especially those which focus on identification and recognition of faces, have underlying impairments of face recognition, often in the absence of impairment of word recognition. Many of these impairments are subtle and only demonstrable on neuropsychological testing. There is much that is yet to be established – why despite having impairments in face processing and also complex visual object processing, only a limited number of individuals in the patient's social network are the focus of the delusional belief, why the phenomena are rarely chronic or protracted and what the relationship is between the discrete psychopathology of delusional misidentification syndromes and the nosology of the psychiatric conditions within which they present. Put simply, how do delusional misidentifications symptoms relate to schizophrenia, mood disorder or Alzheimer's dementia?

2

Othello Syndrome

2.1 Introduction

Romantic jealousy is a set of emotions, thoughts and actions that emerge in a particular social situation (White & Mullen, 1992). It is best to distinguish it from envy, with which it is often conflated or mistaken. Strictly speaking, envy occurs in the setting of a dyadic relationship and refers to the feelings that are aroused by the characteristics or attributes of another person, whereas jealousy occurs in the setting of a triangular relationship and refers to the feelings triggered by the relationship or potential relationship between two other people within the triangle (Klein, 1977). It is also best to make clear at the outset that jealousy is not a basic emotion such as fear, anger or sadness. It is a complex emotion that is a composite of several different emotions triggered by a social situation. The feelings making up this composite include anger, fear, sadness, guilt, envy and sexual arousal. The social setting is usually the perceived potential or real loss of a sexual partner to an imaginary or real sexual rival.

There is little doubt that romantic jealousy is important in human affairs and occurs in all cultures, even though the manifestations and behaviours emanating from the feelings may differ. Its importance is evident in the degree to which it forms the basis of literary fiction and drama in such diverse texts as Euripides' (484–406 BC) *Medea,* Shakespeare's (1564–1616) *Othello* and *The Winter's Tale* and Tolstoy's (1847–1910) *Kreutzer Sonata.*

Medea was first produced in 431 BC. It recounts the story of Medea and Jason. Medea was a princess of Colchis and was married to Jason of Jason and the Argonauts. She responded to information that Jason was going to take as his wife Glauce, daughter of Creon, King of Corinth, by poisoning Glauce and then murdering her own two sons, in order to avenge the shame brought upon her by Jason. The play explores a woman's response to her husband's infidelity and shows the extent of the passion aroused in this social context, including feelings of anger, resentment and the desire to act in a vengeful manner towards both her rival and her spouse. There is a direct link between the fact of her rejection and the violent acts that created the tragic tension in the play. In *Medea* (Euripides, 1963: p. 1) there is a clear and direct link between the real infidelity of Jason and the strong emotions that are aroused. In the opening lines of the play, Medea's nurse says

> Poor Medea! Scorned and shamed,
> She raves, invoking every vow and solemn pledge
> That Jason made her, and calls the gods as witnesses
> What thanks she has received for her fidelity.
> She will not eat; she lies collapsed in agony,
> Dissolving the long hours in tears. Since first she heard
> Of Jason's wickedness, she has not raised her eyes,
> Or moved her cheek from the hard ground.

Medea experiences the pain of rejection, the anguish of loss, the passion and anger that are synonymous with jealousy. And ultimately these feelings lead inexorably to murder.

Shakespeare's *The Winter's Tale* (Shakespeare, 2008) was published in the First Folio of 1623. In this play, Leontes, King of Sicilia, becomes jealous and believes that his Queen, Hermione, has been unfaithful with Polixene, King of Bohemia. This play is important from the point of view of an understanding of the psychology of jealousy and the inherent fears thereof. Leontes is all eyes, watching and observing what he considers the evidence of infidelity. Leontes says

> Is whispering nothing?
> Is leaning cheek to cheek? Is meeting noses?
> Kissing with inside lip? Stopping the career
> Of laughter with a sigh? – a note infallible
> Of breaking honesty! Horsing foot on foot?
> Skulking in corners? Wishing clocks more swift?
> Hours minutes? Noon midnight? And all eyes
> Blind with the pin and web but theirs, theirs only,
> That would unseen be wicked? Is this nothing?   (p. 110)

And then the conjecture that all he has observed are sure signs of infidelity.

> Now, while I speak this, holds his wife by th'arm,
> That little thinks she has been sluiced in's absence,
> And his pond fished by his next neighbour, by
> Sir Smile, his neighbour – nay, there's comfort in't
> Whilst other men have gates, and those gates opened,
> As mine, against their will.   (p. 106)

But the real fear is that his son, Maximillius, might not be his son at all. Hence the question, 'Art thou my boy?'. I will return to this theme when I come to examine the possible explanations for jealousy.

Othello (The Tragedy of Othello, the Moor of Venice) (Shakespeare, 2003) was first published in 1565. It is a story of a Venetian general, Othello, who is of Moorish origin. He is induced to become jealous that his wife Desmodena is having an affair with Cassio, one of Othello's captains, through the machinations of Iago. This particular account of jealousy is exemplary because it is based upon the possibility that an individual might be susceptible to jealousy by being played upon – in other words, that feelings of jealousy can be aroused irrespective of objective facts.

The play also raises the possibility that aspects of a person's character might make the task of triggering jealous feelings more likely to succeed. In Othello's case, he is said to be 'of a free and open nature, that thinks men honest that but seem to be so, and will as tenderly be led by the nose as asses are' (p. 94). Also, there is the possibility that 'jealousy can be so strong that judgement cannot cure [it]' (p. 106), whereas in *The Winter's Tale*, Leontes' fear centres upon the possibility that his son might not in reality be his. In *Othello*, the fear is the loss of sexual exclusivity: 'I had rather be a toad and live upon the vapour of a dungeon than keep a corner in the thing I love for other's uses' (p. 135).

Finally, Tolstoy's *Kreutzer Sonata* was published in 1889 (Tolstoy, 1985). It is a story dealing with jealousy as well as examining the nature of marriage. It is thought to have been based on Tolstoy's own marriage. It is a detailed study of the social context of jealousy, of the psychological effects within the individual and its impact on behaviour and the ultimate destructive effect in the unleashed fatal violence against the partner. The story moves from the husband's inclination to jealousy, to the strained marital relationship following the birth of the children and finally to the introduction in the home of a violin teacher who accompanied the wife who played the piano. There are jealous feelings from the onset of the Introduction.

> He, surveying my wife in the way all debauched men look at pretty women, tried to make it appear as though all he was interested in was the subject of the conversation, which was of course what interested him least of all. She tried to appear indifferent, but the combination of my jealous-husband look, with which she was familiar, and his lustful ogling evidently excited her. I saw that right from the first meeting her eyes began to shine in a peculiar way and that, probably as a result of my jealousy, there was immediately established between them a kind of electric current which seemed to give their faces the same expression, the same gaze, the same smile. (p. 86)

There was also the fact that the protagonist's own past behaviour made him more especially liable to jealous feelings. He said

> If I'd been pure, I wouldn't have understood this, but, like the majority of men, I too had thought this way about women before I'd got married, and so I could read his mind as if it were a printed book. (p. 88)

Jealousy relies on keen observation and the attribution of meaning to innocent and neutral events. This aspect of jealousy is exquisitely described.

> Oh, how well I remember all the details of that evening. I remember how he produced his violin, the way he opened the case, removed the cloth that had been specially sewn for him by some lady or other, took the instrument out and began tuning it. I remember the way my wife sat down at the piano, trying to appear indifferent, while in actual fact she was extremely anxious. (p. 95)

The jealousy ended tragically, and the end was predictable too.

> That same rabid frenzy I had experienced a week previously once more took possession of me. Once again I felt that compulsion to destroy, to subjugate by force, to rejoice in the ecstasy of my furious rage, and I abandoned myself to it. (p. 111)

These literary depictions of jealousy show the triangular contexts in which the feelings arise and indicate the fears that underlie the experience of jealousy, the behaviours that follow on the feelings and the ever-present potential for violence.

The English word *jealousy* is said to have roots in the French *jaloux* and *jalousie*, and both can be traced back to Old Provencal *gilos* and ultimately from the Late Latin *zelus*, meaning 'zeal or ardour' (Shepherd, 1961). Mullen (1991) has argued that in Western culture, a feeling that was originally a socially sanctioned response to infidelity has become transformed into personal pathology, even individual psychopathology, signalling emotional immaturity, undue possessiveness and insecurity. Hence jealousy can be seen as an example of a feeling that was once valued with positive connotations but that under cultural pressure has become transmuted, at least in Western culture, to a feeling with negative connotations. This point emphasizes the degree, given cultural forces, to which a specific feeling responds to nature and expectations of sexual relationships in society.

The other important aspect of jealousy, aside from the influence of culture and social expectations, is the fact that like other emotions and behaviours, it raises questions about the distinction between what is normal and what is abnormal and the degree to which what is abnormal is understandable or a reflection of process abnormalities pointing to aberrations in brain function. In other words, jealousy is a complex of feelings and behaviours that is an understandable response to a particular context. The question is how to determine when it becomes an exaggerated response to an understandable context and when it is a pathological response in a setting in which it is incomprehensible that the feeling should have arisen in the first place. And finally, there is the question of whether there are situations in which the feeling of jealousy arises from abnormal internal processes which are ultimately independent of the social situation of the individual experiencing the feeling of jealousy.

In this chapter, I describe a number of case examples drawn from the original publication by Shepherd (1961), and then I proceed to examine the possible theories of the origins of normal jealousy as well as of pathological jealousy. In the final section, I focus on the emotions, thoughts and behaviours associated with jealousy and conclude by looking at the relationship of jealousy to violence.

2.2 Case Reports

1. Mr. L.P., . . . 49, [was a] wholesale manufacturer. . . . The patient began to accuse his wife of adultery with her former doctor. He justified his opinion by referring to her increasing interest in physical relations which, he said, must have reflected her experience elsewhere. He attempted to buttress his viewpoint by reference to many trivial incidents and events: footprints in the garden, pieces of cotton wool, restless movements. He followed his wife himself and employed a detective to watch her movements but the negative results of these investigations did not alter his beliefs. From time to time he made increasing sexual demands on his wife and when she refused he accused her of having been satisfied elsewhere. He repeatedly requested a confession. At times he appeared very depressed and would bewail his fate, always accusing his wife and never blaming himself. (Shepherd, 1961, pp. 718–19)

2. Mr. . . . 35 [was a] foreman. . . . During the first two years of their married life the patient was out of England on service duty. At this time he received a number of anonymous letters accusing his wife of misconduct. On his return he questioned her closely and she denied the allegations. From then on, however, he rarely failed to dwell on the period of his absence and his attitude towards her was never free of suspicion. Their sexual relations were not satisfactory and from time to time he accused her of consorting with other men. In fact, the patient had had an affair with a friend of his wife's although he had always denied this to her. From time to time, and especially when he was in his cups, the patient behaved in a violent manner towards his wife. . . . For about one year before the consultation the wife had begun to meet a married man with whom she began an affair unbeknown to the patient. She promised the patient that she would stay with him until the children were older and the patient had met the other man; there had been a violent scene on this occasion. Faced with the prospects of marital break-up and also with the realization of what he had feared for so long the patient's conduct deteriorated. He attempted to strangle his wife on two occasions, threatened suicide and became more violent than ever. (p. 731)

3. Mr. E.J., [was] 55 [years of age]. . . . Three years earlier, the patient had noticed that his wife's stockings were torn on one occasion; he became very upset and wondered whether she had been assaulted; he was not reassured for some weeks. One year before he was seen the patient's wife began work in a factory and her physical energy declined; sexual relations consequently became less frequent. After some weeks the patient began to complain of her coldness and he looked increasingly depressed; he complained of pains in the chest, became moody, began to sleep poorly and appeared to be brooding. After several months he suddenly began to accuse his wife of infidelity, supporting his statements by reference to stains on the lining of her coat, a handkerchief which he thought was discoloured and the drawn curtains in the bedroom. He told his wife that he was convinced of her infidelity but that he would forgive her if she would confess that she had been compelled to act in this way. (p. 739)

4. Mrs. G.B., . . . 52, [was a] housewife. . . . Three months before admission, the patient began to become increasingly jealous and suspicious of her husband's behaviour. She alleged that he was being unfaithful and repeatedly questioned him, her accusations continued throughout the day and long into the night. After some weeks she attacked him one evening after a particularly fierce quarrel. She then accused him of homosexual behaviour, citing minor events and observations as 'proof'. The husband became very depressed and after a short episode of hysterical dissociation he made a suicide attempt and was admitted to a general hospital. On his release the patient accused him of trying to take his life because of his guilty feelings; she made increasing sexual demands and the husband was forced to ask his general practitioner for androgens. Eventually the patient became more aggressive towards her husband and threatened to kill him. On examination in hospital the patient was at first uncooperative, claiming that she was not ill and expressing hostility towards her husband. She complained frequently of palpitations and agreed to remain in hospital only because she felt that she required physical investigation and treatment. She maintained at all times that her husband had been guilty of homosexual practices; she referred to the 'evidence' of numerous details, e.g., the alteration in the disposition of objects on the dressing table, stains on the husband's underwear and on the carpets and the cushions, the discovery of pubic hair on the sofa, and the size of her husband's anal orifice when she examined this. (p. 741)

5. Mr. T.N., . . . 50 . . . was admitted to Brixton Prison on a charge of murder, having pushed his wife downstairs with fatal consequences. . . . He stated that he had been worrying about his health for several months and had been off work for about a year. He worried particularly about his stomach, complaining of acid regurgitation, and about his waning libido. During this period he had become convinced of his wife's infidelity. In evidence of her misconduct he stated that he had become aware of his wife's vaginal slackness during intercourse; that the tea which his wife had given him had an unusual taste and that some white sleeping tablets were being added to it; that he had found a pearl ear-ring and bits of curtain in a dug-out; that he had found his wife washing herself at an unusual early hour of the morning; that he had his backdoor unlocked when he felt certain that he had bolted it; that an old man had picked up a blue frock which belonged to his wife and that his wife had been going out secretly at night. He had struck his wife on only one occasion, so he maintained, before the crime. On the morning of the crime he claimed that he had seen his wife waving a handkerchief at someone who was waving back. He said that his wife had then told him to mind his own business, ran downstairs and struck her head in the process. His attitude to recent events was calm and almost indifferent. He claimed that he still loved his wife and that he had himself to blame for not taking her out often enough. He thought that most people thought him innocent. (p. 747)

6. Mrs. C.P., . . . 37, housewife . . . was expressing ideas about her husband's infidelity and admitted to a fantastic series of morbid beliefs on the subject. . . . It appeared that she had

been suspicious of her husband's fidelity at intervals throughout their married life but during the past year she had become certain of his guilt. She had followed him in the streets and had been through his clothes on many occasions; she had on occasion hidden herself in the boot of his car and claimed that she had heard him making love to another woman; she had maintained that her husband's clothes were stained with seminal fluid and that there was lipstick on his handkerchiefs. She also stated that her husband's attitude had changed towards her and that he had admitted his guilt. The relationship between them had deteriorated in consequence of her changed attitude. . . . The essence of the husband's case of cruelty against the wife was that . . . she falsely accused him of carrying on with other women. She made these accusations incessantly, for hours at a time. She checked and kept a record of the daily mileage of the husband's car; she kept a list of phone numbers, and invented names of women with whom she said the husband was associating. On one occasion she told the husband she had been concealed in the boot of his car while she had been making love to a woman in the car. On another occasion she said that she had received a letter saying that one of the women the husband was carrying on with had a venereal disease. When the husband asked to see the letter, she was unable to produce it. (p. 749)

2.3 Explanatory Hypotheses

In order to fully understand the nature of pathological jealousy, an examination of the origins and evolutionary basis of normal jealous is necessary. In this section, I first examine post-copulatory competition in lower animals with a view to drawing attention to the measures, sometimes extreme, that the male animal takes in order to ensure that the progeny carried by its mate is indeed his. Next, I explore how the findings in lower animals pertain to human beings and how far jealous feelings are determined by different cues and concerns between the sexes.

There is considerable evidence of pre- and post-copulatory intrasexual competition in males in the animal kingdom and the links to successful procreation. Pre-copulatory competition includes differential ability in mate selection, territorial exclusion, dominance hierarchy within permanent social groups and dominance during group courtship displays. But it is in post-copulatory competition that the degree of ingenuity and extreme measures to ensure successful procreation is most obvious. These measures include sperm displacement, induced abortion and re-insemination by the winning suitor, infanticide of the loser's offspring and re-insemination by the winning suitor, mating plugs and repellents and prolonged copulation. Other strategies include prolonged attachment to the partner during a period before or after copulation, standing guard but without physical contact after copulation and the mated pair departing the vicinity of competing suitors (Wilson, 2000). Nomadic male langurs, for example, as a matter of routine kill off all the infants of a troop after taking it over. Male mice are able to induce abortion of a pregnant female simply by their odour, thereby rendering her available for re-insemination, the so-called Bruce effect. And male house flies remain in copulation for prolonged periods, up to an hour, even though sperm has been transferred within the first 15 minutes (Wilson, 2000). Wilson (2000) has argued that these aggressive post-copulatory mechanisms are determined by a shortage of a limited resource, namely access to fertile females or, at times, to the availability of males to care for the female's offspring.

There is also a differential in parental investment between males and females. In simple terms, this is best understood as arising from the fact that in females there is anisogamy, in other words, the production of larger gametes which requires more energy to produce than the equivalent male gametes. The female's energetic investment in each act of mating is therefore greater than the male's investment – hence the differential strategy between males and females with respect to mating. Eggs and fertile females are a scarce and limiting resource which leads to competitive drive between males for access to this limited resource. Wilson (2000) discusses the cold calculus underpinning the differential strategies between males and females. Following insemination, the female energetic investment increases exponentially, while that of the male remains small or diminishes. This has implications for how far the male assists in rearing the offspring or deserts. In the circumstances where male contribution to rearing the young is appreciable, then the male's strategy is to make sure that he has exclusive access to the female's unfertilized eggs, and the post-copulatory competitive behaviours described earlier make sense in this context, and pre-copulatory behaviours such as exclusion of other males from territories, controlling other males by dominance systems and prolonged periods between courtship, bonding and copulation all start to make sense.

The fact of the female's concealed ovulation in human beings has been explained as a means to further promote the likelihood that the male will remain close to the female: he is never sure when the female is ovulating in contrast to the situation in other primates, where the fact of the female's oestrus is emblazoned on her rump and is visible for all to see. Concealed ovulation in human females results in her male partner remaining close to her so as to have access to her during her fertile period and also to increase his certainty of the paternity of the children (Chagnon & Irons, 1979; Freedman, 1979; Diamond, 2014). These evolutionary theories frame our understanding of the origins of normal jealousy. In this approach, female fidelity reassures the male that in caring for his female partner he is at the same time fostering the reproductive future of his own genes, and the current thinking is that male fidelity reassures the female partner that enough resources and protection will be available to ensure that her offspring grow up. In other words, the focus of infidelity and jealous concern is different for the two sexes (Stevens & Price, 2015). In the female, the motive for adultery may have to do with the perception that another male is superior to her male partner in status, integrity and loyalty, whereas in the male, it is likely to be a search for sexual novelty and satisfaction. The anger and violence associated with jealousy are also understandable from an evolutionary perspective: Frustration and anger are thought to result when resource access and one's control over resources are threatened, as they are deemed to be in the context of perceived sexual rivals and jealous feelings. Also, anger occurs when sexual reproductive options are constrained, when one is a victim of deception or when one has pursued a high-cost strategy without beneficial results (McGuire & Troisi, 1998).

The preceding discussion is an attempt to explain the evolutionary origins of jealousy. Another facet of the puzzle is to explain not merely the origins of jealousy but also to examine the role and function of jealousy not only as a feeling but also as a complex of feelings, emotions, cognitions and behaviours. The central point here is well expressed by Daly, Wilson & Weghorst (1982, p. 11).

> Homo sapiens [have evolved] certain psychological propensities which function to defend paternity confidence. Manifestations include the emotion of sexual jealousy, the dogged

inclination of men to possess and control women, and the use or threat of violence to achieve sexual exclusivity and control. We will refer to this behavioral/motivational complex as male sexual jealousy.

The evolutionary perspective is not without its critics, but nonetheless there are several studies confirming the general principle as predicted by evolutionary theory of a differential bias in the concerns that males and females have regarding sexual infidelity (Guadagno & Sagarin, 2010; Sagarin et al., 2012), and the differential bias holds true even in egalitarian cultures such as that in Norway (Kennair, Nordeide & Andreassen, 2011). It may be that the extent of these differences is determined by other factors such as attachment style within relationships (Levy & Kelly, 2010), whether the measures of response to hypothetical or real infidelity are continuous or not (Sagarin et al., 2012) and whether the research respondents have experienced real partner infidelity or not (Tagler, 2010). It seems as if prior experience of partner infidelity moderates the responses such that the predicted differential sex-determined bias is markedly reduced. Furthermore, the predicted differential sex-determined bias also influences the inquiries that males and females make about the nature of extra-pair relationships: males inquire about sexual intimacy, whereas females inquire about emotional intimacy (Kuhle, Smedley & Schmitt, 2009). These differential biases also determine the damage-control strategies to mitigate the costs of being caught committing infidelity: males more than females deny emotional involvement, and females deny any sexual involvement (Kuhle, Smedley & Schmitt, 2009).

Intrasexual competition is thought not to be particularly strong in human beings. The evidence for this view is derived from findings that show that compared with other primates, the degree of sexual dimorphism is limited in human beings. For example, height and weight differences between males and females are significantly less prominent in humans compared with other primates (Wilson, 2000). Nonetheless, intrasexual competition exists, and there are features that determine the perceived potential mate value of rivals. Males experience more jealousy than females when their potential rival is more physically dominant, whereas, in contrast, females experience more jealousy when the potential rival is more physically attractive and has more social communal attributes and more social power and dominance (Buunk & Castro Solano, 2011). Height in males is associated with higher mate value, greater perceived dominance and higher social status, and striking height in males, as a measure of high sexual dimorphism, is associated with the lowest levels of cognitive and behavioural jealousy (Brewer & Riley, 2009). Other studies have shown that males demonstrated a preference for their romantic partners to be accompanied on a weekend trip by males whose voices were less masculine and were more jealous in response to males with more masculine voices. In contrast, females rated females with exaggerated sex-typical characteristics as undesirable travel companions for their romantic partners and reported more jealousy in response to imagined flirting from such faces (O'Connor & Feinberg , 2012). These findings are important insofar as they may explain how potential rivals may be identified in the context of pathological jealousy. There is also evidence that jealousy-evoking behaviours may be relevant: a partner's involvement with someone else by means of modern communication devices evokes strong feelings of jealousy, in particular in females, but this response is ameliorated in older people (Dijkstra & Barelds, 2010). This finding makes the point that unintentional jealousy-evoking behaviours may contribute to the provocation and maintenance of feelings of pathological jealousy.

There are other approaches to explaining the psychological origins of jealousy. In the psychoanalytical tradition, primal jealousy arises within the first triadic relationship that an infant experiences that between itself and its two parents. In this scenario, a child identifies with the same-sexed parent and competes for the attention of the other-sexed parent; this competition and rivalry and the feelings and emotions that arise as part of it lay the groundwork for jealous feelings in adulthood. Enoch, Trethowan & Barker (1967, p. 43) summarize the key aspects of psychoanalytical theories as follows:

> A certain event or events may activate … feelings of inferiority, which in turn are always accompanied by anxiety, insecurity, and hypersensitiveness. The threat to the ego becomes real, it must be defended at all costs, and jealousy tends to manifest itself. This in turn is dealt with by the mechanism of projection, and the 'inadequacy' is projected onto the spouse who is accused of infidelity.

There is convergence between psychoanalytical theory and evolutionary biology insofar as both accounts recognize that feelings of possessiveness and the threat of dispossession are important to the emergence of jealousy. But whereas evolutionary biology gives a general account of the origins of jealousy, psychoanalysis attempts to address what it is that renders one person more or less liable to jealousy. Lagache (quoted in Enoch, Trethowan & Barker, 1967) describes a polarity between *amour captatif* and *amour oblatatif*, the former demanding complete surrender and total possession of the sexual partner even in the absence of reciprocation and the other totally giving oneself up to the partner. *Amour captatif* is more linked to jealousy. This description does little to identify what it is that determines exceptional liability to jealous feelings; it merely identifies what pattern of relating is linked to jealousy. The proposition is that the desire to be unfaithful and covert/latent homosexual feelings explain the fact of jealous feelings in individuals. The covert homosexual feelings are intolerable and hence defended against and projected outwards to the partner in the form 'I do not love him; she loves him and not me.' In addition to this formulation is the prior experience of maternal infidelity, which acts to sensitize the patient to the possibility that their own spouse may be unfaithful (Docherty & Ellis, 1976; Hollender & Fishbein, 1979).

The neural underpinning of jealousy is little understood (Marazziti et al., 2013). Research on delusional jealousy provides some evidence suggestive of the neural sites that may be relevant. A patient presenting with chronic delusional jealousy following right cerebral infarct affecting the right temporal and parietal lobes and right frontal involvement confirms the importance of frontal and right hemispheric involvement in various content-specific delusions (Luaute, Saladini & Luauté, 2008,). In a retrospective case series of patients presenting with delusional jealousy, Graff-Radford et al. (2012) showed that delusional jealousy was most likely to be secondary to organic brain disease, most often neurodegenerative disorders. Grey matter loss in the dorsolateral frontal lobes was often present, and there was a preponderance of right frontal lobe pathology. The relative effects of asymmetrical frontal activity were investigated using transcranial direct-current stimulation, which demonstrated that left frontal activity relative to right was associated with greater feelings of jealousy in a modified cyberball paradigm designed to induce jealousy (Kelley, Eastwick & Harmon-Jones, 2015). There is little doubt that there is a need for more investigation of the neural basis of feelings of jealousy as well as of the neurological basis of pathological jealousy.

2.4 Clinical Aspects

The cases described earlier show that morbid jealousy, like jealousy in general, occurs within the context of actual sexual relationships and is accompanied by particular feelings and emotions and specific checking behaviours that are often mundane but that can also be extreme and unusual. In addition, there is the preoccupation with getting the partner to confess to the charge of infidelity. The feelings of jealousy can also occur in the context of real infidelity on the part of the patient or their partner and in some instances both parties. Finally, there is the occurrence of persecutory beliefs taking the form of the erroneous belief that the partner is trying to do away with the patient. As is obvious from these case examples, the risk of violence is very present. In this section, I first draw attention to a community study by Mullen and Martin (1994) which serves to set the context of the range of feelings, cognitions and behaviours reported by a community sample about what constitutes jealousy before going on to elaborate on the feelings and emotions, the behaviours and the effects of jealousy on relationships, and then I discuss the clinical setting of pathological jealousy.

Mullen and Martin (1994) studied a community sample of 351 subjects drawn from a population of 130,000 in the city of Dunedin, New Zealand. They identified 66 subjects (19 per cent) who had high jealousy concerns. In this sample, the most frequently cited jealousy-inducing situations were when a partner showed an interest in someone else (63 per cent) and when the subject did not know the partner's whereabouts (14 per cent). Importantly, 79 per cent of women reported that jealousy had arisen or been exacerbated during periods of menstrual tension. The most commonly reported fear arising from jealousy was the fear of losing the partner (65 per cent), and this was commoner in males. Furthermore, there was also the fear of loss of attention and time (21 per cent), and this was equally common in men as in women. In this community sample, there were no differential fears determined by sex for loss of intimacy, loss of sexual exclusivity, fear of shame and humiliation or loss of financial security. In the subjects scoring highly on jealous concerns, jealous behaviours such as cross-examining of partners, phoning to establish the whereabouts of partners and turning up unexpectedly to check on their partners were more frequent. Searching through partners' possessions, trailing them and examining their clothes for signs of illicit sexual contact were reported exclusively by the more highly jealous group. Strategies for coping with jealousy by women included asking for explanations, open expressions of distress by way of tearfulness or angry recrimination and attempts to make themselves more attractive. Men were more likely to ignore the problem and hope that it would go away. Displacement activities such as spending sprees, drinking excessively and comforting were used by both men and women. The more highly jealous subgroup was more likely to report threatening behaviours and aggression, and a small number reported threatening the rival. A number of subjects (15 per cent) reported having been subjected to physical aggression by a jealous partner, and men and women were equally likely to report this. Low self-esteem was present in 63 per cent of the subgroup with high jealous concerns, and this association was particularly marked in women. Women also were more likely to report responding to jealousy with anger and tearfulness as well as with displacement activities such as excessive eating.

This study in a community sample indicates that the emotions, fears and behaviours associated with jealousy share much with the reported findings from a clinical population. Next, I provide a description of what to expect in a clinical population.

2.4.1 Feelings and Emotions

There's little doubt that a complex of feelings and emotions occurs in pathological jealousy. The most prominent are anger, fear, sadness, envy, sexual arousal and guilt. Jealousy presupposes the belief that the loved object is a possession, and the feelings that occur are understandable once this aspect of sexual jealousy is understood. It is also important to make a distinction between jealousy itself and the fear underlying it, namely the fear or belief that the sexual partner is unfaithful. Strictly speaking, and as White and Mullen (1992) point out, pathological jealousy occurs in the setting of beliefs regarding fidelity of the sexual partner. The anger experienced results from the feeling that one's rightful possession has been appropriated, and the fear or anxiety relates to the possibility that there will be permanent loss of the loved object and also that there may be accompanying shame if it became widely known that the sexual partner had been unfaithful. Socially, this has implications for the sexual desirability or social standing of the jealous person and the possibility of loss of face, loss of status or loss of honour. Sadness rather than anxiety may occur or may alternate with anxiety depending on the degree to which the jealous individual believes that their sexual partner is already lost to them or that their social standing has been unalterably affected. Envy of the attributes of the imagined rival is usually in contrast to the low self-regard of the jealous person. Paradoxically, in many cases the possibility of infidelity serves to increase sexual interest in the partner, and sexual ardour also increases. Finally, feelings of guilt are triggered because of the demanding and often tiresome behaviours that follow in the wake of jealous feelings and the realization that the sexual partner experiences those behaviours in a negative manner.

The feelings and emotions just described are not peculiar to pathological jealousy but occur in jealousy per se. This raises the question of what the distinction is between normal jealousy and pathological jealousy, a subject that I return to later.

Pathological jealousy can occur in the context of other abnormalities of mind, for example, low mood, with associated guilty feelings. The abnormality of mind may then lend to the jealousy particular emphasis or focus. As feelings of worthlessness are not uncommon in depression, the jealous person may come to believe that they are deserving of having an unfaithful partner and that they ought to be deserted and abandoned. Cases where the primary psychiatric condition includes the jealous experience may incorporate persecutory beliefs about malice, beliefs of being unfairly targeted and fear of being poisoned and being in physical or mortal danger. It is also true that the jealous feelings may occur in the setting of emotional vulnerability or physical disability, both of which can influence self-esteem and hence the degree to which an individual believes that they are sexually desirable, and this can obviously feed into the belief that the sexual partner prefers other people and indeed that they are already in a relationship with others.

2.4.2 Behaviours

Checking behaviour that is compelling, totally engrossing and emotionally exhausting is frequent, if not universal, in jealousy. The behaviours include checking the partner's underwear and bed sheets for signs of seminal stain and examining bedding, clothing, curtains and carpets for telltale signs of secret sexual liaisons and intercourse. Diaries, purses, telephone records, motor vehicle milometres and coat pockets can all be subjected to inspection and study. Extreme forms of clandestine investigation, including secretly following the partner, hiring investigative detectives, hiding in car boots and secretly watching the partner from a hideout, are all part of reported behaviours associated with jealousy. These behaviours are all designed to establish the infidelity of the partner, but absence of evidence is rarely sufficient to disconfirm deeply held but erroneous beliefs. Often the result is increasing anxiety and increasing searching and checking behaviours that draw attention to the compulsive aspect of jealousy. It is not unusual for the patient to adduce significance to trivial findings: unusual creases in trousers or bed sheets, depressions on mattresses or car seats, minor changes to the grass on lawns or the manner in which curtains fall when drawn. These are given special meaning, and the patient claims these as evidence of sexual impropriety. In a case reported by Todd and Dewhurst (1955, p. 369), the patient claimed that 'he could hear the windowpane being tapped, and the noise of a car being driven away from outside his house. He would often leave home during the night in search of an "intruder" whom he thought he could hear prowling about outside. Finally, he accused his wife of having a group of lovers and asserted that the noise he could hear at night were signals from her paramours.' There are many reports of inquisitorial cross-examinations and endless pleadings to the sexual partner to confess to their sins and transgressions, and these alternate with naked threats, exhortations and repeated acts of violence. During these periods of checking rituals, surveillance and cross-questionings, the patient may also exhibit a heightened need for reassurance by the partner, asking for kisses, cuddling and increased sexual intimacy. Minor alterations in demonstrations of affection are taken as further signs of infidelity.

In obsessive jealousy, it is argued that the patient does not fully believe in the infidelity of the partner but is assailed by doubt, and the ensuing ritualistic checking behaviours are indistinguishable from compulsive behaviours common in obsessive-compulsive disorder (Batinic, Duisin & Barisic, 2013). This has implications for treatment since the correct treatment is management of the underlying condition.

2.4.3 The Relationship

Sexual jealousy occurs, by definition, within a sexual relationship. The question is whether there are characteristics of sexual relationships that facilitate jealous feelings. Todd and Dewhurst (1955) make the point that significant age difference between the partners might act to trigger jealous feelings and that this can work in both directions. An older man may come to fear that his younger spouse may prefer a younger man. The reverse can also be true – the older woman may come to fear that her husband may have a preference for a younger woman as she ages. In the small series presented by Todd and Dewhurst (1955), there was a preponderance of couples where there was disparity in sexual ardour, and this occurred following a hysterectomy in one case and following childbirth in another case. Much has been made in the literature about the relationship between erectile impotence in a man and subsequent jealousy feelings. The erectile impotence is often secondary to alcohol abuse (Todd & Dewhurst, 1955; Shepherd, 1961). There are also reports of relationships in which either one or both parties have previously openly or secretly engaged in sexual liaisons outside of their relationships. The dynamics of this are multiple and varied. The revelation of sexual impropriety can act to render the partner less trusting, more alert to the possibility of further indiscretions and thereby act to trigger jealous feelings even in the absence of reasonable evidence. Furthermore, an individual who has acted improperly can also come to believe that just as he or she can have sexual liaisons outside their relationship, their partner might also be engaging in such liaisons.

2.4.4 Clinical Setting

Pathological jealousy is best understood as a symptom rather than a condition in its own right. White and Mullen (1992) have created a classification of jealousy and a decision tree to assist diagnostic decision-making. Their approach is to classify pathological jealousy into (1) reactive jealousy and (2) symptomatic jealousy.

Reactive jealousy is characterized by

1. A provoking event such as seeing the partner on their own with a potential rival;
2. A predisposition in the patient that makes them more liable to respond with jealousy in the context of the said trigger and this includes (a) vulnerable personality, (b) prior mental disorder and (c) prior experience of infidelity in a partner or previous experience of abandonment; and
3. An exaggerated jealous response to the trigger involving emotions and behaviours and the nature and quality of the relationship itself.

The notion of a reactive jealousy raises questions about how to distinguish between a normal jealous reaction and pathological reactive jealousy. This question goes to the heart of several issues in defining and characterizing psychiatric disorders. At a simple level, a normal jealous response is one in which the triggering event is factual and would understandably give rise to jealous feelings in most people in the given society under scrutiny. An example would be finding a sexual partner in a compromising situation with another person and where the compromising situation is unequivocal and undeniable. Problems arise in nomenclature when the triggering event is amenable to an alternative explanation, for example, being given a lift in car by a boss of the opposite sex, a scenario that is not definitively a compromising situation. A jealous response in this context needs further elucidation and may become more comprehensible if it becomes apparent that the patient had, as a child, accompanied their mother to visit their paramour in order to throw their father off the scent and had been sworn to secrecy. This context makes clear why with minimal provocation a significant and sustained jealous reaction might occur. In other words, the extent and nature of the triggering event, the presence of vulnerability factors and the extent and severity of the response given the triggering event determine whether the jealousy is regarded as normal or pathological.

In the event that despite evidence to the contrary the belief about spousal infidelity is held with conviction even though triggered by a cue, then the possibility of delusional jealousy must be explored. Delusions can be defined as 'false beliefs that are held with extraordinary conviction and incomparable subjective certainty and are impervious to counter argument' (Oyebode, 2018, p. 105). The key here is the fact that despite the absence of evidence or indeed evidence to the contrary, the patient continues to adhere to the belief of infidelity. There is a distinction to be made between an overvalued idea that is best understood as an acceptable, comprehensible idea pursued by the patient beyond the bounds of reason and usually associated with abnormal personality (Oyebode, 2018) and a delusional belief that is incomprehensible and un-understandable. A good way to conceive of the difference between delusion and overvalued idea in the context of jealousy is illustrated by one of the cases of Enoch, Trethowan and Barker (1967, p. 39).

A 50-year-old man was referred by his own doctor in 1963 because he was accusing his wife of infidelity. There had been a similar episode in 1956–57. Then he had been suspicious for a few months, but he suddenly developed the frank systematized delusion of his wife's infidelity. Eight years later he was able to recount the episode in detail. He stated that his wife had been on a day trip alone, with members of a public-house club. On returning the barmaid made insinuating remarks to him about his wife's behaviour; at that moment the local butcher entered and the patient instinctively 'knew' that this was the man with whom his wife had been associating. This belief became more firmly focused in his mind and he 'went to pieces', becoming agitated and unable to carry on with his work. He believed that 'he knew' that his wife met the alleged paramour at certain times. Minimal clues were misinterpreted as providing definite proof of the liaison, e.g., the change in the appearance of his wife's clothing or behaviour and attitude.

In this case, there is a trigger in the fact of the wife's day trip and the innuendo made by one of the barmaids, yet the pathological belief arose suddenly and fully formed and was then accompanied by a seeking after evidence that no matter how trivial was regarded as confirmatory. The patient's belief can be understood as having arisen in a given context; that is, it is psychologically understandable despite the erroneous belief being held with conviction and hence amounting to an overvalued idea. To reiterate, an overvalued idea is a belief that is understandable but erroneous. A case reported by Shepherd (1961, p. 719), in contrast, illustrates delusional jealousy.

About three months before admission the patient had complained of epigastric discomfort and diarrhoea. About three weeks before admission he had suddenly accused his wife of having had sexual relations with the man in the downstairs flat. He complained of diarrhoea and abdominal pain at this time, and a few days later he again accused his wife and slapped her face. For a few days he appeared to be quite normal, and then he told his wife that he had detailed proof of her infidelity; he had seen her hanging up a sheet to dry which, he claimed, belonged to another man, though it was in fact a sheet from the bed of his own son. On this occasion he struck his wife with a piece of wood and forced a false confession from her; this prevented further violence, and he went to the police maintaining that his wife was poisoning him. . . . In hospital he remained convinced that his wife was unfaithful, citing as evidence the sheet and a code which his wife was supposed to have used for the purpose of communication with her friend; he maintained that his wife was poisoning him and that certain conversations carried a special meaning for him. He was preoccupied with a complex delusional system erected on these beliefs, though at times he appeared to realize that he was mistaken. There was no evidence of hallucinations.

In this case there is nothing that renders the preoccupying belief understandable or comprehensible; the belief is not provoked by a given event that would make the sudden realization that his wife was unfaithful obvious to an independent observer. In a case of this type, we are dealing with a process, a signal event which points to an underlying neurological anomaly rather than a psychologically meaningful and comprehensible reaction to a social event. It could be said that pathology has hijacked neural systems that, in normal circumstances, have adaptive function.

Symptomatic jealousy depends upon the presence of either a primary psychiatric disorder or a neurological disorder, and arguably jealousy is merely a manifestation of the underlying pathology (White & Mullen, 1992). Symptomatic jealousy is said to be characterized by (1) an underlying process that developed prior to or simultaneously with the presenting jealousy, (2) the course and progression are related to the progress of the underlying condition, (3) clinical features of the underlying condition occur simultaneously with the presenting jealousy and (4) there is an absence of any provoking event that can be reasonably related to fears of infidelity.

Pathological jealousy has been reported in organic brain diseases such as epilepsy (Todd & Dewhurst, 1955; Shepherd, 1961), multiple sclerosis (Shepherd, 1961), Alzheimer's dementia (Shepherd, 1961), hypopituitarism (Shepherd, 1961), traumatic head injury (White & Mullen, 1992) and thyrotoxicosis (Shepherd, 1961), and in an study of ex-boxers suffering from a chronic organic brain disease secondary to repeated head trauma during a life of professional boxing, 5 of 17 cases presented with pathological jealousy in the setting of amnestic syndrome (Johnson, 1969) and also as a side effect of treatment with L-DOPA in Parkinson's disease (Poletti et al., 2012). Patients presenting following cerebral infarcts, head injury other than within the context of boxing and meningioma have all been reported (Kuruppuarachchi & Seneviratne, 2011).

Pathological jealousy can also be prominent in schizophrenia (Todd & Dewhurst, 1955; Shepherd, 1961), delusional disorder (White & Mullen, 1992), bipolar disorder (Shepherd, 1961), depression (White & Mullen, 1992) and alcohol-related psychiatric disorder (Shepherd, 1961). It also can be the focus of obsessive-compulsive disorder (Batinic, Duisin & Barisic, 2013).

2.5 Jealousy and Violence

The fictional accounts of jealousy indicate how closely linked are feelings of jealousy and violent anger that too often result in death. In *Medea*, Medea's sexual rival, Glauce, and Medea's two sons are killed as a direct consequence of Medea's sexual jealousy. Othello's induced sexual jealousy results in him killing his innocent wife, Desdemona. And in Tolstoy's *Kreutzer Sonata*, the protagonist kills his wife in a furious rage provoked by jealous feelings. Daly and Wilson (1982) reviewed the literature and showed clearly that male sexual jealousy is a systematized set of behaviours that serve as coercive constraint on female sexuality and that this pattern of behaviour is universal. To put it more explicitly, the claim is that male sexual jealousy is part of a propensity to defend paternity confidence, and it involves sexual jealousy and a dogged inclination to control women and includes the threat of the use of violence to achieve sexual exclusivity. This proposition relies on ideas derived from evolutionary biology and makes the case that violence against wives is largely to be understood as a reflection of sexually differentiated mental mechanisms of sexual proprie-tariness which evolved in an ancestral milieu in which assaults and threats functioned to deter wives from pursuing courses of action that threatened their husbands' fitness. The adaptive cognitive and emotional systems respond to cues indicative of a risk of usurpation of a valued sexual relationship by rivals, cues that vary from indirect and probabilistic indicators of such risk to irrefutable evidence (Daly & Wilson, 1997).

Daly and Wilson (1982) show from their examination of homicide data from Detroit in 1972 that a substantial number of homicides resulting from social conflict were ultimately motivated by sexual jealousy. However, the data set shows that of 47 cases precipitated by male jealousy, 16 female were killed for infidelity, whereas for 11 cases precipitated by female jealousy, 6 males were killed for infidelity. This suggests that many more cases are provoked by jealous males, but nonetheless more females respond violently in the context of sexual jealousy. The importance of the jealousy motive is also confirmed in other studies of homicide (Gibson & Klein, 1961; Chimbos, 1978), and there is further evidence that the risk of spousal homicide is increased by the fear of being abandoned by the spouse (Wilson &

Daly, 1993). The risk here is mainly of violence against women, and the recurring male declaration is often 'If I can't have her, nobody can' (Wilson & Daly, 1993). In this multinational study of spousal homicide in Canada, Australia and the United States, Wilson and Daly (1993) show that in Canada and Australia it was three times more likelihood that the victim was female rather than male, whereas in the United States there was no bias towards females being victims. In addition, the likelihood of the victim being female was significantly greater if the victim was already separated from the male partner at the time of the killing. In other words, the likelihood of the female partner being a victim of homicide was greater if she was not only estranged but also separated from her male partner. The risk was greatest in the period immediately following estrangement (Wilson & Daly, 1993). These findings about spousal homicide and jealousy are replicated in Russia, where the risks to female spouses appear to be greater than in the United States (Gondolf & Shestakov, 1997) and in Ghana (Adinkrah, 2008). In other words, the increased risks to females in spousal homicides appear to have pan-cultural generality.

The risk factors predicting lethal violence including spousal homicide include a history of previous domestic violence, cohabiting, childhood victim of family violence, large age disparity, drug and alcohol misuse, sexual jealousy, threats of separation by the female spouse and personality disorder (Aldridge & Browne, 2003). There is some uncertainty about the strength of previous history of domestic violence as a predictor of lethal violence (Dobash et al., 2007) in the sense that there seems to be a distinction between males who use non-lethal violence compared to those who use lethal violence, but for practical purposes, it is probably best to consider previous history of domestic abuse and history of violence against a previous partner as suggestive of the risk of lethal violence in the context of sexual jealousy.

Spousal homicides tell us something about the motivation for homicide within intimate relationships, and it is clear from the foregoing that sexual jealousy plays a considerable role in spousal homicide. Familicides, the killing of families, share characteristics with uxoricides, the killing of wives: firstly, familicide is almost exclusively perpetrated by a male, and the victims are his spouse, children or stepchildren. There are two distinct varieties of familicide, one involving a male with a grievance directed at his spouse and the other a despondent male faced with imminent financial ruin. In the first variety, coercive control and sexual jealousy seem to play a role (Wilson, Daly & Daniele, 1995).

Evolutionary theory suggests that spousal homicide should be more likely in situations where the female spouse has children by previous partners and also that in cases of familicide, stepchildren ought to be over-represented. There is limited support for this hypothesis in the study of familicide by Wilson, Daly and Daniele (1995) insofar as stepchildren were over-represented as victims in comparison to their numbers in the wider population and less so than in filicides. Brewer and Paulsen (1999) showed that females with stepchildren residing with them compared with females with children fathered by their current male partners were four times more likely to be victims of spousal homicide. In a retrospective study carried out in Belgium, De Koning and Piette (2014) reported that specifically in murder-suicides, males (86 per cent) were most likely to be the offenders, and sexual jealousy was the motivation in 56 per cent. These murder-suicides included spousal murder-suicides, filicide-suicides and familicide-suicides. Sexual jealousy was particularly predominant in young couples, whereas 'mercy killing' was commoner in older couples. Familicides in this series were exclusively male offences.

The pattern of killing in sex-related homicides, predominantly in cases where the motivating cause is jealousy, has been reported to be characterized by multiple stabbings, defined by stabbings of three or greater stab wounds (Radojević et al., 2013). In Scandinavia, homicide by firearms where the victim is female has been reported as being the result of jealousy, and the victim is shot in their own home with a shotgun rather than with a handgun in a different location for male victims (Hougen, Rogde & Poulsen, 2000).

Sexual jealousy also has a role in domestic violence. Studies from women's refuges show that sexual jealousy was one of the reasons why their husbands assaulted them, and Wilson and Daly (1993) in their study reported that 55 out of 362 cases (15.2 per cent) were precipitated by accusations of infidelity and where police intervention was precipitated by an assault, and 29 out of 118 cases (24.6 per cent) were due to accusations of infidelity. The role of sexual jealousy in partner violence is also reported in a population-based survey from China in which 7.2 per cent of females reported that they were hit by their partners in the past year (Wang, Parish & Laumann, 2009).

Looking specifically at cases of jealousy including pathological jealousy (coded as insane homicide), Gibbens (1958) reported that 22 out of 80 sane murders (27.5 percent) and 21 out of 115 insane murders (18.3 per cent) are due to jealousy. The majority of the victims were either wives or mistresses. Shepherd (1961) reported on 81 cases of pathological jealousy, and of these, 1 man had killed his spouse and 3 had attempted to kill their spouses. It is notable that 32 of the 63 men (51 per cent) had assaulted their female spouses compared to 1 female of 18 women (16 per cent). These findings have to be taken with caution given that Shepherd's series is not a consecutive series and is inherently biased. Nonetheless, it gives us an idea of the risks of spousal violence and homicide attendant on pathological jealousy.

2.6 Conclusion

Pathological jealousy, especially the delusional jealousy variant, provides us with the opportunity to further our understanding of how a complex emotion that arises within intimate romantic relationships that has evolutionary biological underpinnings develops into pathology. The set of feelings, cognitions and behaviours that occur within a normal setting can become exaggerated or disassociated from the usual cues such that they can said to be pathological not merely on account of being extreme variants but precisely because they can no longer be understood as comprehensibly arising from shared and psychologically meaningful contexts. The link to violence is also important because it draws attention to the biology and anthropology of male-derived lethal violence directed at female victims and speaks to motivations that are tractable to basic animal behaviours.

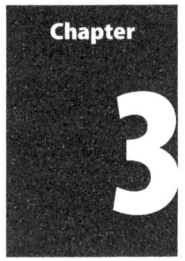

Folie à Deux

3.1 Introduction

In Chapters 1 and 2, I dealt with delusional misidentification syndromes and morbid jealousy, respectively. Delusional misidentification syndromes are, in the main, conceived as explicit manifestation of underlying implicit neurological abnormalities and morbid jealousy as explicable in the light of sociobiological processes. In this chapter, I turn to folie à deux and related conditions that signal the importance to our understanding of delusions of how beliefs and attitudes are formed, how they are amenable to change and how they are transmitted within society.

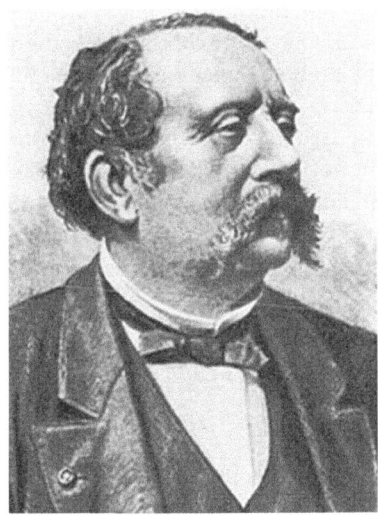

Charles Lasegue 1816–1883

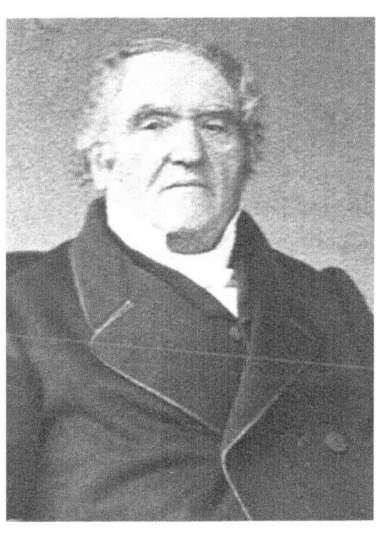

Jean Pierre Falret 1794–1870

Folie à deux was first described by Lasègue and Falret (Lasègue & Falret, 1877/1964). This condition was characterized by the transmission of abnormal beliefs, namely delusions, to another person who in the classic description is usually psychologically normal but lives in close proximity to the ill patient. Where the delusion is transmitted to two people it is termed *folie à trois*, and further extensions to three people (*folie à quatre*) and to whole families (*folie à famille*) have also been described. Subtypes have also been described: *folie imposée* (the mentally ill person imposes their abnormal beliefs on another person), *folie simultanée* (simultaneous but independent psychosis in two people), *folie communiquée* (two related people independently develop psychosis with similar delusional content at the onset but soon become autonomous), and *folie induite* (enrichment of the content of the delusions of another person by a primary case). See Gralnick (1942) and Enoch, Trethowan and Barker (1967) for a full examination of these subtypes. Enoch, Trethowan and Barker (1967) conclude that even though these subdivisions are in common usage, they are of limited value, for not only is their theoretical basis uncertain, but they are also difficult to differentiate in practice (Enoch, Trethowan & Barker, 1967).

Although the first acknowledged descriptions were those by Lasègue and Falret, in fact, case descriptions go back at least to Primrose, who described a case in 1635, to William Harvey in 1651 and to Sir Kenneth Digby in 1685 (Enoch, Trethowan & Barker, 1967). Various other terms have been applied to these conditions, including *communicated insanity*, *induced psychosis*, *infectious psychosis*, and so on.

The essence of these conditions is the fact of delusional beliefs being transmitted from one person to another. It is never surprising that ideas are communicated between people or that beliefs are taught in school. Rhetoric and persuasion are tools for convincing others of notions that they do not already subscribe to. Nonetheless, at face value, it is surprising that false beliefs can also hold sway and be transmitted much in the same way. This means that mechanisms that underpin the transmission of normal beliefs and attitudes may equally be relevant for the transmission of false beliefs. The closest we get to the transmission of patently false beliefs with dire consequences in society are the cases of mass suicide in the context of religious beliefs. These tragic events include the Heaven's Gate mass suicide event of 1997, which occurred in San Diego involving a UFO religious movement; the mass murder/suicide of the Order of the Solar Temple in France, Canada and Switzerland in 1994, 1995 and 1997; and the murder/suicide event in 2000 of the Movement of the Restoration of the Ten Commandments of God in Uganda. Perhaps, the best-studied mass suicide event is the Jonestown event of 1978 in northwestern Guyana, in which 918 people died. These events illustrate the capacity for unusual beliefs, if not outright false beliefs, to be propagated and then to have such force as to persuade ordinary people to take their own lives.

3.2 Case Descriptions

These case reports are drawn from the original cases by Lasègue and Falret (Lasègue & Falret, 1877/1964).

1. Two elderly spinsters were given sole custody, by one of their sisters, of a small, frail, . . . 8-year-old orphan girl. Financial conditions among the three were poor. With the death of one sister and the subsequent lowered income, the economic difficulties increased. The remaining sister developed a common delusion of persecution. . . . She felt the neighbourhood to be leagued against her, heard insulting voices and different noises which she considered to be threatening. The mental deterioration increased gradually and after four years grew to such an extent that other occupants in the house became alarmed. The aunt remained behind locked doors and allowed the child to go out only when absolutely necessary. Questioning the girl, we were told that someone had tried to poison her and her aunt. Both had experienced serious accidents; kidnappers had tried to break into the house to seize the child. . . . The spinster was placed in a mental institution and the child in an orphanage where she is no longer troubled by the parasitic illness of her former guardian.

2. The woman, X, . . . 66-years-old, practices as a midwife in her town. A premature aging process restricted her intellectual capacity as well as her practice. . . . The daughter is 28-years-old; of medium stature, but of limited intelligence. She has studied a bit and even attained a diploma of the lowest degree, as a teacher but has never succeeded of making use of her knowledge. . . . The two women are expelled from their poor apartment without resources [and] arrived in the city. . . . The daughter, X . . ., had, as a matter of fact, an aim with which she acquainted her mother. There existed a Dubois inheritance, or as the mother said . . . a legacy from a certain Dubois. The origin and title of this heritage were unknown, but they were sure it existed. A relative, the daughter's uncle, brother of the mother, was supposed to be the inheritant, but she could not explain the reason because he did not have the name of the pretended testator; he had, so to say, assembled all the papers and made arrangements which were suddenly cut short by his death. . . . Here, after prolonged examination, one begins to trace a web of delusional ideas, imagined by the daughter and reflected by the mother who sanctions them by the wisdom of her age, the sobriety of her statements and the apparent sincerity with which one relates the events of a romantic novel. The two women arrived [in Paris] . . . and lived in a house managed by a Mrs. X. . . . They sought work but found none. The daughter was offered a teaching job in Poland, which she refused because her absence would compromise the success of the enterprise. The landlady seemed to be a little taken in with the delusion which could possibly have become a communication of insanity involving three persons, if the relationship had been more intimate and of longer standing. However, they are more and more reduced to necessity. They sell the little they possess, a ring, linens, and so on until only a few clothes remain. . . . Once the delusion begins it progresses step by step; thus we understand how easy it is to resort to a delusion of persecution, when all effort is powerless, every resource exhausted and one is left, as the mother says, to die of hunger.

3. L . . ., the widow of S . . ., 46 years old, no profession and M . . ., 49 years old, a working woman living together in the same house, were arrested at one o'clock in the morning for sleeping on a bench in the train arrival section, in the Orléans railroad station. They confessed they had passed four nights thus, obliged to hide from mysterious police who desired valuable papers which they possessed. They had arrived together from the south, in Paris, the fifth of December 1872. They went directly to Versailles demanding to see the President of the Republic to obtain justice for thefts of which Mrs. M . . . (we will call her Jeanne) is the victim. The widow, Marie S . . ., had the money necessary for the trip and for their modest upkeep in Paris, during the six months there resided there. She stated the police were incessantly after them and although they were becoming despondent, she hoped to regain some of her money. Without being particularly self-seeking, nevertheless she was certain that when Jeanne becomes a millionaire she would receive a share of the wealth. . . . The interrogation of the commissioner of police, in charge of the first investigation, is explicit enough for us to reproduce now: The woman M . . . related the affair to the parish in which she lived in 1857, at the time of her grandfather's death. He, before dying, knew of the existence of a treasure in a certain house he described with no mention of the location. The priest discovered the hiding place and stole the treasure and it was only in 1866 that the theft took place. She came to Paris to seek the protection of Mr. Thiers. She declared, besides, to have had in 1868, a serious illness brought on by a powder which momentarily paralysed her and her son. . . . At night, on many occasions, strange apparitions have appeared in her room; they do not speak, but make menacing gestures; shiny daggers in the shadows, odd sensations which give her the belief that she was the object of shameful violence, being first put to sleep by odours or drinks, and then abused. During this time someone takes away heavy loads of precious things, and the next day, she awakens in such pain and suffering that she believes she must have a priest. Her friends charitably assume that she is possessed by

the devil and, therefore, should be exorcised. Later the obsession occurs both day and night; the conspirators are disguised, some as merchants, others as salesmen or farm women. They are, of course, able to act more freely. Unknown carriages drive about in the street; some conversations, of the insane woman knows the meaning, are going on. There is a conflict of stories, of enigmatic conversations, of aborted steps to arrive at the truth, of complaints addressed to authorities of the country, one time well-received, another skilfully repulsed. The answers of the widow S . . . during the medical interrogation are both explicit and naïve enough to be worth being mentioned: 'I've known Mrs. M . . . since April or May 1872. The widow of a captain whose ship made long voyages; I met her at the house of one of sailor-friends; I immediately tool interest in her troubles. I am not too familiar with her misfortunes and do not wish to delve into them. . . . I have spent money for her and if she attains her fortune, she will repay me. I started to help her and I won't back-down now, even if I miss my children terribly. I don't expect to make any profit. She always said she will repay me generously, but I don't count on it and in any case, it's nobody's business. I left more than willingly and I don't regret anything because I've done a noble thing; I know she was treated unjustly. My husband saved a fortune like that; the ship burned; they found hidden gold in the desert; I said to myself, "I will be able like him to save a fortune."' . . . The widow S . . ., after a short separation, asked to return to her children. Upon request, they came to Paris to pick her up. The woman Jeanne M . . . was put in a mental institution.

3.3 Explanatory Hypotheses

Lasègue and Falret (1877/1964) in their original paper argued that the following conditions must be met in order for folie à deux to occur. These conditions were, firstly, the presence of an active individual who is more intelligent than another and who creates the delusion and gradually imposes it on the second, more passive individual. The second, passive individual resists the pressure of his or her associate by reacting to modify, correct and coordinate the delusion until it becomes a common cause. Although it is not explicitly stated, a power relation exists that allows the communication of the false belief to occur. Secondly, it is essential that both individuals live a close-knit existence, in the same environment, for a long period of time, sharing the same feelings, the same interests and the same apprehensions and hopes and be isolated from outside influences. Thirdly, the delusion must be kept within the limits of the possible, based upon past events and an apprehension or hope for the future. The condition of probability makes the belief communicable and allows for the conviction to take place (Lasègue & Falret, 1877).

Earlier attempts to grasp the underlying mechanisms focused on psychoanalytical theory and added to the conditions identified by Lasègue and Falret's notions of identification of the secondary case with the primary case, notions of imitation and sympathy and, finally, the shock and strain of caring for a person with a psychiatric disturbance (Gralnick, 1942). Specifically, identification referred to an unconscious mechanism by which an individual seeks to pattern his or her own ego after the image of another. And the proposition that the shock and strain of caring for someone with a psychiatric disorder suffers the same difficulty as that of identification as a mechanism because not all who care for psychiatric patients go on to develop a psychiatric disorder. The mediating factor that is often advanced as of potential interest is heredity or personality vulnerability (Gralnick, 1942).

The conditions that Lasègue and Falret stipulate and the further adumbrations of these factors presuppose the possibility that beliefs and attitudes in general are communicable within culture – and that the same factors or features of communication that operate within the normal sphere must, by definition, also have force in the context of the transmission of abnormal beliefs. Culture can be thought of as sets of traditions, rules and symbols that shape and are enacted as feelings, thoughts and behaviours of groups of people. Thus, culture can be regarded as all the artefacts including ideas, beliefs and practices that are produced by human beings and passed from one generation to another. Our interest is specifically in what counts as belief, and this is often set against what counts as knowledge since the transmission of knowledge, factual knowledge, is also an aspect of culture.

Abelson (1979), without defining exactly what beliefs are, characterized the typical features of beliefs in contrast to knowledge. His characteristic features include (1) lack of consensus, (2) concern with the existence or non-existence of certain conceptual entities, (3) representations of alternative worlds, (4) evaluative and affective components of beliefs, (5) the need for episodic material from personal experience or cultural beliefs, (6) openness and (7) the fact that beliefs are held with varying degrees of certitude. In this schema, Abelson is referring with respect to the term *lack of consensus* the fact that the term *belief* carries the connotation that the content of a particular belief is disputable. Concern with the existence or non-existence of certain conceptual entities is best illustrated by the idea of belief in witches or aliens. This concern draws attention to the fact that the dispute does not depend on facts as such. Insofar as representation of alternative worlds is concerned, here we are dealing with the possibility of, for example, utopian or idealized solutions to the present world. Abelson refers to the evaluative and affective components of beliefs, stressing how beliefs serve to appraise concepts as either 'good' or 'bad' and, on the basis of the resulting judgement, organize and motivate behaviour. The beliefs are sustained by episodic memory (i.e., beliefs are justified by events or personal experiences), whereas it is not the case that knowledge claims are justified by personal experience but rather by objective non-personal facts. Abelson makes the important claim that beliefs are 'open', and he means by this the fact that there is an unclear boundary between belief systems that excludes as irrelevant concepts lying outside their framework and that this is the case because beliefs require the self-concept of the believer at some level. Finally, beliefs are held with various degrees of certitude, whereas it would be unusual to make the claim that one knows a fact to be true strongly. Now it is important to emphasize that Abelson makes a distinction between belief and knowledge but that this distinction is not without criticism (Österholm, 2010).

In many respects, these features of beliefs are as important for our understanding of delusional misidentification syndromes and morbid jealousy as they are for our understanding of folie à deux and for delusions in general. It is the case, though, that given the degree to which folie à deux behaves like ordinary beliefs that are liable to cultural transmission, the characteristic features of beliefs in opposition to knowledge statements become even more important.

I want now to turn to the evaluative aspect of beliefs. Usually, *attitude* is defined as an evaluative response to an antecedent stimulus or object. The stimulus may or may not be observable and can best be thought of as an independent or exogenous variable. It is thought to have three components, the so-called tripartite theory, including cognitions, affect and behaviour. An illustrative example is as follows: a person responds to the presence of a Mercedes-Benz car by thinking that it a prestigious object (cognition), he or she then experiences a pleasurable feeling in response to the cognition (affect), and this provokes the purchase of the car (behaviour). In this account, there is an assumption that all three component parts of an attitude cohere as an entity, whereas empirical evidence does not wholly support this view but rather suggests that these components can operate in partial or with complete independence from one another (Breckler, 1984). What is important for our purpose is that there is an inter-relationship between our notion of beliefs and attitudes insofar as beliefs have an evaluative aspect to them and attitudes express our evaluative stance towards objects in the environment and determine how we behave towards those objects. But of prime interest is the degree to which we understand the factors that determine how attitudes can be influenced because these factors may be relevant to how we conceive of the process underlying the transmission of abnormal beliefs in folie à deux.

So what are the factors that are recognized as being important in persuasive communication and that are influential in changing attitudes and hence altering beliefs? Persuasive communication is best understood as the use of verbal messages to influence attitudes and behaviours. It is unique in the sense that it relies on and appeals to reason as a means of accomplishing change and compliance by convincing an individual of the validity and legitimacy of an advocated position (Ajzen, 2005). It is recognized that aspects of the source of information, features of the recipient of information, characteristics of the message and the social context of the communication all matter. Physical attributes of the source of the information such as age, ethnicity, facial expressions and social status, including income, power and self-confidence, are important. Credibility and attractiveness are the most often studied factors in the source of information. The personality traits, gender, intelligence and social status of the recipient of information influence the degree to which the individual is likely to respond to persuasive communication. Finally, the context of the communication, whether or not there is distraction or forewarning, determines how the message will be received. Broadly speaking, the factors described are well established, and there is consensus regarding their importance. But, in addition to these factors, there is a role for other motives for agreeing with others: attitude change can result from the wish to ensure social coherence and a favourable evaluation of the self and making sure that satisfactory relations with others are maintained given the rewards and punishments they can provide. There is also the pressure to fully understand the issues described in the material that is the subject of an influence appeal (Wood, 2000).

Persuasive communication theory and empirical findings that derive from it have yet to be systematically studied or applied to folie à deux. However, the original suppositions of Lasègue and Falret, as described earlier, can be understood in the light of persuasive communication theory – namely that factors in the source of the delusional belief and in the recipient will determine whether or not the false belief comes to be transmitted at all. The nature of the belief, the degree to which it is plausible and amenable to logic and reason and the context of the communication and the fact that the individuals live in close proximity and have a degree of mutual dependence contribute to the successful transmission of the false belief from one to the other.

3.4 Clinical Aspects

Gralnick (1942) reviewed 103 cases that had been reported to date at the time of her publication in 1942. She confirmed that folie à deux was a rare condition occurring in 0.028 to 1.7 per cent of hospital admissions. Most often the condition occurred within sister-sister dyads followed in frequency by mother-daughter dyads. The inducer was more likely to be an older than a younger person. The abnormal belief was predominantly persecutory in nature, and the psychiatric condition in the inducer was schizophrenia. The role of dominance and submission within the relationship was not always clear. The fact that folie à deux occurs in individuals who are closely associated and live together makes the distinction between hereditary and environmental causation difficult to disentangle as the pair are very often blood relatives.

Silveira and Seeman (1995) studied case reports published between 1942 and 1993. They concluded that males were as likely to be affected as females. There was equal prevalence in younger and older patients, and the majority of shared psychoses were equally distributed among married couples, siblings and parent-child dyads. Hallucinations were also common, and the individuals were socially isolated.

A more recent review of 42 cases by Arnone, Patel and Tan (2006a) showed that even though the mean age for primary cases was older than for secondary cases, this was not statistically significant. There were more female primary and secondary cases too, but the differences between males and females were not statistically significant. The cases occurred almost exclusively within nuclear families, and the largest proportion was within married or common-law couples and the second largest between sister-sister dyads. In married couples, there was no difference between husband-wife and wife-husband dyads with regard to who was the primary or secondary case. There was evidence of social isolation, substantial periods of association between the primary and secondary cases and substantial duration of exposure to the abnormal beliefs. Delusional disorder and schizophrenia accounted for over half the primary cases, and persecutory beliefs were most prominent. Nonetheless, there were reports of cases with affective disorders. Separation as a form of treatment for the secondary case, on its own, was only used in 19 per cent of cases, and 62 per cent requited medication alone. This suggests that separation is probably not the treatment of choice in secondary cases. There are notable changes between the original review by Gralnick (1942) and the latest review by Arnone, Patel and Tan (2006a), and this suggests that with improved clinical diagnosis, the pattern of presentation may be changing such that the original preponderance in females and female pairings may no longer be true. Furthermore, the established consensus that separation is likely to be beneficial in the secondary case may be optimistic.

A review of 97 cases reported in the Japanese literature confirmed many of characteristics already established in Western cases except that mother-child dyads are commoner and sister-sister dyads less frequent. The primary case is more likely to be young compared to Western countries, and religious delusions are said to be commoner (Kashiwase & Kato, 1997).

It is of interest too that the communicability of delusional parasitosis is unstated in the literature on folie à deux, perhaps because the emphasis has been on the transmission of persecutory beliefs. Nonetheless, there is increasing appreciation of the liability of delusional parasitosis to be transmitted to others (Bourgeois, Duhamel & Verdoux, 1992; Kim et al., 2003; Friedmann et al., 2006; Gönül et al., 2008; Daulatabad et al., 2017), and Cordeiro, Corbett and Cordeiro (2003) report that 5 to 25 per cent of cases present as folie à deux (see also Evans & Merskey, 1972). In a series reported by Musalek and Kutzer (1990), 9 cases of folie à deux occurred in a sample of 107 patients (8.4 per cent) with delusions of infestation. Females were more likely to be primary cases, and there was a suggestion that genetic factors were less likely to be involved as mechanisms.

The emphasis in reports of folie à deux is often on delusional beliefs, but there are reports of induced hallucinations, such as that by Dantendorfer, Maierhofer and Musalek (1997) in which the inducer required a combination of drug and psychotherapeutic treatment, whereas the secondary recovered solely with psychotherapeutic treatment. Indeed, Arnone, Patel and Tan (2006b) reported in their review that hallucinations were shared in 59 per cent of cases, predominantly auditory hallucinations in 45 per cent of cases, but not exclusively so. There were also cases of induced somatic, visual, tactile and olfactory hallucinations.

It is also true that the clinical setting of folie à deux is almost exclusively schizophrenia, affective psychosis and delusional disorder. However, it has been reported in the context of Alzheimer's dementia (Draper & Cole, 1990) and intellectual disability (Meakin, Renvoize & Kent, 1987; Ghaziuddin, 1991; Mazzoli, 1992).

The condition is not restricted to dyads as many cases involving three, four or more individuals have been reported, including cases involving whole families (Dewhurst & Eilenberg, 1961; Sims, Salmons & Humphreys, 1977; Fernando & Frieze, 1985; Glassman, Magulac & Darko, 1987; Dippel, Kemper & Berger, 1991; Guisado Macías et al., 2001; Ilzarbe et al., 2015).

3.4.1 Twins

Descriptions of folie à deux in monozygotic twins raises the question of how to distinguish between the coincidental onset of psychiatric disorder in two people who are twins and therefore liable to develop a psychiatric disorder given the genetic vulnerability that exists for conditions such as schizophrenia and the possibility of a disorder that is induced in one of a pair of twins by a primary case. Shiwach and Sobin (1998) report a case of folie à deux in two elderly twins and make the claim that on review of the published literature, delusional disorder rather than schizophrenia is more likely to be the psychiatric disorder in the primary case in folie à deux in twins and, furthermore, that neither separation nor drug treatment was particularly helpful.

It is true that some cases reported as folie à deux in monozygotic twins, on review, seem more likely to be cases of coincidental schizophrenia in individuals with a genetic propensity (Craike & Slater, 1945), whereas others, such as the report by Lazarus (1986), demonstrate the complexity of the interaction between genetics and a symbiotic social life in generating and sustaining folie à deux in twins. In another report (Adler & Magruder, 1946), both twins acutely developed the delusional belief that their father was dead, on the same day, and both responded well to electroconvulsive treatment. However, the familial genetic loading for schizophrenia was considerable, and the degree to which this case report could be said to exemplify folie à deux is weak. Kendler et al. (1986) introduced the concept of a positive-feedback loop in which two genetically vulnerable individuals develop psychosis simultaneously, and because of their social symbiosis, their psychopathology becomes involved in a positive-feedback loop that both intensifies and maintains their psychosis. This view is echoed by White (1995), who commented that progression of the delusion appears to be fuelled by resonance mechanism. To complicate matters further, Ohnuma and Arai (2015) reported on a case of *folie à quatre* that involved a primary case who was a twin and the transmission of his beliefs and visual hallucinations to his monozygotic twin and their parents. This case report underlined the complexity of disentangling the biological from the social in cases of folie à deux in twins.

3.4.2 Suicide Pacts

Suicide pacts and folie à deux are both rare phenomena. It is estimated that death by suicide pact is a mere fraction of the overall suicide rate: in England and Wales, it is reported as 0.6 per cent, in Germany as 3.6 per cent and in Japan as 4 per cent. In contrast, folie à deux comprises 1.7 per cent of consecutive admissions to psychiatric hospitals (Salih, 1981). The subject is of interest because of the occurrence of events such as the Jonestown mass suicide in which 912 members of the People's Temple took their own lives at the instruction of their leader Jim Jones, where we see an intersection between erroneous but firmly held beliefs allied to mass suicide. Salih (1981) reports a case of two women who jointly decided to die by suicide in the context of shared and identical delusional beliefs against a backdrop of a close social association. He argues that the report demonstrates that the factors determining the development of folie à deux also facilitate suicide pacts, and this is supported by other reports (Lange & Ficker, 1976). Rosen (1981) makes the point that dyadic, family and collective suicides have a lot in common, including exclusivity and isolation, the threat of dissolution and the presence of a powerful initiator – the main distinction from folie à deux being the threat of dissolution of the relationship. In a study by Brown, King and Barraclough (1995), there were 9 suicide deaths (2.5 per cent) by pacts in 722 consecutive suicides. In none of these deaths was folie à deux a factor. The motivations included the need for relief from mental disorders and pain.

3.4.3 Violence and Crime

It is not always well recognized that folie à deux may be associated with violent crime. Grenberg (1956) reviewed the literature on folie à deux and crime and drew attention to the association between folie à deux and murder. His review included case reports going back to 1821 and examined cases of suicide pacts, murder by individuals and murder or mass suicides within cults. Kelly (2009) wrote of two cases of homicide in nineteenth-century Ireland. He reported that both cases occurred in the context of *folie à plusieurs*. The first was a case of three brothers who became suddenly mentally ill with pyrexia and tachycardia and who killed a fourth brother. The second was a family of five including a mother, three daughters and a son who killed another son. The father was present but was not charged with any offence. In both cases, there was a sudden development of mental illness in several individuals who then acted jointly to murder another family member. This relationship of homicide and violent action to folie à deux is further developed in the paper by Kraya and Patrick (1997), in which they describe five New Zealand cases in all of which there was association of a fatal or potentially fatal outcome with shared religious delusions. They make the point that the religious beliefs may appear normal such that other relatives may be unaware of the ominous risks that attend these beliefs. Finally, the courts found it difficult to consider the notion of 'communicated insanity' as equivalent to 'a genuine case of insanity'. This issue of the psychiatric status of the beliefs that facilitate or indeed determine the violent actions that lead to death is once again referred to in a paper by Rahman et al. (2013) in which they describe a case of infanticide. The mother had a history of schizoaffective disorder, whereas the father had no significant psychiatric history but had come to share in his wife's abnormal religious beliefs, which subsequently led to the death of their infant by starvation. In this case, in order to satisfy the courts, it was argued that the husband's abnormal beliefs were examples of overvalued ideas.

Folie à deux in forensic psychiatry contexts highlights the problem of comprehending the nature of abnormal beliefs in general and in folie à deux in particular. How far can an induced belief in an individual without prior psychiatric illness and whose abnormal beliefs are transitory be regarded as occurring out of an abnormality of mind? Even though secondary cases in folie à deux can be shown to have impairments of belief evaluation, the source of these impairments seemed to be due to motivational rather neuropathological mechanisms. This was contributed to by social isolation (Nielssen, Langdon & Large, 2013). In other words, the degree to which an induced delusional belief can be said to be evidence of mental illness for forensic purposes is currently moot.

In an unusual case report, Caribé et al. (2013) describe *folie à trois* associated with the murder of a son by his mother and brother. The primary case appears to have occurred, acutely, in the context of systemic lupus erythematosus, but the abnormal beliefs were influenced by widely shared cultural beliefs in other family members. The role of sleep deprivation in augmenting the extent and severity of the disorders was notable. These cases, including those described earlier, invariably involve the murder of family members within the context of widely shared religious beliefs. In this latter case report, even the family members, after the event, continued to explain the tragic outcome through religious and mystical understandings.

Folie à deux can also be involved in court decisions to rule on parental custody cases as it can on criminal cases (Newman & Harbit, 2010). In custody cases, the prominent question is whether or not the shared parental or family beliefs put the children at risk of harm. The essential issues are the same, namely whether or not the shared beliefs contribute to the behaviours that are under consideration. There is a risk of therapeutic paralysis as the clinical decisions can be confounded by legal issues and families may flee, in pursuit of social isolation, thereby rendering the children even more at risk (Ulzen & Carpentier, 1997).

Where the alleged crimes are by cult members, there is the thorny issue of how to distinguish between abnormal shared beliefs and culturally normative but sub-cultural beliefs. Joshi, Frierson and Gunter (2006) make the point that a cult may resemble mass shared psychotic disorder and that in determining whether a cult member has folie à deux, three questions may be helpful: (1) when does the teaching of a few become mainstream, (2) when do false beliefs become delusional, and (3) how many people have to participate for a group to become a cult?

In a case described by Newman and Harbit (2010), *State v. Ryan*, the defendant was accused of torturing and killing a fellow cult member. The group lived on a remote farm and believed that their leader could communicate directly with God, or 'Yahweh'. The victim fell out of favour and was demoted to 'slave' after his first year. The cult leader, who was also the father of the defendant, instructed subordinates to torture and kill the victim. The victim was chained, forced to sleep on the porch and was subjected to whipping, having a shovel pushed into his rectum and being forced to have sex with a goat. It was reported that the defendant bragged about the killing, showed no remorse and deriving pleasure from sadistic behaviour. This case graphically exemplifies the principle that killings that are apparently driven by shared but erroneous beliefs may not be recognized by the courts as demonstrating evidence of insanity precisely because the defendants can be shown to understand the nature and quality of their actions and know that the actions were wrong and punishable.

3.5 Conclusion

Folie à deux cases illustrate the fact that abnormal beliefs can be induced in people with no prior history of psychiatric disorder. It is well established that the primary case and the secondary have to be in a close and intimate relationship and that social isolation facilitates the development of folie à deux. It is no longer a given that separation of the individuals necessarily results in improvement in the secondary cases. Furthermore, the role of hereditary factors in the secondary cases cannot be ruled out as a considerable number cases occur within families. An understanding of the social psychological literature on persuasive communication may help to further our understanding of the processes and mechanisms that underpin folie à deux. The risks of suicide pacts, violent behaviour and murder must be recognized by clinicians and properly assessed.

Chapter 4

Couvade and Pseudocyesis

4.1 Introduction

In Chapters 1–3, I explored the differing origins of delusional beliefs with the express purpose of arguing that the underlying mechanisms of delusional beliefs are what distinguishes different sets of delusions from one another. This notion is a departure from the now well-established demarcation of delusions into primary and secondary delusions and overvalued ideas. It emphasizes underlying mechanisms, pointing to the role of impairment of face processing, for example, in delusional misidentification syndromes and the place of the evolutionary biology of mate selection and the differential energetics of mating strategies in morbid jealousy. Finally, I argued that in folie à deux, the social psychology of persuasive communication and the normative mechanisms for transferring beliefs between people and in social groups are a prerequisite for understanding its origins.

In this chapter, I examine couvade and pseudocyesis, two distinct but conceptually related conditions. I demonstrate that social and cultural contexts can influence bodily experiences and sometimes belief formation, including abnormal beliefs, and that beliefs too have a propensity to determine subjective experience of the body. In this section, I distinguish between belief acquisition driven by the features that are known to influence belief acquisition in the presence of another person (as described in Chapter 3) and the development of beliefs in the context of social expectations and norms. In the one, it is intimate relationship with a person displaying emotional and psychiatric disturbance that provokes in another disturbed thinking and abnormal beliefs. In the other, the abnormality of thinking influences bodily experience but is set in the context of social and cultural beliefs that make the abnormal belief ponderable. In order to exemplify these points, I draw attention to couvade and pseudocyesis. Couvade, as I describe in the next section, is the physical experience of features of pregnancy, parturition and lactation in males without the accompanying erroneous belief of pregnancy. This condition is comprehensible in the context of the normative sociocultural couvade ritual. In contrast, pseudocyesis is false pregnancy in a female combining the false belief of pregnancy with the physical manifestations of pregnancy. This is once again a condition that is comprehensible in a cultural context, namely one that places premium on fertility and childbearing.

4.2 Couvade

Couvade is defined as the custom in which a father at the birth of his child makes a ceremonial pretence of being the mother, nursing and taking care of the newborn and performing other rites such as fasting and abstaining from certain foods and occupations in order to protect the newborn from harm. It is the father who experiences fatigue and the discomfort of childbirth, while the mother continues with her daily occupations (Doja, 2005). To be more specific, this is a birth custom characterized by the confinement and restriction of the father for a period after the birth of the child. This cultural practice is said to be prevalent worldwide but particularly so in South America and Southeast Asia. The term *couvade* is attributed to Edward Burnett Tylor (1832–1917), an English anthropologist, and is said to be a variation on the French word *couver* meaning a 'hatch or brood of hens'. Later work has demonstrated that the origin of the term was in fact an error, since it never meant a brood of hens but simply a covey of chickens. Whatever the case, the term is now established. The social function of this rite is still in dispute. Some authorities believe that it is a means of legitimizing the father's social role, a means of strengthening conjugal bonds in societies with fragile and unstable conjugal bonds or as a certificate of legitimacy and recognition of the child as the father's (Doja, 2005). There are psychoanalytical explorations of the role of ritual couvade, including viewing the practice as a consequence of conflicts about penis envy, castration anxiety, womb envy and unconscious aggression directed at the female progenitor of children.

More modern examinations, exemplified by the works of Laura Rival (1998) and Karen Middleton (2000), focus on the performative aspects of couvade and emphasize the way that a ritual acts to announce the arrival of a new human being and reform the originally established configuration of affiliations. Doja (2005, p. 929) puts it like this: '[i]f procreation is a quintessentially creative act, the birth of a child represents an essential moment of the life transfer process, which involves the recognition of both a new person and the web of relationships without which she or he would not exist as a full social being.' In other words, 'the natural birth is counterbalanced by a cultural birth. . . . What is called couvade is part of a public means of confirming or creating classificatory relations, of rearranging the cognatic universe into the idiom of substances, objects and behaviours' (p. 946).

This discussion about couvade sits within the context of our ambivalence regarding the possibility of males giving birth or indeed about males enacting a ritual of being in labour or delivering a child. Various myths have male characters giving birth, such as Athena springing fully formed from Zeus's forehead and Loki, the shape-shifter, turning into a mare to avoid a stallion and giving birth to Sleipnir. But these myths only serve to accentuate the prevailing tendency to look at the possibility of male pregnancy or childbirth with suspicion, if not with outright derision, as pregnancy and motherhood are synonymous with being a woman. It is within this context that I examine couvade syndrome.

4.2.1 Case Reports

The original case descriptions are from Trethowan and Conlon (1965).

1. A 26-year-old Australian soldier was admitted, while on active service, to a military hospital with a swollen abdomen resembling that which might have been caused by a fairly advanced pregnancy. There was occasional dry vomiting but no pain or tenderness. Investigations showed no evidence of intra-abdominal disease. On being anaesthesized his abdomen became quite flat and no mass or abnormality could be felt on deep palpation. Once consciousness was regained tumefaction returned. He had married while on leave and learned after returning to duty that his wife was pregnant. It was at this point that his abdominal swelling occurred. His wife suffered greatly from morning sickness and importuned him by letter to return home. He worried greatly over this and at

the irregularity of mail. Altogether his abdominal swelling persisted for 22 months; then he returned home, for the first time since his child was born, and the swelling at once subsided. Twelve years later the swelling recurred, on this occasion not in relation to a pregnancy (there were no subsequent children) but following separation from his wife. Once again, all investigations were negative.

2. F.L., a 29-year-old man who earned his living as an itinerant house-painter, presented to the casualty department of a general hospital immediately after his wife's admission to the obstetric wards for her first confinement. He complained of 'labour pains', which he said consisted of a sensation of pressure in his pelvis and tightness in his abdomen. Retrospectively it was discovered that he had suffered various symptoms throughout his wife's [pregnancy], including nausea, a feeling of distension and quickening sensations. As her labour proceeded, so did his symptoms progress. When he learned that his wife had undergone an episiotomy, he developed perineal soreness. During the first part of her lactation he complained of bilateral breast discomfort. Then, during her involution, all his symptoms receded. Despite the bizarre and prolonged nature of these complaints, and although no physical abnormality was evident, to him his symptoms were undoubtedly real ones.

4.2.2 Explanatory Hypotheses

As described earlier, anthropology uses the term *couvade* to define the different ritual behaviours fathers-to-be must follow in various societies in order to be initiated into paternity. In some cultures, the man will also go to bed as labour begins, take limited amounts of food and water and simulate labour pains and pelvic movements as though giving birth himself. He will sometimes receive concerned attention from other community or family members, much like his 'labouring wife'. This whole sequence of ritual couvade has been observed in many racial and national groups and extends far back into antiquity. One of the earliest descriptions is from 60 BC by Diodorus Siculus about the phenomenon he observed in Corsica. Anthropologists have noticed many rituals surrounding pregnancy and childbirth and have been interested in the way the husband's role was tightly woven into many of the rituals. The couvade rituals in which men wore special clothes, ate certain foods and acted out a mock labour were believed to be a way for the father either to assert his paternity or to protect the pregnant woman from evil by acting as the decoy and posing as the expectant one. Frazer distinguishes between two forms of ritual couvade, prenatal or pseudo-maternal couvade and postnatal or dietetic couvade (George, 1910). Frazer's own view is that couvade is not a ritual intended to transfer or confer parental rights over the children to the father. Rather, the aim is by sympathetic magic through a strict diet and regimen prenatally to protect the newborn or by simulation of childbirth by a man to relieve the mother of the pangs of childbirth by transferring them to the pretended mother, that is, the man. Frazer cites examples of pseudo-maternal couvade among the Dyaks of Sarawak, who perform a pantomime of obstructed labour on the husband when his wife is in difficulty. There are other examples among the Gujaratis and Erukalavandlu of Southern India and in Ireland, France, Germany, Estonia and Scotland. A vestige survived in Europe, where it was a custom for the woman in hard labour to wear her husband's trousers or hang them round her neck or creep between his legs when he is asleep. In Guiana, it has been reported that the husband leaves his occupation prior to the delivery and follows a strict diet. He avoids weapons because he believes that he is united to the child by such an intimate bond of physical sympathy that the child might otherwise be hurt or even killed (Bogren, 1983).

These customs are different from postnatal couvade, where the intention is to protect the child from disease, caused by the father's behaviour, by imposing a regimen upon him (Brockington, 1996). There are examples of first-time fathers among the Caribs undergoing a severe ordeal of fasting and absenteeism from work and hunting in South America from seventeenth-century travellers' tales (Brockington, 1996). This has been attributed to the natural bond and sympathy of father and child among peoples who deny the physical separation of individuals. These customs are worldwide and present among many peoples in South America, Borneo, Greenland, California, West Africa, China, northern Spain, and Corsica (Bogren, 1983).

The clinical phenomenon of couvade has been widely documented and is reported as occurring at rates of 20 to 80 per cent in the United States (Schodt, 1989). It is defined as a wide range of symptoms that expectant fathers may display or report during the pregnancy of their partners. The salient feature is said to be the timing of the symptoms – they have their onset with the pregnancy, are not explained by injuries or illnesses and resolve with birth of the child. It has also been observed in societies where ritual couvade is not practiced.

Wainwright (1966) noted that psychopathological reactions to fatherhood probably occur with more frequency than is commonly recognized. Since the illness is attributed by the patient to other stressors, the importance of the recent birth of a child may be overlooked initially; therefore, a careful enquiry is necessary to establish the relationship. Clinton (1986) makes an observation in her 'developmental crisis theory' that transition to fatherhood is as dramatic as that to motherhood. This has been put forward as an explanation for the experiences of expectant fathers. Transitional stresses that have been aetiologically linked to pregnancy symptoms in Western men include an increased sense of economic and social responsibility, anxiety about what parenthood means for future job prospects, feelings of alienation and abandonment as attention is centred on the pregnant partner and guilt and fear about the mate's impending delivery ordeal. Such a hugely complex issue definitely deserves more exploration than what it currently has managed to attain.

There is a distinction to be made between understanding the basis and origin of ritual couvade and clinical couvade. A number of theories have been put forward, and it is sometimes difficult to distinguish between theories exploring the meanings of ritual couvade and the underlying dynamics of clinical couvade. To put it more precisely, ritual couvade is best understood as a cultural practice that serves particular purposes, whereas clinical couvade serves no cultural end, and even if understood in the light of what we know about ritual couvade, in the individual reported cases there is no denoted cultural meaning.

The proposed theoretical explanation for clinical couvade includes (1) a man's psychological reaction to his wife's pregnancy arising from envy of the wife's ability to bear children and create life (Wilson, 1977; Radhakrishnan, Satheeshkumar & Chaturvedi, 1999), (2) empathy existing between husband and wife and their intense sharing of emotional experience and physical sensation (Wilson, 1977), (3) ambivalence about fatherhood and perception of the foetus as a rival (Tényi, Trixler & Jádi, 1996; Budur, Mathews & Mathews, 2005b), and (4) expression of the anxiety in men stemming from the psychological crisis of childbirth in the form of somatic symptoms.

The first theory explains the phenomenon by viewing it as a psychological reaction of a man to his wife's pregnancy, which symbolizes expression of frustrated creativity and deep-rooted infantile envy of his wife's ability to bear a child. However, there is no empirical evidence that patients with couvade have explicitly claimed that they are envious of their wife's pregnancy. The explanation that the husband wants to intensely share the emotional experience of the wife had been put forward by Marco Polo as early as the thirteenth century when he described vicarious suffering in Oriental countries, and he considered that it was only fair that the husband should share in the pains of childbirth. It is true that there must be identification with the wife to have certain symptoms, and a constellation of explanations based on the idea of empathy and identification with wives' situations has been recorded (Wilson, 1977). These explanations appear to be reasonable but do not go far enough to explain the mechanism underlying how empathy or identification provokes physical sensations. There is a conviction that dissociation or conversion processes are at play, but even if they are, we are still at a loss to explain the mechanism that transforms emotional distress to physical symptoms in these cases. The third explanation is the idea that the father is ambivalent about fatherhood and perceives the foetus as a rival. In this model, clinical couvade is thought to reflect unexpressed underlying aggressive impulses. It is unclear whether the couvade is a defence against aggressive impulses or an expression of aggressive impulses. Some authors have observed that men in their effort to suppress their own worries about the pregnancy and childbirth converted them to somatic symptoms. This theory to an extent is drawn from Reik's propositions that pseudo-maternal couvade occurred in the setting of an ambivalent relationship between sexual partners and that ritual couvade was a protective measure against aggressive tendencies and impulses from the man towards his partner (Reik, 1974). Furthermore, in this scenario, dietetic couvade is designed to protect the newborn from the aggressive impulses of the father. These theories do not help to explain how unconscious aggressive impulses towards the spouse or child are converted to physical symptoms.

A novel approach to explaining the transmission of physical features of distress from one to another is encapsulated in the term *compathy*, which is described as occurring when one person observes another person suffering a disease or injury and experiences in one's physical body a similar or related distress. Compathy is said to be the physical equivalent of empathy. Triggers for the compathetic response include observing the suffering or hearing, reading or thinking about descriptions of the symptoms (Morse & Mitcham, 1997). Use of the terms *empathy* and *compathy* does not exactly assist an understanding of mechanisms and systems underpinning the physical features of distress from one person to another. For that we need to appreciate the physiology of mirror neurones. These neurones appear to underlie action understanding in monkeys and in human beings too. In human beings specifically, there is evidence of activation of mirror neurone systems during observation of actions, including gestures and intentional and meaningless movements. Furthermore, imitation of actions that are in the observer's repertoire of movements also activates mirror neuronal circuits. Finally, there is a suggestion that oral movements may have a role in the evolutionary development of language (Rizzolatti & Craighero, 2004). The finding that mirror neurones have a role in imitation and mimicry, together with a greater understanding of how imitation facilitates empathy, allows convergence between cognitive models, social psychology and the neuroscience underpinning the basic infrastructure and function of mirror neurones. These emerging findings indicate the role of perceptual and motor mechanisms in imitation and also in action and gesture understanding (Iacoboni, 2009a, 2009b).

4.2.3 Clinical Aspects

Trethowan and Conlon (1965) were the first to collect a large number of cases to see if couvade syndrome existed. They investigated 327 men immediately after their wives' deliveries and compared them with 221 married men whose wives had not been pregnant in the past nine months. In a questionnaire they were asked about symptoms occurring during the preceding nine months. Indigestion or colic, attacks of nausea or sickness, increased appetite, decreased appetite, diarrhoeas, constipation, toothache, backache and other aches and pains were enquired after. All these symptoms (55.7 vs 43.4 per cent), with the exception of backache, were more common among the expectant men, but there were statistically significant differences in poor appetite, toothache and nausea or sickness between the groups. There were no differences between those who were first-time fathers and those who had been fathers before. The peak incidence of symptoms occurred in the third month of pregnancy and diminished steadily thereafter. Symptoms cleared before labour began in a third of cases, and a further third became symptom free directly after their wives had given birth. There was an apparent direct relationship between anxiety and the somatic symptoms, but the content of the anxiety was not directly related to a real obstetrical concern. A third of fathers with these symptoms had been similarly affected during their wives' other pregnancies.

In an American study by Lipkin and Lamb (1982), a random systematic sample of 267 couples was studied. The operational definition used to identify couvade was fresh occurrence in the mates of pregnant women of symptoms related to pregnancy for which they seek medical care and which are not otherwise objectively explained. The authors looked superficially for symptoms of nausea, vomiting, abdominal pain and bloating, appetite changes, weight or bowel change, toothache, concern about skin lesions, leg cramps, faintness and lassitude. Of the 267 men in the sample, 60 (22.5 per cent) had couvade syndrome. This translates to a prevalence rate of 225 of 1,000 husbands at risk. The men who sought care tended to be less well educated, of lower socioeconomic class and have less experience as fathers. They had a twofold increase in visits to health care, a threefold increase in reported symptom and were more likely to receive medication. There was no significant difference in age, race, complications of the wife's pregnancy and attendance at childbirth education classes.

Schodt (1989) studied 110 couples attending New York childbirth education classes in a New York City hospital. Prospective fathers and their pregnant partners in the third trimester reported their perceptions of attachment to their unborn children, and prospective fathers reported their couvade phenomena during the preceding one-month period. Although this study did not demonstrate an association between father-foetus attachment and couvade, these findings did suggest that a certain level of couvade among some fathers may be observed. Symptoms reported by at least 20 per cent of the groups studied were considered significant, and they included tiredness, difficulty sleeping, headaches, restlessness, irritability, backache, difficulty concentrating, nervousness, weight gain and cold. These findings were in line with previous reports (Clinton, 1986; Strickland, 1987).

Masoni et al. (1994) studied 73 couples where all the women were in the last month of pregnancy and had 73 men as a reference group from acquaintances and patients' escorts. The authors had a 37-item questionnaire divided into seven classes which was scored from zero (absent) to three (severe). No difference in age or school level of education was seen. Pregnancy was desired by both partners in 72.6 per cent. The women were more emotionally demanding, had more fear and anxiety but were happier than the males, who were more curious. Sexual habits changed dramatically, with the men being more afraid of indelicacy and hurting their spouses. Women had more somatic symptoms, including more gastrointestinal and dermatological symptoms, whereas men had more sleep problems. However, this study was unable to statistically confirm the existence of couvade syndrome with its own physical symptoms.

Bogren (1983, 1984) randomly selected 112 women and their partners and interviewed them on three occasions through the pregnancy and postpartum. Sixteen men (20 per cent) fulfilled the criteria for couvade syndrome, which was defined as new occurrence of two or more symptoms. The commonest symptoms were weight gain, gastrointestinal symptoms, toothache and decreased appetite. The authors made some interesting observations, including that couvades syndrome was commonest among older men and men with older parents. These men were more attached to their mothers, and birth of the child seemed to be associated with a greater change in everyday life. They worried about parturition and the health of child at birth, but during the early pregnancies, they suppressed their own worries and converted them to somatic symptoms.

In a study in expectant Thai fathers in Bangkok, Khanobdee, Sukratanachaiyakul and Gay (1993) used the conceptual framework that the presence of somatic symptoms can be used as a reflection of the males' attempt to cope with or adapt to the focal stimulus of their partner's pregnancy. The authors proposed that the regulator subsystem, which was an innate coping mechanism, could be observed in any one of four modes: the physiological, self-concept, role function and interdependence modes. They used a 22-item somatic symptom checklist modified to 25 symptoms to retrospectively identify the occurrence of couvade in the Thai fathers. The final sample studied was 172 fathers, of whom 105 (~61 per cent) had two or more somatic symptoms, 50 had two to four symptoms, 44 had five to ten symptoms and 11 had more than ten symptoms. The most frequently reported symptoms were increased appetite, nausea, decreased concentration and fatigue in the first trimester; increased appetite, fatigue and increased sleep in the second trimester; and fatigue, frequent urination, decreased food digestion, decreased concentration and increased sleep in the third trimester. The commonest symptoms at any time were increased appetite, fatigue, increased sleep, decreased concentration, decreased appetite, nausea, diarrhoea, frequent urination, food cravings and nasal congestion.

These reported studies all deal with symptoms that male patients present with or that are elicited on inquiry in the context of their partner's pregnancy or parturition. Even though it is important to recognize these aspects of the mental welfare of males with pregnant partners, these complaints are unlike the cases described by Trethowan and Conlon (1965), as described earlier, where very specific symptoms that are more akin to mimesis of the female condition during pregnancy and also during childbirth occurred.

However, there are also reports in the literature that deviate from the expected. It is then arguable whether these case reports fit the accepted nomenclature. Tényi et al. (2001b) reported two cases of 'psychotic couvade', and Budur, Mathews and Mathews (2005a) reported one case. Here the definition of couvade was accepted as occurrence of somatic and/or psychiatric symptoms including psychotic phenomena in expectant fathers or another relative including a sister during a woman's pregnancy. In my view, these cases probably stretch the accepted definition of couvade. Classically, couvade does not involve the erroneous belief of pregnancy, merely the experiencing of symptoms that mimic pregnancy or labour. In addition, couvade derives from descriptions of mimesis in husbands within a cultural context. Hence, description of couvade in a twin sister falls outside the usual definition, even though the phenomenon in a twin sister probably has the same underlying mechanisms as in the husband.

4.3 Pseudocyesis

Pseudocyesis is a diagnosis from medical antiquity in which the physiological and psychological concomitants of pregnancy develop in the absence of the true gravid state (Cohen, 1982). It has decreased in frequency in recent years, and the manifestations, too, are said to have changed over time. It is hypothesized that this could be because of a lessening in the procreative imperative which leads to a reduction in the psychological determinants of pseudocyesis (Cohen, 1982). Certain sociological factors may also have contributed to this change, including trends towards smaller families, decreased fear of infant mortality and more widespread knowledge of and increased familiarity with medicine, sexuality and reproduction. One of the effects of this decrease in reported cases is the gradual disappearance of the condition in standard textbooks of obstetrics and the real possibility that cases are being missed or unrecognized as a consequence (Gaskin, 2012).

The term *pseudocyesis* (*pseudes*, 'false', and *kyesis*, 'pregnancy') was introduced in 1823 by John Mason Good (Cohen, 1982). It is a distinctive condition that was observed by Hippocrates in 300 BC, who reported 12 cases of women 'who imagine they are pregnant seeing that the menses are suppressed and the matrices swollen' (Brown and Barglow, 1971, p. 221), and has been recognized to affect all peoples, all nations and all strata of society. It has been referred to as the oldest known psychosomatic condition, and a famous case mentioned in the literature is that of Mary Tudor in the sixteenth century (Medvei, 1987, pp. 767–8). She is said to have had recurrent pseudocyesis, having symptoms of pregnancy lasting nine months with two episodes of false labour.

> On 25th July 1554, Mary and Philip [Prince of Spain] were married. Mary believed herself to be pregnant on two occasions during her short married life. As early as September 1554, one of the Queen's physicians thought that she was very probably with child. Count Langosco, the Duke of Savoy's ambassador with Charles V, confirmed it on 19 September: 'The Queen is with child. I have personal reason to believe it, as I have noticed her feeling sick.' . . . On 30th December, Queen Mary wrote, 'As for that child I carry in my belly, I declare it to be alive'. . . . On 21st April 1555, Simon Renard reported to the Emperor: 'The Queen has withdrawn, and no one enters her apartments, except the women who serve her and who have the same duties as court officials. . . . However it is believed that she will be delivered before the 9th day of the next month'. Philip and the Queen had indeed gone to Hampton Court in Easter for her confinement. . . . A series of letters, with the dates left blank, from Mary to the Pope, the Emperor, King of France and other princes, informing them of a safe deliverance are preserved in the Public Record Office. . . . On 26th June Renard wrote to the Emperor 'Her doctors and ladies proved to be out of their calculations by about two months'. . . . On 29th June, he wrote '. . . one can not doubt that she is with child. A certain sign of this is the state of her breasts and that the child moves. Then there is the increase of the girth, the hardening of the breasts and the fact that they distil'. On 6th July, however, the Queen Dowager of Hungary wrote to Simon Renard from Brussels 'The Queen's deliverance is delayed and it is doubted whether she is really with child'. By September it was all over. The Emperor wrote to his ambassador in Portugal on 14th September 1555 from Brussels: 'The King, my son

arrived, here four days ago, in good health, God be praised! The Queen was well also, although there is no longer any hope of her being with child.'

In the autumn of 1557, Mary once again believed herself to be pregnant, and the next six months were a repetition of the experiences of 1555. She died of dropsy on 17 November 1558.

Mary Tudor's life, including her childhood and later adult life, and situation demonstrate the complexities and psychological and physical dimensions of pseudocyesis that will be discussed later in this section. Medvei (1987) makes the point that Mary Tudor suffered paternal deprivation in childhood; experienced recurrent unexplained amenorrhoea from age 19 years; complained of 'racking headaches'; had attacks of palpitations, recurrent indigestion and impaired and severely deteriorating vision; during the periods of presumed pregnancy had amenorrhoea, swelling of the abdomen, morning sickness, swelling of her breasts and lactation; had recurrent episodes of melancholia; and died at the age of 42 years. This combination of physical and psychiatric symptoms is not unusual in pseudocyesis. Equally important in Mary Tudor's case was the pressure put upon her and expectation that she would have a child, preferably a boy but at worst a girl, and that this would all transpire quickly.

The commonest definition of the term requires both a false belief that one is pregnant and the presence of some somatic changes characteristic of pregnancy. The definition contains an organic aspect consisting of a cluster of signs and symptoms associated with the gravid state and a psychological aspect centring on the belief that one is pregnant. This belief ranges from a conviction tenaciously maintained in the face of contrary medical evidence and societal pressure to a fleetingly considered idea. It has also been described as an entirely unconscious thought process introduced by social influence. Given the foregoing, it is not surprising that there is overlap with delusion of pregnancy, and this is reflected in the literature.

It is possible to subdivide pseudocyesis into pseudocyesis vera (the so-called true pseudocyesis), delusional pseudocyesis, simulated pseudocyesis and erroneous pseudo-cyesis (Bolakale, Ibrahim, & Amusa, 2015). These divisions are, of course, problematical. The standard way to distinguish between pseudocyesis vera and delusion of pregnancy is to argue that in pseudocyesis vera there are accompanying features of pregnancy, namely abdominal distension, breast enlargement and tenderness, and amenorrhoea, whereas in delusion of pregnancy these ancillary features of pregnancy are not present. Seeman (2014) makes the important point that even in cases arising in the context of schizophre-nia, the erroneous belief of pregnancy is often either provoked or at least facilitated and maintained by amenorrhoea, that is, secondary to drug treatment with antipsychotic agents. This calls for a far more nuanced understanding of the interrelationships between pseudocyesis vera and delusion of pregnancy. In any case, in circumstances where the physical manifestations of pregnancy coincide with a false belief of pregnancy, the correct psychopathological term is overvalued idea as opposed to delusion. What is unusual in pseudocyesis is that both the false belief and the physical manifestations occur contem-poraneously, and it is unusual and rare for delusional disorders in general to be accom-panied by physical confirmation of the erroneous belief. In some cases, clinical exploration might reveal a less than fixed incorrigible conviction; hence a somatoform condition might be a more suitable explanation. Despite the difficulties just described, it is still important to attempt to distinguish between pseudocyesis and delusion of preg-nancy not only to establish a clinical distinction but also to attain a better understanding of the aetiology and phenomenology of the two conditions but also to proceed to appropriate treatment.

One of the first attempts to differentiate pseudocyesis from other forms of false pregnancy such as hallucinations of pregnancy stemming from a psychosis, simulated pregnancy in which the woman pretends to be pregnant and pseudopregnancy occurring when a tumour or other structural defect causes endocrine changes simulating pregnancy was made by Flanders Dunbar in 1938 (Murray & Abraham, 1978). Dunbar defined pseudocyesis as a condition in which a woman firmly believes herself to be pregnant and develops objective pregnancy signs in the absence of pregnancy. However, authors such as Bivin and Klinger (1937) have preferred to classify it under a psychoneurotic condition, whereas Brown and Barglow (1971) defined pseudocyesis as those psychic or somatic manifestations which on psychological investigation appear to originate from two intimately connected components: (1) the awareness of a recent bodily change or disturbance linked to (2) a conscious fantasy about some aspect of a pregnancy wish, fantasy or fear. Modern classifications tend to regard pseudocyesis as a somatoform disorder. However, one needs to note that there are recently described physical conditions that mimic pseudocyesis. In galactorrhoea-amenorrhoea-hyperprolactinemia syndrome (GAHS), a combination of galactorrhoea with amenorrhoea is associated with hyperprolactinemia in 50 to 70 per cent of all cases and with prolactinomas in 35 to 60 per cent of all cases (Cohen, 1982; Barrett, 1988). In common with pseudocyesis are the two cardinal symptoms of GAHS: menstrual disturbance and abnormal lactation. Other common findings that have been noted are abdominal enlargement due to obesity or water retention and a dramatic response to brief psychotherapy. In contrast, patients diagnosed with GAHS do not usually believe they are pregnant. The authors argue that examples of every subtype of GAHS are discernible among the cases that have been labelled in the literature as pseudocyesis. These include cases which result from medications that lower serum dopamine, from lesions that stimulate neural control pathways and from brain tumours involving the pituitary or hypothalamus.

4.3.1 Case Reports

William Harvey (1578–1657) reported two cases (Hunter & Macalpine, 1970, p. 132).

1. I am acquainted with a young woman, the daughter of a physician with whom I am very intimate, who experienced in her own person all the usual symptoms of pregnancy; after the fourteenth week, being healthy and sprightly, she felt the movements of the child within the uterus, calculated the time at which she expected the delivery, and when she thought, from further indications, that this was at hand, prepared the bed, cradle, and all other matters ready for the event. But all was in vain. . . . [T]he motions of the foetus ceased; and by degrees, without inconvenience, as the abdomen had increased so it diminished; she remained, however, barren ever after.
2. I am acquainted also with a noble lady who had borne more than ten children, and in whom the catamenia never disappeared except as the result of impregnation. Afterwards, however, being married to a second husband, she considered herself pregnant, forming her judgment not only from the symptoms on which she usually relied, but also from the movements of the child, which were frequently felt both by herself and her sister, who occupied the same bed with her. No arguments of mine could divest her of this belief. The symptoms depended on flatulence and fat. Hence the best ascertained signs of pregnancy have sometimes deceived not only ignorant women, but experienced midwives, and even accurate physicians.

4.3.2 Explanatory Hypotheses

Several hypotheses have been postulated for pseudocyesis in females. These include (1) physical or mechanical causes, (2) psychological factors arising from different psychodynamic processes, and (3) neuroendocrinological hypothesis.

There is a long tradition explaining the origin of pseudocyesis as purely physical or mechanical (Murray & Abraham, 1978). The abdominal distension has been attributed to bowel gas, excess intra-abdominal fat, faecal impaction, urinary retention and contraction of abdominal muscles. However, it is obvious that this cannot be the sole explanation for the origin of the symptoms. A number of psychological explanations have also been put forward (Murray & Abraham, 1978). These include intense desire for having children, guilt of an illicit sexual relationship leading to fear of pregnancy, manifestation of attention-seeking (histrionic) behaviour and depression in women, in whom pseudocyesis is seen as a means of protection against abandonment by securing the affection of the imagined child. This again does not fully explain the associated physical changes in this condition.

More recently, neuroendocrinological hypothesis have been described (Murray & Abraham, 1978). Most influential of these are alteration in pituitary-ovarian function leading to elevation of prolactin levels, lowered luteinizing hormone releasing factor (LHRF) and follicle-stimulating hormone releasing factor (FSHRF) leading to lowered luteinizing hormone and follicle-stimulating hormone. But this still does not explain the pathological belief that is involved in the process. There is no consensus about the aetiology of pseudocyesis in males.

4.3.3 Clinical Aspects

Fischer (1962) has described the most common physical symptoms of pseudocyesis as being hypo- or amenorrhoea; gradual abdominal enlargement; breast changes consisting of enlargement, tenderness, secretion of milk or colostrums and areolar pigmentation; sensation of foetal movement; morning nausea and vomiting; and increase in appetite and/or weight gain.

Azizi and Elyasi (2017) reported from their comprehensive narrative review of the literature that the incidence in the United States decreased from 1 per 250 pregnancies in 1940 to 1–6 cases per 22,000 deliveries in 2007. The frequency of cases in Nigeria is 1 per 344 pregnancies and in Sudan 1 per 160 pregnancies (Ouj, 2009). A number of biological factors have been reported in association with pseudocyesis, and these include neuroendocrine disturbances involving the hypothalamus-pituitary-axis; hormonal changes; treatment with psychotropic medication, obstetrical issues such as recurrent miscarriages, imminent menopause and sterilization surgery; and gynaecological pathologies such as hydatiform mole, ovarian cysts, uterine fibroids, ectopic pregnancy and morbid obesity. Rarely, gonadotropin-secreting adenocarcinomas of the lung may present with false pregnancy and manifest as cessation of menses, breast tenderness and raised β-human chorionic gonadotropin compatible with pregnancy (Byrd & Roy, 1993; Manzi et al., 1995). A 17-year-old female patient presented with pseudocyesis in the context of use of Depo-Provera (which is known to cause amenorrhoea) that the patient then interpreted as sign of being pregnant despite evidence to the contrary. She had abdominal distension, linea nigra and breast fullness and said that she had felt foetal movements. The pseudocyesis terminated abruptly once the

Depo-Provera was discontinued, and she had a spontaneous menstrual period (Flanagan & Harel, 1999).

In addition to these biological factors, psychological factors and psychiatric disorders have been identified as important factors. These include ambivalence about the existence of a pregnancy; intense desire to have children, fear of pregnancy or history of infertility; grief reaction following tubal ligation or hysterectomy; and severe psychiatric disorders such as bipolar affective disorder or schizophrenia. A case report from Morocco illustrates the intersection of infertility, psychological distress and the societal pressure to have children (El Ouazzani et al., 2008). The 49-year-old female patient had been married twice and had no children. She presented with recurrent pseudocyesis (six episodes) manifesting with abdominal distension, amenorrhoea, mammary tenderness, nausea, vomiting and weight gain on each occasion. There was also associated polydipsia. The difficulty in the distinction between pseudocyesis and delusional pregnancy is illustrated, albeit imperfectly, in the report by Fennig et al. (1993) of a patient with a previous history of postpartum psychosis and previous presentation with pseudo-hallucination. The authors attempt a distinction between delusion as presented in postpartum psychosis and over-valued idea of pregnancy in pseudocyesis.

The important social context is illiteracy or low educational attainment. Marital difficulties and relationship instability are also relevant (Ibekwe & Achor, 2008). Pseudocyesis is said to be commoner in rural communities, and there is evidence that communities where fertility status is associated with the attributed social value of a woman or where infertility usually results in divorce or a second marriage are more closely linked to the development of pseudocyesis. The psychological distress associated with involuntary childlessness is well described in a qualitative study from South Africa by Dyer et al. (2002). These authors describe feelings of anger, sadness, bitterness, guilt, loneliness and desperation. To illustrate the intensity of feeling and associated low self-esteem, one woman said, 'I cannot be anybody in the world.'

There is literature on pseudocyesis in males. Reported cases have often been categorized as delusions of pregnancy, even though they manifest with either one or more physical symptoms, and the reported phenomena may not fall under the rubric of delusion. One of the earliest reports was a case of a 30-year-old man reported by Evans (1951). During his early childhood, he had shared his parents' bedroom and was a witness to their sexual intercourse and his mother giving birth to his siblings. At 12 years of age, he provoked a man to seduce him but later married and became a father. During the first stage of his wife's labour, he imitated all her movements, and it was a description of couvade. His fantasies of being pregnant were enacted on the analytical couch when he started having abdominal pains and rumblings and described having a noisy child inside him. He started playing the part of a pregnant woman in his everyday life. His fantasized pregnancy came to an abortive end on a self-chosen day when during mentalizing the labour he watched his flatus disappear on the surface of the water.

In a case reported by Knight (1960), a 33-year-old merchant marine seaman who was uncertain of his own background always felt inadequate and unaccepted by his father and his numerous partners. He had both heterosexual and homosexual experiences but felt more secure and contented within same-sex relationship, as he thought men were the most desired and stronger of the two sexes. He looked upon himself as a woman in a man's body and believed that the female hormone was dominant in him. While at sea, one of his close friends had spoken about getting married and having a child, which made him feel rejected. He intensely wished to be able to give his friend this child and shortly after started having symptoms of abdominal distension and experienced foetal movements, morning nausea and increased appetite. His abdomen became enlarged and protuberant, and he expressed the belief, 'I think there is life in my abdomen. This may be a pregnancy' (p. 261). He believed that he had been chosen by God in a special way and that a miracle had happened. After four months of psychotherapy, his psychophysiological symptoms and the abdominal distension and movements disappeared.

In another account (Barrett, 1988), a 40-year-old man who was receiving hypnotherapy for smoking cessation was asked in his last session to imagine himself as the person he would like to be, and he visualized himself as a pregnant woman. Several hours after the session, he noticed that his abdomen was enlarging, and he subsequently developed morning nausea, a watery secretion from his nipples and a throbbing like a heartbeat in his abdomen. He continued to visualize himself as a pregnant woman and presented to the hospital as he was going through a false pregnancy. He was exclusively homosexual, having lost his partner 2½ months prior to the onset of his symptoms. He had consciously wished to have a child by this man and wished himself to be a woman inside a man's body, received oestrogen injections and dressed in a woman's clothes to fulfil his fantasy. Though he was familiar with the term *transsexual* and identified himself with it, he never had any interest in pursuing gender reassignment surgery.

Pseudocyesis has also been reported in a 40-year-old man with pre-existing chronic undifferentiated schizophrenia co-morbid with depression (Evans & Seely, 1984). The patient became sad when his daughter grew up and his wish to have another baby was refused by his wife. He started expressing his wish to impregnate his wife and felt sexual. Later he reported nausea, vomiting and something moving in his stomach like a baby but retained insight to the extent that he realized that he couldn't be pregnant because he was a man. With continuation of antipsychotic agents, his mental state improved, but it was only on stopping the antipsychotic agent and starting lithium that his increased weight and abdominal girth started to reduce. The important thing in this case is to recognize the role of antipsychotic medication in causing quasi-symptoms of pregnancy.

These cases of pseudocyesis in males only go to show how difficult it is to sustain a judgement of pseudocyesis in males given the unlikelihood of physical manifestations of pregnancy in males.

4.4 Delusion of Pregnancy

Delusion of pregnancy is by definition the false and incorrigible belief of pregnancy. It is widely reported in both women and men (Michael, Joseph & Pallen, 1994). The wish to bear a child in men is common in the psychoanalytical literature, where it goes by the name of *parturition envy* (Brockington, 1996). By definition, in this condition, the delusion should occur in the absence of any somatic symptoms of pregnancy in order to strictly differentiate it from pseudocyesis. Michael et al. (1994) also mention that it is useful to also distinguish it from organic pseudopregnancy, where pregnancy symptoms occur as a consequence of an endocrine tumour–related illness and simulated pregnancy when the person is aware that he or she is not pregnant.

The first case of delusion of pregnancy is attributed to Esquirol in the nineteenth century (Chaturvedi, 1989). It is rarely reported and is seen in a wide variety of conditions including schizophrenia, dementia, general paralysis of the insane and depression (Chaturvedi, 1989).

4.4.1 Case Report

The first case is attributed to Esquirol (Brockington, 1996).

> A 31-year-old woman studied botany under a famous and elderly professor: she believed herself pregnant by him, although she had never spoken to him: there is no description of the signs of pregnancy, except that her periods stopped: she stopped eating and, when after all her efforts to induce were in vain, she died (still deluded) 18 months later.

4.4.2 Explanatory Hypotheses

Delusion of pregnancy is not a homogeneous condition but is unified merely by the singular content of the delusional belief, namely the false belief of pregnancy without any accompanying physiological changes. As described next, it occurs in a variety of psychiatric conditions and does not have a singular pattern or underlying mechanism.

4.4.3 Clinical Aspects

There are very few reported cases of delusion of pregnancy in the literature. The descriptions are complicated by the overlap with pseudocyesis. By definition, if physical symptoms of pregnancy accompany the erroneous belief of pregnancy, then pseudocyesis is the more accurate term for the presentation. A number of reports are best regarded as pseudocyesis (Bitton, Thibaut & Lefevre-Lesage, 1991; Adityanjee, 1995; Radhakrishnan et al., 1999; Varma & Katsenos, 1999).

Delusion of pregnancy is reported in schizophrenia and delusional disorder (Bitton et al., 1991), as well as in bipolar affective disorder (Miller & Forcier, 1992). In a report of a number of unusual cases, Chowdhury et al. (2003) reported delusion of pregnancy with a puppy in both male and female patients. Delusion of pregnancy was part of postictal psychosis in two patients (Chaturvedi, 1989; Tényi et al., 2001a) and was a consequence of an abdominal malignant lesion in one (Aronson, 1952). Learning disability was associated with delusion of pregnancy in some of the case reports (Jenkins, Revita & Tousignat, 1962; Bhate, Spear & Robertson, 1989; Chaturvedi, 1989; Varma & Katsenos, 1999). Homosexuality has been reported in association with delusion of pregnancy (Aronson, 1952; Bitton et al., 1991; Miller & Forcier, 1992; Michael et al., 1994).

However, it is hard to discern any pattern to the presentations or common underlying aetiological factors in these case reports. The consistent finding was a short duration of symptom manifestation and a good response to antipsychotic medication.

4.5 Conclusion

There is apparent overlap between the clinical features and pathogenesis of the conditions of couvade, pseudocyesis and delusion of pregnancy, but it is possible to make a clinical distinction between the three conditions. Couvade is comprehensible in the context of our understanding of ritual couvade and the greater recognition and awareness of the stresses attendant on becoming a father and the associated responsibilities of fatherhood, a role which in modern society may demand more involvement and participation in the upbringing of offspring. But clinical couvade insofar as it demonstrates the imitative aspects of behaviours deriving in a man from the observation of his mate raises fundamental questions of how observing the partner's pregnancy and/or labour can come to induce similar, if not identical, physical experiences in the man. In couvade, we see how the role of mirror neurons in imitative behaviour and mimicry can come to begin to explain the induction of mirror experiences. It is important to emphasize that the man in couvade, despite his experiencing of the symptoms and features of pregnancy and parturition, never makes the claim that he is pregnant or in labour.

As for pseudocyesis, there is ample evidence of decreasing incidence in developed countries with demonstrable less emphasis on the maternal role of women and the status and worth of women being less tied to procreation and fertility. This condition is demonstrably understandable in the context of a social climate in which childbirth is privileged. The patient believes that she is pregnant, and this belief is sustained by the physical features of pregnancy. The conundrum here is how to explain the development of physical manifestations of pregnancy in the absence of a foetus. Here the physical manifestations of pregnancy coexist with the erroneous belief of pregnancy.

Finally, delusions of pregnancy are of interest insofar as they appear, superficially, to relate to the two foregoing conditions, namely couvade and pseudocyesis. It confirms what should already be obvious, that thematic convergence on pregnancy and labour does not mean that distinct conditions are structurally or conceptually related.

Erotomania or de Clérambault Syndrome

5.1 Introduction

Erotomania can be understood as a condition in which a person believes that he or she is in an amorous (romantic) relationship with a person of higher social rank who is the first to fall in love and to make advances. There are a number of associated but ancillary themes, namely that the object of the love is unable to be happy or to have a sense of self-esteem without the subject; the object of love is free or his or her marriage is invalid; the object attempts to make contact with the subject, has indirect communication and exerts continuous surveillance and protection of the subject by means of significant resources; there is universal support for the relationship; and the contradictory or paradoxical responses of the object of love towards the subject can be explained away (de Clérambault, 1942). It is also thought that the affective triad of hope, love and pride is always present.

The term *erotomania* has a long pedigree, having first been used by Jacques Ferrand in 1640 in the title of his book, *Erotomania or Treatise Discoursing of the Essence, Causes, Symptoms, Prognosticks, and Cure of Love or Erotic Melancholy* (Hunter & Macalpine, 1970). The idea that there are corporeal effects of unrequited love is described in Jerome Gaub's *De Regimine Mentis*, first published in 1747 and 1763 (Gaub, 1767; Rather, 1965). Gaub wrote

> How often do beautiful maidens and handsome youths, caught in toils of love, grow ghastly pale and waste away, consumed by melancholy, green-sickness, or erotomania, when delays occur or the hope of possession is lost? These ailments become worse and so much the more difficult for the physician to cure since the underlying affection commonly hides behind the mask of disease and the true source of origin is often difficult to discover. . . . Let Perdiccas come forth: inflamed by love of Phila, the concubine of the king his father, he had abandoned all hope of ever possessing her and, having restrained his ardour within, is said to have fallen seriously ill. Nor did he recover until Hippocrates shrewdly observed that as often as Phila came by the pulse beat of the invalid altered, and having thus uncovered the cause of the disease and prevailed upon the father, rendered him at last partaker of the desire.   (Gaub, 1767, p. 151)

The correspondence between unrequited or unfulfilled love and irregular pulse is also a subject in the tale of the king and the servant girl written in *The Masnavi* (Rūmī, 2007). And this effect of desire upon the pulse is only one example of the bodily effects of desire and unfulfilled love. Gideon Harvey (1637–1700) listed 'amorous consumption' as a differential diagnosis of wasting disease.

An Amorous Consumption implies a rapid extenuation occasioned through love, whose passions, affrights, fear, anger, jealousie and despair do so extreamly disperse and consume the vital and animal spirits, that we see its ordinary for young Wenches to be reduced to faintings, swoonings, and extream weakness, to the admiration of their parents, whence such subitous and efforoyable accidents should source. (Hunter & Macalpine, 1970, p. 197)

Jean Etienne Dominique Esquirol (1772–1840) regarded erotomania as an example of monomania. For him, monomania was

of all maladies, that which presents to the observer, phenomena the most strange and varied, and which offers for our consideration, subjects the most numerous anomalies of sensibility, all the phenomena of the human understanding, all the consequences of the perversion of our natural inclinations, and all the errors of our passions.

(Hunter & Macalpine, 1970, p. 735)

Furthermore, for Esquirol, erotomania was

a chronic cerebral disease, characterized by an excessive love for an object either known or imaginary; it is a disease of the imagination and is accompanied by an error of judgment. Amorous ideas in this mental disorder are as fixed and dominant as religious ideas will be in theomania or religious lypemania. Erotomania differs essentially from nymphomania and satyriasis. The latter originate from an irritation of the reproductive organs that reaches the brain; in erotomania love is all in the head; the nymphomaniac and satyromaniac are victims of a physical disorder; the erotomaniac is the victim of his imagination. (Berrios & Kennedy, 2002, p. 389)

Berrios and Kennedy (2002) provide a conceptual history of the term *erotomania* and argue that there are four historical developments in the evolution of the term. The first, lasting from the Classical period to the eighteenth century; the second, lasting well into the nineteenth century; the third, holding sway in the twentieth century; and the fourth, currently depicting erotomania as a delusional belief. In the Classical period, the term referred to a general disease caused by unrequited love and demonstrable by irregular pulse when the subject sees the object of his or her love or hears her name or receives messages about him or her. However, by the eighteenth century, erotomania came to mean the practice of excessive physical love, namely nymphomania, and the origin of this malady was located in the genital organs. This localization later came to be used as a rationale for surgical treatments such as amputations of the clitoris and labia minora. From the early nineteenth century onwards, erotomania came to be regarded as a type of mental disease, a form of monomania. As Berrios and Kennedy (2002) put it, even though erotomania was conceptualized as being part of monomania, it survived the demise of monomania and was reformulated as a delusion in the early twentieth century, with the writings of Sérieux and Capgras, Ernst Kretschmer, and Kraepelin foreshadowing de Clérambault's contributions. De Clérambault's major contribution was that he systematized a condition that was previously well known but poorly described and even less well characterized by precise symptoms.

5.2 Case Reports

The original cases reported by de Clérambault have been translated and summarized by Singer (de Clérambault, 1921, 1942; Signer, 1991). This section provides four case descriptions.

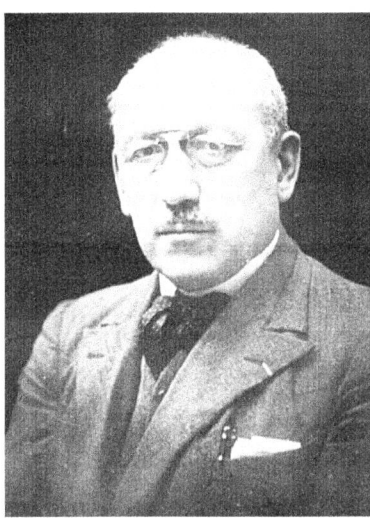

Gretan Gatian De Clerambault 1872–1934

1. Léa Anne B., a 53-year-old milliner, was premorbidly overbearing and suspicious. From age 22 to 40, she was supported by a well-placed lover, and immediately after his death she took up with a younger man. During this time, while living in the countryside, Léa Anne complained of her isolation and at 43 years began to complain of organised persecution by the peasants, whom she believed accused her of sexually corrupting a young man. Five years later, in the early part of World War I, believing herself denounced as a spy, she claimed to have destroyed foreign government documents during a fit of 'spite' that had lasted 6 weeks. In 1917, she believed an American general was in love with her. On each of her many extravagant trips, she thought that she was the object of silent advances, by officers of many ranks, and regretted not having taken advantage of the situation. She claimed the King of Belgium wrote letters to her, and thought that English and Russian nobility were among her past lovers. She came to believe that King George V was in love with her, that he watched over her with secret emissaries under various disguises, and that all of London knew of their affair and wanted it to succeed. She often expressed grandiose plans concerning him. She spent large sums of money to travel to England, prowling around royal residencies, often in a state of ardent anticipation. Léa Anne occasionally doubted these ideas or thought that the King put up obstacles or caused her difficulties. Several months of increasing preoccupation, flamboyant behaviour, agitation and assaults on strangers brought her to the attention of the authorities and led to her incarceration.

2. Over a 37-year period Henrietta H., a 55-year-old fashion designer, had the recurrent belief that a priest loved and persecuted her. She was thought to have a precocious and strong sexual drive. The erotic delusion began suddenly during a Mass, and thereafter she completely beleaguered the priest. The family tried to deal with this behaviour by marrying her off, but less than a year she began a series of affairs. Tranquil periods were followed by reawakenings of her love, when she would return impulsively to Paris to again pursue the priest. After a divorce, she established herself there and continued by ambushes, scenes, letters and calls. Over the years, she showed many remissions and relapses. Her descriptions of her encounters were accompanied by strong sexual imagery, including consideration of a 'ménage à trois' with a priest and another woman. She may have suffered a depressive episode at the time of her presentation.

3. Clémentine D., a 50-year-old fashion designer, had erotic, grandiose and persecutory delusions. She believed that a vicar wanted to marry her, was paying a large sum of money for an apartment, and thought he smiled, signalled, and communicated secretly with her. In the stage of 'spite', she was jealous when he spoke to other women, as she thought they were trying to influence him against her. Clémentine was angry because he did not support her properly, and completely disrupted his life. She held grandiose, extravagant ideas about the origin, position and possessions of her life, believed plots were engineered against her by another priest and neighbours, and that hostile references appeared in the newspaper. Auditory hallucinations, possibly commenting on her actions, and her beliefs, were present. Clémentine had a haughty, superior, coquettish attitude. She was often in an 'exalted' state and decorated her hospital uniform with ribbons and knots. She refused food believing it poisoned. The patient misrecognised a physician consistently as another person.
4. Louisette, 30 years of age, maintained for four years that her aged, married employer was young, single and in love with her. She maintained an exalted, euphoric air in spite of disappointments and tests of her love. The usual evolution of the delusion was inverted with a preceding brief period of persecution. (Signer, 1991, pp. 81–4)

5.3 Explanatory Hypotheses

Erotomania is conceptualized as a delusional disorder. It is different from the disorders described in Section 1 insofar as it concerns a belief that an identified love object loves the patient. Although there is often no explicit statement that the patient loves the love object in return, this is implicit in the behaviour of the patient. This raises the issue of the relationship between beliefs and emotions and the degree to which there is primacy of belief over emotions or vice versa.

The story of Marie Bashkirtseff (1858–1884), a Russian diarist, painter and sculptor who assiduously kept diaries from 1873 till her death in 1884, illustrates the complex interactions between belief and emotions. It also illustrates how little we know about the actual experience of love and of the motivating drive. It is estimated that Marie wrote at least 104 substantial exercise books and thousands of pages. Her diaries are of interest to us because they document her avowed love for the Duke of Hamilton, describing the throes and agonies of love, the yearning, the pining, the envy of the love object's other relationships and the despair and sometimes anger that follow upon the unreciprocated love. The thorough account of Doris Langley Moore (1966), based on the unexpurgated diaries, allows us to understand the development of love, albeit not of erotomania, and its effects on thinking, mood and behaviour.

Moore believed that Bashkirtseff 'as good as certain ... started to keep a diary chiefly to have an outlet for her overflowing feelings about the Duke'. The Duke 'was a large and robust young man. ... [H]is mother was a princess and his maternal grandmother the adoptive daughter of Napoleon I and the Empress Josephine.' Moore says of his wealth '[h]is income was by any standards, enormous. The reference books of the day estimated that he owned nearly one hundred and sixty thousand acres in the British Isles and, scattered over them, several mansions and castles of antiquity. Over and above all this grandeur, he was skilful with yachts, horses, and guns, good looking, unmarried and not yet twenty-eight.' Even though, the Duke of Hamilton was unmarried 'he could be seen with a beautiful and exquisitely dressed Italian [Gioia] who was spoken of as his mistress'. So this was the context of Marie Bashkirtseff's love.

Bashkirtseff wrote on 3 March 1873: 'Oh God, give me the Duke of Hamilton and I shall love him and make him happy! I shall be happy myself too. I shall do good to the poor.' On the 4th March, she wrote: 'He has one whom he loves [Gioia]. Oh, I believe he doesn't love her but he prefers to be free. To have a woman since it's necessary for *le chic*; horses, a woman, the pigeon-shooting, all those are the attributes of a young English great nobleman who has fallen into bad company.' On 5th March, she wrote: 'He appeared young, handsome, rich, free, noble, – what a happy man! Having an enormous income, he distributes it with prudence – which I believe he doesn't do but, I don't know why, all these thoughts passed in my imagination. He appeared to me so handsome, so noble, so agreeable.'

These comments demonstrate very clearly how romantic love develops in the context of erotomania. The psychiatric literature says little, if anything, about how the patient feels about the object of love; the emphasis is usually upon their erroneous belief that the object of love loves them. On 8 February 1873, Marie wrote: 'All of a sudden I hear someone whistling behind me. It was the Duke. He was whistling on the first evening when I saw him at Baden. He whistled. (Even in writing it my heart throbs.) I turned round, he saw me, then I blushed and my heart started to beat like a hammer. He had a coat of the type of my casaque, a blue shirt, a maroon hat. He remained near me a moment, never did I imagine so great a happiness! My God, grant that he remains like that, always near me!' She went on: 'What I want now is that he should know I love him. He spoke of beautiful ladies, but he returned to my side. Our eyes have met again. What happiness!'

Moore (1966) makes the following point:

> The difference between Marie and a normal girl of fourteen was the durability of an emotion which was never at any time stable. It veered to all points of the compass like a weathervane, but, like a weathervane, it had a firm pivot – her delight in wealth and grandeur.

There was yearning by Marie for the Duke: 'Dear – dear, I love you so much. You will be dazzled by my splendour, and you will love me. You will see the triumph that surrounds me, and this is true, you are worthy of a woman such as I hope to be.' There was despair: 'I used to see him every day and now he follows the proverb, "When one wishes to be adored, one must make oneself wanted". I'm bored without him. I'm sad, sometimes my face takes on a pensive and languishing expression, today especially.' There was preoccupation with her imagined rival, Gioia: 'I find her beautiful because he finds her beautiful.'

In May 1873, Marie made the decision to follow the Duke wherever he might go: 'I hope this winter we will know him, and then I shall know where he passes the most of his time and there we shall go', and Moore comments, 'The Duke, all unknowing, had begun to exercise an influence that was invading and pervading the lives of a family entirely alien to his world.'

On learning that the Duke had left his paramour, Gioia, Marie wrote

> Nevertheless I can't believe it because it would give me too much pleasure. She alone is worthy of envy. If she's finished I'm happy. I see now that I envy her and that I detest her, the sentiment that follows envy, and if it's true that the Duke is no longer her protector, and that she's finished, passed out of fashion, I'm very glad. But no, such happiness couldn't be! I'm not worthy of it.

On Monday, 13 October 1873, Marie discovered that the Duke of Hamilton was going to marry the Duke of Manchester's daughter. She wrote

> I lift the book nearer my face, for I am red as fire. I felt as if a sharp knife were plunged into my chest. I began to shake so that I could scarcely hold the book. My breath grew heavy and

came out of my chest trembling like a sound [yet] it was only breath. I was afraid of fainting but the book saved me.

In 1880, seven years after the event, she wrote: 'All this for a gentleman whom I'd seen about ten times in the street, whom I didn't know, and who was unaware of my existence!'

But in real time, her distress and continuing preoccupation with the Duke did not end in October 1873. The Duke's wedding was fixed for 10 December 1873, and on that day, her diary entries included 'I am angry with him, and I would willingly do him some harm.'

Enoch, Trethowan and Barker (1967) have argued that narcissism was the fertile ground on which Marie Bashkirtseff's love for the Duke was based, and they cite an extraordinary diary entry that illustrates her extreme self-preoccupation as support for their supposition.

I am capable of remaining for hours together in my dressing room quite naked in front of the glass. Never has anyone seen such whiteness, fineness and elegance of modelling. After having admired, I feel kind to everyone, esteeming them sufficiently unlucky for not having been able to see me. . . . Happy those who will see me! I swear to you that you can't even have an idea of how I'm formed, and the whiteness and fineness of my skin. I often stay an hour in contemplation instead of bathing, and I only leave the mirror with difficulty.

Enoch, Trethowan and Barker (1967) move from this extreme self-regard to propose that narcissism underpins erotomania. I will return to this issue later. What Marie Bashkirtseff's account does is to underscore how little we know about love, about its relationship to infatuation, about how passion and sexual intimacy intersects with romantic love.

In order to fully comprehend erotomania, there is a need for further understanding and clarification of the nature of love itself. Beall and Sternberg (1995) make the case for a social constructionist notion of love. Their case is that both the definition and subjective experience of love are determined by context and that context varies across time and across cultures. This view is distinct from the view that love is a universal experience that is defined in the same way irrespective of time and place. Or the view that love is a universal experience that is culturally structured, meaning that the subjective experience is the same across cultures but differently defined. The case for the changes over time is supported by the fact that love has been construed as a romantic, sexual or interpersonal phenomenon at varying periods, and the current conception of love as romantic in nature, in Western culture, only started at the beginning of Romanticism in the modern world (Singer, 2009). Indeed, Beall and Sternberg (1995) make the point that in the Classical Greek period, the proper object of masculine love was an adolescent boy and that wives were treated with contempt. Furthermore, there are disparities between contemporary Western notions of love as the basis for a marital relationship compared to, for example, Chinese notions that apply the term *love* to describe an illicit liaison that is not socially respectable.

The triangular theory of love described by Sternberg (1986, 1988) includes three components, namely intimacy, passion and commitment. In this account, intimacy is the feeling of being close and being connected with another person; passion is the feeling of sexual attraction and the desire for sexual consummation; and commitment refers to the belief that one is in love and is committed to a romantic relationship. But this is not the only conception of love. What all conceptions of love appear to have in common is the sense that love involves behaviours, thoughts and feelings, and central to this constellation is some notion of the love object, the feelings that accompany love, thoughts that are associated with love and actions or relations between the subject and object of love.

The proposition that both the experience and definition of love vary over time and place is problematical insofar as it implies that something as fundamental as personal emotional experience is determined by context. This proposition is not arguing that the determinants of the experience of love are culturally determined but that the actual experience of love is context bound. It is not simply stating that the object of love for a male can be female, male or God but that the inner subjective experience is not universal but has both a diachronic dimension as well as a cultural dimension.

I want now to turn to what we know of the biological underpinnings of mating behaviour. Sexual mating is a ubiquitous human characteristic and seems to be comprehensible given what we know about mating in other animal species. Sexual dimorphism, a term that refers to the differences in the physiques of males and females, is recognized as indicating the degree to which there is intrasexual competition. For example, if there is competitive drive between males, manifest in intrasexual aggression, then males are likely to be considerably larger than females (Wilson, 2000). In humans, males are 5 to 12 per cent larger than females, that is, less dimorphic than chimpanzees, for example, and this has implications for the varying reproductive strategies and success between males and females (Chagnon, Irons & Association, 1979). The physical characteristics that signal the extent of dimorphism in males, namely size (height and girth), may be identified as evidence of genetic fitness by females. And the reverse will be true for males, too. And there is a role for ornamentation as a sexual signal. Ornaments appear to signal to the opposite sex either (1) genetic ability to produce vigorous, highly competitive and successful offspring or (2) availability or quality of parental effort on the part of the bearer (Chagnon, Irons & Association, 1979). However, there are other issues of relevance here; the likelihood of reproductive success is different between the sexes. In other words, not all males are reproductively successful, whereas practically all females who wish to have offspring are able to do so. As Buss and Schmitt (1993) point out, most human societies practice polygyny, permitting men to take multiple partners, but in fact, very few males acquire multiple mates, thereby rendering other males mateless.

The differential sexual strategies between males and females has implications for predicting what formal features may be seen as signalling sexual fitness in the context of erotomania, namely which male partners will female patients be attracted to and which female partners will male patients be attracted to. Buss and Schmitt (1993) argue that the mating strategy problems that males in the ancestral environment had to solve were (1) identifying a reproductively available female, (2) ensuring certainty in paternity, (3) identifying females with good parenting skills and (4) identifying females who are willing and able to commit to a long-term mating relationship. In contrast, females had to solve (1) identifying males who have the ability to invest resources in her children on a long-term basis, (2) identifying who demonstrates a willingness to invest resources in her and her children on a long-term basis, (3) identifying males with good parenting skills, (4) identifying males who are willing and able to commit to a long-term relationship and (5) identifying males who are able and willing to protect her from aggressive conspecifics. Males are thought to utilize physical attributes as cues to identify female fertility and reproductive quality, and these include features of physical appearance such as full lips, clear skin, smooth skin, clear eyes, lustrous hair, symmetry, good muscle tone and absence of lesions. Observable behaviours such as sprightly youthful gait, high activity level and, finally, social reputation are all also important. Age and physical features are, in contrast, less reliable cues of male reproductive value, and male reproductive value is tied to the degree that males are able to demonstrate that they are able to accrue, defend and monopolize resources and that they are indeed willing to invest these resources in a woman and her children. Females therefore depend on demonstrable evidence of control of territory, money and goods. In summary, it is likely that male patients will be attracted to females who are young, have high social worth as fertile and have high reproductive value. Females will be attracted to males who have high social status and who can be seen as having control of resources predicated on their access to territory, money or goods.

Martin Brüne (2001), in his review of 246 cases worldwide, argued that the behavioural characteristics of erotomania were consistent with the sexual strategies theory as enunciated by Buss and Schmitt (1993). Brüne (2001) proposed that erotomania is likely to be an aberration of long-term mating strategy and that this is manifest in the fact that erotomania is commoner in females and that the onset is limited to adults. Furthermore, subjects with erotomania will be less likely to be involved in satisfactory relationships and will therefore be more likely to be unmarried, divorced or in ambivalent relationships. Female subjects with erotomania will be more likely to focus on socially high-ranking (older) men of high mate value, whereas males will focus on physically attractive and younger females. Finally, long-term mating strategy in males is likely to activate mechanisms to detect sexual infidelity; thus males with erotomania are more likely to exhibit sexual jealousy, including aggression and violence directed towards the love object, and stalking is more likely to be part of the behavioural manifestations. And, indeed, Brüne (2001) reported that his analysis revealed findings consistent with his predictions.

Sexual strategies theory only provides an underpinning theory for mate selection. It does not comprehensively describe the underlying neurobiology of mate selection, affiliation and establishment and maintenance of bonding. This is a complex subject that is only starting to be investigated. Young (2009) argues that the emotional connection between a ewe and her lamb or a female macaque monkey and her offspring is similar to human motherly bonding and hence must demonstrate that these relationships share evolutionarily conserved neural mechanisms. There is evidence that oxytocin is released during labour, delivery and nursing, and infusion of oxytocin in ewes results in rapid bonding with a foreign lamb. And, in female prairie voles, infusion of oxytocin causes rapid attachment pairing with the nearest male in the vicinity. This raises the question of the role of oxytocin in human mating. Stimulation of female nipples and the cervix during sexual intimacy releases oxytocin and may therefore strengthen the emotional bond between sexual partners. In male prairie voles, vasopressin stimulates pair bonding, aggression towards potential rivals and paternal behaviours such as grooming of offspring. In human males, the *AVPR1A* receptor gene appears to be associated with pair bonding and relationship quality. These findings confirm that pair bonding and the emotions underpinning it are under the influence neurochemistry.

Bartels and Zeki (2004) have shown that romantic and maternal love both activate similar regions, namely the medial insula and the cingulate gyrus dorsal and ventral of the genu. Subcortical activity was also found in the striatum and the head of the caudate nucleus and additionally in the posteroventral part of the thalamus. There was deactivation of the middle prefrontal cortex, the parieto-occipital junction and the medial prefrontal/paracingulate cortex. The implications are that romantic and maternal love are subserved by neurocircuitry that overlaps with that involved in reward systems and that both oxytocin and vasopressin have receptors at these same sites. The role of deactivation appears to be to reduce the influence of the social judgement network on maternal and romantic love, thereby inoculating love from negative emotions, critical social judgement and the assessment of intentions. This finding may be relevant for erotomania since it will predict that both the love object and the subjective experience of love itself will be less under critical scrutiny. This may be the link between poor insight and the social notion that 'love is blind'.

I have focused on the evolutionary underpinnings of mate selection and the neurobiology of romantic love, but, of course, there are other approaches to understanding erotomania. Enoch, Trethowan and Barker (1967) take a psychoanalytical perspective. They explored the possibility of the patient seeking after an 'ideal father' or after a safe and unattainable love object or of the patient being subject to self-love that is projected onto another person or, alternatively, of a defensive manoeuvre which substitutes delusional heterosexual attachment for unconscious homoerotic desires and narcissism, which is a form of self-rescue attempt from self-contempt and social insignificance and in which the attributed love of a high-status individual is merely an ancillary effect. Finally, in de Clérambault's original analysis, erotomania resulted from an affective triad comprising hope, love and pride, and in this model, pride was the most singularly important, and de Clérambault's terms pride the 'generator' of the syndrome (Signer, 1991).

5.4 Clinical Aspects

The original notion of de Clérambault's syndrome was that the subjects believed that they were in an amorous union with a person of high social rank who was the first to fall in love and to make advances. There are ancillary themes, including (1) the love object is unable to be happy or have a sense of self-esteem without the patient, (2) the love object is free or their marriage is invalid, (3) the love object makes attempts to contact the patient, has indirect conversations, and exerts ongoing surveillance and protection of the patient by means of extraordinary resources, (4) there is universal support or sympathy for the relationship and (5) the love object demonstrates paradoxical or contradictory attitude towards the patient (Signer, 1991). In the original description, the syndrome could present as a 'pure' case or as an 'associated' case, in which the symptoms were a prelude to or associated with other delusions and/or hallucinations (Signer, 1991). Most of the commentators since then have taken this same approach, namely that erotomania is divisible into a pure form, where the disorder is singular and primary, and a secondary form, where it is associated with other conditions such as schizophrenia, bipolar disorder and depression (Hollender & Callahan, 1975).

Ellis and Mellsop (1985) propose operational criteria for erotomania derived from de Clérambault (as described earlier), and these are (1) delusional conviction of amorous communication; (2) a love object of higher rank; (3) the love object being the first to fall in love; (4) the love object being the first to make advances; (5) sudden onset within a seven-day period; (6) the love object remaining unchanged, and if other love objects occur, they are only of transitory significance; (7) the patient rationalizes the paradoxical behaviour of the love object; (8) there is a chronic course; and (9) there is an absence of hallucinations. Kennedy et al. (2002) report on 15 patients. In their series, erotomania predominantly occurred in the context of schizophrenia, schizoaffective disorder and bipolar disorder. Only 20 per cent of their cases could be described as primary in nature. In 13 of 15 subjects, the love objects were of higher social status. The primary erotomania cases were more likely to have love objects who were celebrities. Nearly half the subjects (7 of 15) had a history of a psychiatric disorder in their first-degree relatives. Six of the 15 subjects had never had a sexual relationship. The chronicity of erotomania seemed to depend upon the psychiatric context. In patients with schizophrenia and schizoaffective disorder, the outcome paralleled the outcome of the primary diagnosis and was predictably poor, whereas in bipolar disorder, the outcome was full resolution in between episodes.

In the series of cases reported by Mullen and Pathé (1994a), there is a focus on the notion of *morbid infatuation*, which is defined as an intense infatuation without the need for any accompanying conviction that the affection is currently reciprocated. In addition, the object of the infatuation does nothing to encourage the feelings or clearly and repeatedly rejects any continuing interest or concern, but in the patient, the infatuation is preoccupying to the exclusion of other interests, resulting in serious disruption to their lives. In addition, the patient insists on the legitimacy and possible success of the quest. There is often severe accompanying distress and emotional disturbance in the love object. For Mullen and Pathé, symptomatic (secondary) erotomania owes its origins and evolution to an underlying mental disorder which emerges before, or with, the features of erotomania. The features of erotomania occur alongside the features of the underlying disorder and resolve as the underlying disorder resolves. In contrast, in pure erotomania, the features of erotomania constitute the totality of the clinical picture, and the onset and emergence of the features of erotomania are understandably related to the patient's personal and social situations as well as to their underlying personality. Furthermore, there may be a provoking, triggering event. In Mullen and Pathé's (1994a) series of 16 cases, 11 had demonstrable personality disorders, namely avoidant, narcissistic, paranoid, antisocial and schizoid types. The pure cases were more likely to be associated with aberrant personalities.

Mullen and Pathé (1994a) also draw attention to the relationship between erotomania and normal love. They argue that the boundary between the normal and the pathological is ill-defined. They also make the point that pathological love is similar to pathological jealousy insofar as both form a continuum with the normal experiences but that there is a tendency to under-diagnose pathological love because it is hard to distinguish it from excessive and exuberant manifestations of love, whereas there is a tendency to over-diagnose pathological jealousy because pathological jealous feelings annex much of the territory of the normal, probably because jealous feelings are less acceptable in modern culture. I will deal with stalking and violence associated with erotomania in the next subsection.

There is a considerable adverse impact upon the life and relationships of the love object, who can properly be regarded as a victim. The love object's life is disrupted by phone calls, letters and repeated face-to-face approaches. In some cases, physical and sexual assaults take place, and some love objects are killed (Mullen & Pathé, 1994a).

Erotomania coexists with other syndromes such as Capgras syndrome or Frégoli syndrome in the context of schizophrenia (Sims & White, 1973; Brüggemann & Garlipp, 2007) and Frégoli syndrome in the context of Down syndrome (Collacott & Napier, 1991; Mann & Foreman, 1996). In a case report from Dubai, the coexistence of erotomania and Capgras syndrome was distinct in the sense that the patient did not make any attempts to contact the love object but maintained that the love object secretly visited her at night and had sexual intercourse with her and that she was pregnant by him. She expressed the view that her husband was an impostor and a stranger to her. Both the erotomania and the Capgras syndrome occurred in the setting of schizophrenia (Zarrouk, 1991).

There is some evidence that erotomania is more likely to be associated with affective symptoms, in particular manic symptoms, and with schizoaffective psychosis and bipolar disorder (Rudden, Sweeney & Frances, 1990). Alongside the fact that secondary erotomania occurs in the context of schizophrenia, schizoaffective psychosis, bipolar disorder and psychotic depression, it can also arise in the context of organic brain disease. It has been reported in association with epilepsy and traumatic brain injury (Signer & Cummings, 1987; John & Ovsiew, 1996), dementia (Cipriani, Logi & Di Fiorino, 2012), following subarachnoid haemorrhage (El Gaddal, 1989; Suárez-Richards & Fournes, 2002) and as the presenting feature of frontotemporal dementia–motor neurone disease (Olojugba et al., 2007). The prevalence of erotomania is unknown but estimated to be 0.3 per cent in a case series of 1,802 patients consecutively admitted to hospital (Retterstøl & Opjordsmoen, 1991).

5.4.1 Stalking and Violence

Stalking and violence are two of the possible actions that derive directly from erotomania (Kamleiter & Laakmann, 2003). In Mullen and Pathé's (1994b) series of 16 cases encountered in forensic practice, all patients indulged in stalking behaviours that included following, loitering in the victim's vicinity, approaching, telephoning and sending letters. The love objects were threatened in five cases, violently assaulted in five cases with one death and sexually assaulted in seven cases. There was also risk of violence directed at those perceived by the patient as standing in the way of consummation of their pathological love. Stalking in the context of erotomania is a subset of stalking in general, a typically male behaviour that affects 1 in 20 women during a lifetime and involves surveillance, threatening behaviour and aggressive and violent behaviours. The victims are liable to suffer anxiety, depression, guilt, helplessness and features of post-traumatic stress disorder (Abrams & Robinson, 1998). In Colombia, the expression of violence can take the form of deliberate burning with acid (Restrepo-Bernal, Gómez-González & Gaviria, 2014), and the violent behaviour is attributed to rejection of sexual or love advancements. These behaviours have been reported from Southeast Asia, Africa and the Middle East. The emphasis is on violence-prone males suffering from erotomania whose violent actions derive from their delusional beliefs.

Cyberstalking is a variant of stalking that has come into prominence in the age of the internet. The term is used to refer to repeated threats or harassment via email or other computer-based communication that make a reasonable person fear for his or her safety. It is relatively common behaviour, with upwards of 23 per cent of the general population indicating that they have been victims of stalking. Strawhun, Adams and Huss (2013) have shown that cyberstalking behaviours are related to past measures of traditional stalking and are associated with prior attachment, jealousy and significant prior violence within relationships. In this study, more females admitted to cyberstalking behaviours, a change in the previously established association of stalking behaviours with male gender.

By definition, the love object in erotomania is a person of high status, often unattainable, and not unusually medical practitioners can be the focus of a patient's desire and the love object in erotomania (Hardeman, 1970; Pathé & Mullen, 1993; Kok, Cheang & Chee, 1994). The love object can be a child (Remington, 1997), a person of the same sex (Giannini, Slaby & Robb, 1991; Mann & Foreman, 1996) or indeed an imaginary lover (Seeman, 1971; Goldwert, 1993).

The outcome of erotomania is best regarded as the outcome of the primary condition when it is secondary to a primary condition such as schizophrenia, and in the pure type, there is limited evidence, but the outcome is often chronic and poor (Gillett, Eminson & Hassanyeh, 1990; Retterstøl & Opjordsmoen, 1991), with enduring difficulties in establishing relationships and lifelong social isolation, although not altogether hopeless because of the possibility of response to treatment.

5.5 Conclusion

Erotomania is a condition that draws attention to the intimate relationship between beliefs and emotions. It underscores how little we understand about love itself, its underlying mechanisms and the relationship between normal love and pathological love. Finally, the links between unrequited and unconsummated love and the propensity to stalking and violence are manifest in erotomania.

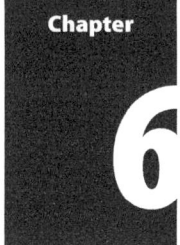

Chapter

6

Charles Bonnet Syndrome

.

6.1 Introduction

Charles Bonnet (1720–1793) was born in Geneva to a wealthy French family who had settled in Switzerland in the sixteenth century. He was a scholar, naturalist and philosopher who is best remembered for the syndrome that is named after him. He described in 1860 in his book, *Essai Analytique sur les Faculties de l'Ame*, the visual hallucinations of his 87-year-old grandfather, Charles Lullin (Hedges, 2007, pp. 112–13).

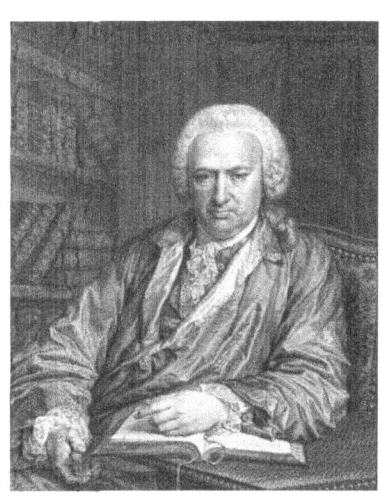

Charles Bonnet 1720–1793

> I should tell about a strange case that would be considered fabulous if not supported by testimonies of the highest credibility. However, the release of this psychological phenomenon would deserve a writing of its own. I will simply say that I know a respectable man full of health, of ingenuousness, judgment, and memory, who, completely alert and independently from all outside influences, sees from time to time, in front of him, figures of men, of women, of birds, of carriages, of buildings . . . etc. He sees these figures make various movements: getting closer, fleeing, diminishing or increasing in size, appearing or disappearing; he sees the buildings rise in front of his eyes and a display of all the outside construction material. The tapestries in his apartment appear to change suddenly; these tapestries cover themselves with paintings displaying different landscapes. Another day, instead of the tapestries and furniture it is only the naked walls with an assembly of raw materials. All these visions appear to him in perfect clarity and affect him as strongly as if the objects themselves were present. However, these are only paintings because the men and women do not talk and no noise comes in his ear. All of this appears to have its seat in the part of the brain that commands the sense of sight. The person I am talking about was subject at different times and at an advanced age to cataract operations on the two eyes. The great success of this operation would never have been challenged if a less ardent desire to read had enabled this elder to better manage his sight as it deserved.

In order to emphasize the integrity of his grandfather's cognitive function, Charles Bonnet added the following in a footnote:

> He still had a remarkably good memory for his age. He read a great deal, retained most of it and loved entertaining his friends and lectures. He particularly enjoyed history and politics. I was among those who often attended his lectures and frequently interrupting the description of some historical event to pay attention to a vision that he experienced at that

particular moment. 'There it is', he would say to me, 'the tapestry is covered with paintings; the frames are gilded etc. . . .' Immediately after, he would describe in detail another decoration or some other vision; and, after having jested over these fictions of his brain, he would calmly resume his discourse.

(Damas-Mora, Skelton-Robinson & Jenner, 1982, p. 251; see also)

This account is regarded as the first full and accurate account of visual hallucinations. The description of his grandfather's experience also allowed Charles Bonnet the opportunity to speculate on the possible mechanism underlying this experience. He wrote

All of this appears to have a seat in that part of the brain involved with sight. It is not difficult to imagine physical causes, strong enough to shake sensitive bundles of fibres that will produce in the mind, the picture of various objects with as much veracity as if the objects themselves had stimulated the fibres. And if the fibres used for thought are not involved but remain in their natural state, the mind will not confuse vision with reality. (Hedges, 2007)

Charles Bonnet himself later suffered from severe visual impairment from an unknown cause. His visual loss is said to have commenced shortly after the age of 20 years and became severe by the age of 40 years. In his later years, he too experienced visual hallucinations in the context of blindness but with preserved cognitive functions. The discovery by Flournoy (1923) of a lengthy manuscript written by Charles Bonnet but dictated by his grandfather, Charles Lullin, cast some doubt on the accuracy of Bonnet's prior descriptions of his grandfather's experiences.

Lullin said that his visions only appeared when standing or sitting but not when he was lying down and that the visions were clearer on his left visual field but disappeared when he turned his eyes to the right. (Berrios, 1996)

Morsier, in 1936, coined the eponym *Charles Bonnet syndrome* and later reported 18 cases, 5 of whom had visual hallucinations in the absence of visual loss. He concluded that the term *Charles Bonnet syndrome* should be restricted to visual hallucinations in elderly patients without evidence of cognitive impairment and unrelated aetiologically to peripheral problems of vision (Berrios, 1996). This set the scene for the ongoing debate about the provenance of Charles Bonnet syndrome, as Morsier implied that the primary cause lay in the brain and was not necessarily associated with visual impairment. Hence visual hallucinations in the elderly in whatever setting or context became liable to be labelled as Charles Bonnet syndrome.

In addition to the questions of provenance and of the conceptual boundaries of the syndrome, the psychopathological classification of the actual subjective experience of the visual phenomena is subject to intense debate. It raises fundamental questions about what counts as a hallucination and what the relationship of the so-called pseudo-hallucination is to true hallucinations and whether there is any value in retaining the term *pseudo-hallucination*.

The term *hallucination* refers to the abnormal experience of perceiving an object in the absence of a stimulus. It is distinguished from an illusion, a false perception in which a real stimulus is transformed and hence misinterpreted as another object, and also from a pseudo-hallucination. In order to fully grasp the nature of a pseudo-hallucination, it is perhaps best first to understand the formal characteristics of a real perception since a true hallucination is conceived as being indistinguishable from a real perception except with regard to the absence of an object, a stimulus. A real perception is characterized by a sense of concrete or objective reality, occurs in external objective space, is clearly delineated (the sensory elements being full and fresh) and remains constant and invariant. Real perceptions are independent of the subject's will and conceptually are received with a sense of passivity. These characteristics are said to underpin true hallucinations too and to contribute to the veridical aspect of true hallucinations since in essence true hallucinations have all the compelling immediacy of real perceptions.

Jaspers (1997) made a distinction between the formal characteristics of real perceptions and images. In his scheme, images were figurative in nature, appeared in inner subjective space, were often incomplete in detail and poorly defined (the sensory elements being insufficient and dissipating easily) and, finally, depended on the subject's will since they are created with an effort of will. In Jaspers' terms, pseudo-hallucinations were indistinguishable from real perceptions or true hallucinations except insofar as they occurred in inner subjective space. In other words, pseudo-hallucinations had a sense of concrete reality, were clearly delineated (full and fresh in their sensory elements) and were experienced independent of the subject's will. This characterization of pseudo-hallucinations relied on Victor Kandinsky's (1849–1889) account of his own experiences as 'subjective perceptions which in vividness and character are real hallucinations except that they do not have objective reality' (Berrios, 1996, p. 56). This characterization of pseudo-hallucination is termed *pseudo-hallucination of the imagistic type.*

It is worth noting that the term *pseudo-hallucination* was introduced into the literature by Friedrich Hagen (1861, 1868) and at the time was used to describe 'errors of the sense or illusions' (Berrios, 1996, p. 55). Kräupl Taylor (1966, 1981) gave an account of pseudo-hallucinations that distinguished between the imaged type as described earlier and the perceptual type in which the hallucinatory experience is identical to true hallucinations except that the subject has insight into the falsity of the experience. Given that Charles Bonnet's first account privileged insight in his conceptualization ('And if the fibres used for thought are not involved but remain in their natural state, *the mind will not confuse vision with reality* [emphasis added]'), then it is reasonable to conclude that the abnormal visual experience in Charles Bonnet syndrome is in the form of perceptual-type visual hallucination, namely a pseudo-hallucination.

It is important, though, to emphasize that as Berrios has said about the term pseudo-hallucination,

> unrestrained usage has strayed even wider, pseudo-hallucinations being sometimes applied to (i) phenomena which meet criteria for hallucinations or illusions, (ii) hallucinations in people without mental illnesses (e.g., the bereaved), (iii) the false perceptions of people recovering from psychotic illnesses, (iv) factitious hallucinations in malingerers, and (v) occasionally normal but unusual perceptions which initially seem to be hallucinations (e.g., radio reception in dental amalgam or intracranial shrapnel fragments).
>
> (Berrios, 1996, p. 50)

This means that classifying the visual experiences in Charles Bonnet syndrome as pseudo-hallucinations may not necessarily clarify the provenance of the abnormal experience, nor of the syndrome itself.

Finally, Charles Bonnet syndrome demands our attention not merely because it is an example of a psychopathological curio but precisely because it is an example of an abnormal phenomenon, namely visual hallucination, that occurs in the absence of neurological or psychiatric disorder and for which the subject recognizes the abnormality of the phenomenon. It therefore offers the opportunity to investigate the nature of visual perception and, by extension, the nature of perception itself by focusing on the neural and cognitive mechanisms that underlie visual experience in this condition.

6.2 Case Reports
The two case examples in this section are excerpts from Damas-Mora et al. (1982).

1. W.W., aged 86, [is] a widower living alone in a second-floor flat. He suffers from bilateral cataracts, visual acuity reduced to hand movements in the R.E. [right eye] and 6/12 in the L.E [left eye]. He was initially seen at an out-patient department where he had arrived after travelling alone by bus. At the interview, he was well orientated for time, place and person. He showed no signs of marked impairment of memory for recent and remote past. He appeared to be mildly euphoric and spoke quickly. He wore a clean, old, two-piece dark suit. He complained of having had visions for 4–5 years. He had seen figures of men marching through his bedroom. As he went out shopping or for a walk, he could see flowers 'of all colours' covering the ground. As he walked, the ground would become covered by flowers up to a few hundred yards in front of him. He was aware of the unreality of these images. He frequently stopped his discourse to point to the walls and ask: 'Can't you see the wallpaper with flowers?' But, before any reply could be given, he added: 'Of course, you cannot see it! ... Two years ago, I saw soldiers marching past the bedroom window. They were dressed with proper soldiers' clothes. There were four of them. They marched outside the window. ... Sometimes, when I look through the window, all the park, through and up the wood, is crowded with people. The more I look the more they come. I bet it must be more than a thousand people. ... I thought they were coming from a football march, just like that ... and then there are all these soldiers marching past. (pp. 253–4)

2. M.D. [is a] 69-year-old housewife [with] no history of psychiatric disorders. She did not present signs of psychotic or affective disorders at the interview, nor did she show any signs of intellectual deterioration. In September 1979, she was submitted to left intracapsular cataract extraction. She was readmitted days later with severe pain; she then showed prolapse of the iris and raised intraocular tension. She relates the onset of the pain to having carried a heavy bag. She was submitted to surgery for left excision of iris prolapse. In May 1981, visual acuity on the right was 6/18, while on the left it was limited to hand movements, even with contact corrective lenses. There was raised intraocular tension and optic atrophy in the left eye. 'I saw something like little black specks moving up and down before the operation. They were like little flies. At first I thought they were flies and I tried to catch them with my hand. They came and went and moved all the time. ... And they continued, I knew that they were not there. I still see them now. ... Only recently, for the past three months or so, at night, when I go to the toilet, as I come back to bed and before I drop off to sleep, I close my eyes and I see, I have seen, these optical illusions. I see them almost every night. I am awake. First, it was like the head of a lion, like those you see on doorknobs. ... A little small knob. ... [Its colour] is more like brown. It appeared and then went away. Later I saw faces of people, like a crowd in a football match or even like you see on TV. ... Men's faces and heads or busts of people; then, on other occasions, women's faces, individual faces. It is like looking at a picture, a photograph, and it passes on and another face comes on and passes on. They follow one after the other unless I see a group of people sitting down. They are bright and very, very clear. They are mostly middle-aged women. These are all white people, not in colour but in black and white. ... It is perhaps we do not have a coloured TV ... only black and white television set. ... And another thing is the wallpaper. I do not have wallpaper apart from the bathroom and that is blue. When I walk to the front of the bedroom, going to the toilet ... I do not put the light on but I can see because there is

a street light on and I know the way. . . . It is like that the whole from where I am walking until I get to the bathroom is covered by the same wallpaper of a flower design. This is in black and white. As I am walking, all the walls are full of this wallpaper. (pp. 256–7)

6.3 Explanatory Hypotheses

In the original description of visual hallucinations in his grandfather, Charles Bonnet proposed that the seat of the disorder was in the brain.

All of this appears to have a seat in that part of the brain involved with sight. It is not difficult to imagine physical causes, strong enough to shake sensitive bundles of fibres that will produce in the mind, the picture of various objects with as much veracity as if the objects themselves had stimulated the fibres. And if the fibres used for thought are not involved but remain in their natural state, the mind will not confuse vision with reality.

(Hedges, 2007, p. 113)

This view, that privileged the role of the brain in the causation of visual hallucinations, only made sense in the context of the visual impairment of the individual subjects. Nonetheless, visual impairment of the subjects raised questions about the role of peripheral eye pathology in determining the development of abnormal visual experiences of the kinds reported in Charles Bonnet syndrome. Damas-Mora et al. (1982) provide an excellent review of the older literature. They make the point that the main explanatory models were based upon (1) peripheral ocular pathology, (2) central neurophysiological disturbances or (3) psychological mechanisms. And these models followed the increasing understanding of the mechanisms underpinning visual hallucinations in general. Thus, for example, complex visual hallucinations, such as vision of snakes or spiders, in normal subjects were thought to possibly reflect underlying simpler forms such as 'wave-lines' or 'radiating lines' or elementary forms such as tunnels, spirals or cobwebs. With respect to Charles Bonnet syndrome, the chronological relationship between the visual hallucinations and sudden decrease in visual acuity, the effect of eye movement on the visual phenomenon and its disappearance on the restoration of vision all pointed to the importance of optical pathology. However, de Morsier (1967, 1969) argued that it is not uncommon to find Charles Bonnet syndrome in individuals without sensory loss, and even where Charles Bonnet syndrome is associated with sensory loss, the temporal relationship between the sensory loss and the development of visual hallucinations can be quite substantial, sometimes upwards of 20 years. And in any case there is significant rarity of visual hallucinations in the totally blind. This suggested the importance of central neurophysiological disturbance, which de Morsier located in the diencephalon. Finally, the role of psychological mechanisms in the form the conversion of memory-based fantasy into reality is exemplified next.

'The apparitions [vision of his mother and wife] at breakfast time', he wrote in a letter, 'illuminate the moment that was once the most pleasant. It is to me a very happy hour in which I can meet in spirit with those two beloved ones.' . . . One morning, a few weeks before his death, he woke up and regretted that he did not have flowers because that was his son's birthday. But, when he went down for breakfast, he saw the figure of his wife holding a bunch of flowers. She was also surrounded by three baskets of flowers. He was happy to show this spectacle to his son but disappointed because he realised that his son could not see it. (Flournoy, 1923)

6.3.1 Peripheral Ocular Pathology

Charles Bonnet syndrome occurs in 0.47 to 0.5 per cent of samples of patients attending either a neuro-ophthalmic unit or an ophthalmological or optometric outpatients department (Shiraishi et al., 2004; Santos-Bueso et al., 2014a). In individuals with low vision, the prevalence rose to 11 to 15 per cent (Teunisse et al., 1995; Vukicevic & Fitzmaurice, 2008; Santos-Bueso et al., 2014a) and was particularly prevalent in neurovascular age-related macular degeneration, and the prevalence in this population was established in a systematic review as 15.8 per cent (95 per cent confidence interval [CI] 11.0–21.2 per cent; Niazi et al., 2019), including diabetic retinopathy and glaucoma (Gordon, 2016). In neurovascular age-related macular degeneration, the areas of geographical atrophy, as estimated by detailed optical coherence tomography and autofluorescence, was significantly greater in patients with Charles Bonnet syndrome than in those without it (Singh & Sørensen, 2012). However, Shiraishi et al. (2004) showed that in individuals in whom the mean corrected visual acuity was 1.1, a relatively good visual acuity, the prevalence of Charles Bonnet syndrome was 0.8 per cent, probably reflecting the importance of the severity of visual acuity in determining the development of Charles Bonnet syndrome visual acuity. To emphasize the relationship between visual acuity and Charles Bonnet syndrome, Gilmour, Schreiber & Ewing (2009) demonstrated that Charles Bonnet syndrome was likely to occur in individuals with visual acuities between 20/40 and 20/1,600 but twice as likely to occur if visual acuity was between 20/301 and 20/800. This finding underlined the connection between severity of visual loss and Charles Bonnet syndrome. In a study specifically investigating neurovascular age-related macular degeneration, the prevalence of Charles Bonnet syndrome was 9 per cent, and this prevalence rate was doubled when the patient was also on proton pump inhibitors, with an odds ratio of 2.154 (Leandro et al., 2017). This relationship between visual acuity and Charles Bonnet syndrome was given even more credence by the findings of the National Comorbidity Survey analysing hallucinations in visually impaired individuals: the prevalence of visual hallucinations in this sample was 12.8 per cent, and the odds ratio of this association was 3.09 (95 per cent CI 1.06–8.99). This finding was only true for individuals aged 60 years and over.

Thus, reduced visual acuity is a predictor of Charles Bonnet syndrome, but the relationship between partial or total visual loss and Charles Bonnet syndrome is shown by the case report of a 78-year-old man with a visual deficit moving toward end-stage glaucoma. The complex visual hallucinations ceased once he lost all his vision (Santos-Bueso et al., 2014b). Patients with low vision due to central scotoma following laser photocoagulation or photodynamic therapy for macular degeneration have also been reported with complex visual hallucinations in the immediate aftermath of treatment (Cohen & Le Gargasson, 2006).

The eye complications of leprosy can cause Charles Bonnet syndrome, and this occurs in 0.4 per cent of patients with leprosy (Adachi, 1996). This is, of course, still an example of sensory loss due to abnormality attributable to the eye directly. Marked ptosis as a cause of visual sensory loss has been reported as a cause of complex visual hallucinations (Hashmi, Ogra & Madge, 2019). This suggests that occlusion of the eye may be associated with Charles Bonnet syndrome and is confirmed by a report that monocular complex visual hallucinations can attend surgical occlusion of the eye as part of treatment (Hughes procedure) for eyelid basal cell carcinoma (Wilson et al., 2016). Similarly, acute complex visual hallucinations have been reported to occur in craniomaxillary surgery for unilateral orbital floor fracture followed by eye patching with a Frost suture (Gander et al., 2014). These reports go to show how important it is to recognize the role of eye patching as a causative factor in

Charles Bonnet syndrome, especially in cases where the syndrome is easily reversible (Beaulieu et al., 2018). Other causes include temporal arteritis (Sonnenblick et al., 1995).

6.3.2 Central Neurophysiological Disturbance

In the preceding section, I drew attention to the role of visual loss in the development of Charles Bonnet syndrome. I now turn to cases in which peripheral lesions leading to visual impairment are not present, but central lesions are demonstrable and putatively of relevance to the development of complex visual hallucinations.

There are reports of complex visual hallucinations in the context of normal cognitive function and intact insight into the unreality of the visual experience but not always with ocular pathology. These reports include complex visual hallucinations in the hemianoptic visual field following occipital infarction (Ashwin & Tsaloumas, 2007), visual impairment following bilateral occipital infraction in the context of cardiac surgery (Cook et al., 2017) and another following trans-sphenoidal adenomectomy without optic nerve damage (Park et al., 2016). In this latter case, the visual hallucinations were only present during eye closure. In another case report of Charles Bonnet syndrome developing in the context of hemianopsia, the patient had anteromesial temporal lobectomy for drug-resistant epilepsy. The complex visual hallucination was restricted to the hemianoptic field and was of static or dynamic 'Lilliputian' human figures or of countryside scenes (Contardi et al., 2007). And, in another case report, Charles Bonnet syndrome occurred in the setting of occipital cortical resection for treatment-resistant epilepsy (Choi et al., 2005).

Visual hallucinations with the characteristics of Charles Bonnet syndrome have been reported in epilepsy (Miyaoka et al., 2005; Ossola et al., 2010; Brown-Vargas & Cienki, 2012). Mocellin, Walterfang and Velakoulis (2006) reported on three cases presenting with complex visual hallucination in the setting of thalamic infarction, pontine infarction and temporoparietal epileptiform activity, respectively. Their view was that there is considerable overlap between peduncular hallucinosis and Charles Bonnet syndrome and that complex visual hallucinations can arise from any lesion that alters or reduces input into the retino-geniculo-calcarine tract or ascending brainstem modulating structures (see the next section for a discussion of the conceptual and theoretical explanations for the genesis of Charles Bonnet syndrome).

Arai et al. (2014) reported on a case of transient Charles Bonnet syndrome in an individual with established diabetic retinopathy. The visual hallucinations followed resection of a right occipital meningioma. The hallucinatory experiences were associated with recovery of the occipital lobe from the compression caused by the tumour and shown by initial hypoperfusion of the right parieto-occipital lobe. Cases of Charles Bonnet syndrome in the context of intracranial tumours often demonstrate the complex relationships between the locus of the tumour and the influence of additional factors such as seizures, ablative surgery, radiotherapy and chemotherapy (Boyer, Devlin & Boggild, 2018). These cases and others underline the importance of seeking more than one remediable cause of Charles Bonnet syndrome. Chatterjee et al. (2018) reported on a patient with a combination of cataract and normal-pressure hydrocephalus in whom both conditions demanded treatment in order to resolve the Charles Bonnet syndrome.

The role of optic neuritis in Charles Bonnet syndrome is indicated in the reports of associations with multiple sclerosis (Alao & Hanrahan, 2003; Tan & Au Eong, 2007), retrobulbar neuritis (Paradowski et al., 2013) and syphilitic optic neuritis (Ogata et al.,

2011). Complex visual hallucinations associated with neurosarcoidosis have been reported in an individual with right seventh nerve palsy, right facial paraesthesia and bilateral progressive visual loss, once again emphasizing the fact that the any lesion impairing the integrity of the visual pathways may cause Charles Bonnet syndrome (Zhang et al., 2013).

The role of specific loci and functional connectivity in Charles Bonnet syndrome is only starting to be explored. Martial et al. (2019) reported that decreased grey matter volume was observed in the middle occipital gyrus and cuneus in patients with Charles Bonnet syndrome compared to individuals who developed late blindness, in whom there was decreased grey matter volume in the middle occipital gyrus and the lingual gyrus. In Charles Bonnet syndrome there was increased functional connectivity between the precuneus and secondary visual cortex, whereas in late blindness there was reduced connectivity between the DMN and the fusiform gyrus, areas known to support hallucinations. In the similar vein, Adachi et al. (2000) reported on hyperfusion in the lateral temporal cortex, the striatum and the thalamus during the experience of complex visual hallucinations in five subjects presenting with Charles Bonnet syndrome. They argue that this is a result of excessive cortical compensation in the context of eye disease. In another report, they demonstrated, using a serial single photon emission computed tomographic study, that visual hallucinations were associated with hyperperfusion in the left temporal region and basal ganglia and hypoperfusion in the right temporal region and concluded that asymmetrical blood flow in the temporal regions may be correlated with visual hallucinations in Charles Bonnet syndrome (Adachi et al., 1994).

In an elegant study, Painter et al. (2018), using a stimulus-driven electrophysiological response paradigm, showed that in patients with macular degeneration with Charles Bonnet syndrome, there was good evidence of elevated visual cortical responses to peripheral field stimulation, confirming the likelihood of visual cortical hyperexcitability in Charles Bonnet syndrome and indirectly confirming the key theory about Charles Bonnet syndrome, namely the retinal deafferentiation theory (see next section for a fuller description).

6.4 Explanatory Hypotheses

The current consensus is that Charles Bonnet syndrome results from deafferentation of certain structures in the brain, primarily the cortex, or from the effective silencing of principal afferents to these structures. The idea is that the reduced sensory stimuli resulting from deafferentation leads to an excessive neural response by way of increased excitability or association with an increase in spontaneous neural activity (Burke, 2002). This phenomenon was previously referred to as a *release* phenomenon. The liability for visual hallucinations to occur in normal subjects exposed to sensory deprivation is already well established, and the relationship between relative sensory deprivation and well-formed hallucinations and total sensory deprivation and an absence of visual hallucinations is also known (Thorpe, 1961). To emphasize this point: perceptual isolation that allows a slight amount of light stimulation produces hallucinations of flashes of light, flickering light and geometric shapes, including squares and circles. In circumstances of total absence of visual stimulation, only a minimum of visual hallucinations occurred. Highly structured visual hallucinations of integrated scenes only occurred during lengthy sensory deprivation in which the subjects wore translucent goggles in an illuminated room.

Burke's (2002) contribution is to explain the mechanisms in detail. Burke, himself an Australian professor of physiology, had experienced and described his subjective experiences of visual hallucinations in the context of macular degeneration. He had experienced brief flashes in his right eye lasting 1 second and complex visual hallucinations in his left eye, including (1) a type resembling a brickwork (tessellation or tesselopsia), (2) round objects or spots arranged in an egg-crate fashion, and (3) a lozenge-shaped object arranged in a 45-degree angle. Burke's proposal is that denervation or deafferentation is followed by hyperexcitability and that there are microscopic and neurochemical structural changes underpinning this hyperexcitability: increases in the size of boutons, in the number of vesicles, in the size of the release zone, in the size of the readily releasable pool and in the release probability. Biochemically speaking, there is an increase in the glutamatergic N-methyl-D-aspartate (NMDA) response and a decrease in gamma-aminobutyric acid (GABA). In addition to hyperexcitability, there are also reports of increased spontaneous activity following deafferentation. Perhaps the most radical hypothesis put forward from Burke is that the pattern of the hallucinations, namely the tessellation including size, configuration and pattern, was strikingly like the pattern created in areas V_1 and V_2 by staining for cytochrome oxidase or by functional magnetic resonance imaging (fMRI). This suggests that the geometrical patterns reflect underlying structural patterned systems which become visible in the context of deafferentation. Finally, Burke (2002, p. 539) says that 'the more extensive the visual loss, the more complex the hallucination; second, the more extensive the visual loss, the longer the visual hallucinations persist; and third, that in the disappearance of hallucinations the more complex hallucinations should disappear first, followed by other simpler images progressing back to very simple images that may originate in the thalamus'. The advantage of this proposition is that it is testable.

If we accept that the visual hallucinations that patients experience in Charles Bonnet syndrome are understandable given visual impairment or lesions within the visual pathways, the question is how far we can understand the neural basis of not only the form of the visual hallucinations but also the content. Earlier I described how the geometrical patterns may speak to the underlying structure of the visual cortex. I turn now to examine our current understanding of the mechanisms underpinning both the form and content of visual hallucinations. As a preamble, I make the point that in clinical psychopathology, the distinction between form and content is such that form is given precedence; it is privileged because it is considered that content is idiosyncratic to the individual, whereas the form is saying something about universal principles. The discussion that follows undermines some of this notion since it emphasizes both form and content and tracks content down to specific brain regions.

Santhouse, Howard and Ffytche (2000) identified phenomenological correlates of cerebral functional architecture within Charles Bonnet syndrome. Their findings are important for several reasons. Firstly, they had shown in a previous paper that the visual hallucinations described, predominantly in patients with macular degeneration, were remarkably consistent and were classified into the following groups: tessellopsia (brickwork patterns, tiles), hyperchromatospia (vivid colours, fireworks exploding in vivid colours), prosop-metamorhopsia (misshapen and mutilated heads, faces with distorted features), dendropsia (lines of trees or hedges), perseveration (visual persistence on looking away), illusory visual spread (the spread of an isolated feature across the visual field), polyopia (numerous and repeated items and objects in the visual field) and micro/macropsia (see Ffytche & Howard, 1999). Next, they showed that these anomalous experiences could be clustered into three groups: (1) extended landscapes scenes, vehicles and small figures in costumes with hats, (2) hallucinations of grotesque, disembodied distorted faces with prominent eyes, and (3) visual perseveration and delayed palinopsia located in the peripheral visual field. They concluded that the typical Charles Bonnet visual hallucination was a single constant and solid object appearing in the central visual field, seen in a flash and in more detail than a veridical object. Commonly, it was a complex grid (see Burke earlier), a disembodied and distorted face or a small costumed figure with a hat or a branching structure. They contended that the first cluster of visual experiences, namely landscapes, figures, vehicles and trees/shrubs, along with emotional content, derived from lesions affecting the anterior temporal projections of the ventral visual pathways. In addition, the second cluster of phenomena, namely distorted faces that evoke no emotional response, derived from lesions in the superior temporal sulcus, and finally, the third cluster, namely of perseveration and delayed palinopsia, derived from functional impairments within the visual parietal lobe, an area responsible for representations of space in a variety of different reference frames. I have concentrated on the form and content of the visual hallucinations. Now I turn to the colour of the hallucinated perceptions. Madill et al. (2009) showed that deafferentation and secondary cortical hyperexcitability in Charles Bonnet syndrome have a correlate in psychophysical threshold for colour perception and indicated that the change in sensitivity relates specifically to the hallucinated colour axis rather than across all colours. This means that hyperexcitability leads to a decrease in colour contrast thresholds.

This development, the possibility of linking both the form and the content of visual hallucinations to specific neural correlates, brings into focus the view that psychopathological objects, the phenomena that constitute psychopathology, can in their own right be at the centre of our attention as valuable in determining the mechanisms and nature of brain function, as well as the relationship between neural correlates and events in the mind. To emphasize this point, as Ffytche (2007) points out, hallucination of an object is associated with spontaneous activity in object-specialized cortex and hallucination of a face is associated with spontaneous activity in face-specialized cortex. In contradistinction, visual imagery, a distinct phenomenon from visual hallucination, is associated with activation in visual areas as well as in frontal and parietal lobes (Ffytche, 2007). Furthermore, there is the importance of appreciating the emergence of different paradigms for understanding the neural basis of psychopathology. The original and more established approach, which is to identify the localization of dysfunction in specific brain regions, is the so-called topological approach, and the newer approach, which is to explore how dysfunction relates to connections between brain areas, is the hodological approach (Ffytche, 2008; see Martial et al., 2019, for fuller details on this approach). Finally, this evolution in our thinking about psychopathology, what Ffytche terms 'neurophenomenology', is likely to refine our understanding of the boundaries and affiliations of differing phenomena. Ffytche suggests that the traditional distinctions between hallucinations and illusions may become de-emphasized, whereas the links between the groups of phenomena described earlier may become emphasized.

6.5 Clinical Aspects

Damas-Mora et al. (1982) defined Charles Bonnet syndrome as a syndrome in which persistent or recurrent visual pseudo-hallucinatory phenomena of a pleasant or neutral nature occur in a clear state of consciousness. Despite its vividness, clarity and impelling character, the visual experience is recognized as unreal (this is why it is labelled as a pseudo-hallucination). The condition tends to occur in the elderly with clinically preserved intellectual function and is often associated with ocular pathology. This definition was subtly modified by Gold and Rabins (1989) to de-emphasize specific clinical context and bring to the fore the nature of the visual hallucinations, namely that they were well formed visual hallucinations that were complex in nature, persistent or repetitive, stereotyped with full or partial insight and in the absence of primary or secondary delusions and the absence of hallucinations in other modalities (Gold & Rabins, 1989).

The mean age of onset was reported as 81 years, even though younger cases have been reported (Schwartz & Vahgei, 1998; Santos-Bueso et al., 2017). The previously reported preponderance in females has been shown to be untrue (Damas-Mora et al., 1982). The onset is reported as variable from sudden onset of highly organized and complex visual hallucinations to initially simple and elementary forms that progress to complex figures and scenes. The experiences can be episodic, periodic or continuous. The visual hallucinations are in external objective space, and the distance from the observer may vary from time to time (Damas-Mora et al., 1982). Characteristics of the visions as already described earlier include faces, well-proportioned human figures, animals, flowers, Lilliputian images and various scenes. The perceptions are clear, well defined, bright, multicoloured or in black and white. The scenes, when present, may change continuously. The patients may be indifferent to the experience or may evidence surprise, amazement, curiosity, delight and rarely fear. There is usually insight into the unreality of the experience despite its being vivid, compelling and appearing in three dimensions (Damas-Mora et al., 1982).

There is literature suggesting that in patients attending a low-vision and glaucoma clinic and presenting with Charles Bonnet syndrome, mild cognitive impairment, partial insight and the visual hallucination of familiar figures may predict increased risk of the subsequent diagnosis of dementia (Russell & Burns, 2014; Russell et al., 2018). In a small study of individuals with Charles Bonnet syndrome, all had ocular pathology and abnormal visually evoked potentials. In comparison to a matched control group, the individuals with Charles Bonnet syndrome were reported to have abnormal neuropsychological scores derived from the Weschler Adult Intelligence Scale–Revised, the Mattis Dementia Rating Scale, the Weschler Memory Scale and the Auditory Verbal Learning Test. The authors concluded that subtle cognitive deficits accompany the onset of visual hallucinations (Pliskin et al., 1996). In a retrospective study of a sample of patients with a diagnosis of Charles Bonnet syndrome, it was reported that there was significantly increased mortality compared with the background Minnesota population, and 26 per cent of the sample went on to develop dementia, most often of Lewy body type (Lapid et al., 2013). It is probably wise to exclude the possibility of Lewy body dementia in patients presenting with complex visual hallucinations (Walker & Keys, 2008).

Despite the fact that Charles Bonnet syndrome mostly occurs in the setting of ocular pathology, there are social factors that seem to be important in determining whether or not an individual with limited vision will develop complex visual hallucinations. Teunisse et al. (1994, 1999) showed that social isolation, loneliness and shyness were risk factors.

In a sample of cases reported by Berrios and Brook (1984) drawn from consecutive referrals to an old age psychiatrist and presenting with visual hallucinations, there was also evidence that ocular pathology was significantly associated with visual hallucinations. Insight as to the unreality of the experience was absent in 27 per cent of cases. The characteristics of the hallucinations were described as 'fleeting, ghostly and mundane' but typically were of people, animals and formless. There is good reason to recognize that the presence of dementia in individuals with visual hallucinations in the context of ocular pathology does not necessarily invalidate the neurobiological underpinning of the experience.

In a survey of 1,254 individuals with macular degeneration, 39 per cent had experienced hallucinations, mainly of patterns (63 per cent), faces (39 per cent), objects (39 per cent), figures (36 per cent) and animals (22 per cent). In this sample, typically the hallucinations were of short duration, lasting minutes or seconds. At their worst, the hallucinations occurred weekly (30 per cent), monthly (21 per cent), daily (22 per cent) or constantly (13 per cent). At the outset, 38 per cent found the experience startling, terrifying and frightening, which decreased to 8 per cent by the time of the survey. The experience affected daily activities in 46 per cent: television watching (24 per cent), moving about (14 per cent), cooking (8 per cent) and sleeping (14 per cent). Practically all the respondents had told someone about the experience. The outcome was as follows: 88 per cent had the experience for two years or more, and it had resolved in 25 per cent at nine years. The factors associated with poor outcome were (1) frequent fear-inducing, longer-lasting hallucination episodes, (2) one or more daily activities affected, (3) attribution of hallucinations to serious mental illness and (4) not knowing about Charles Bonnet syndrome at the onset of symptoms. The authors concluded that Charles Bonnet syndrome may be longer lasting than previously thought (Cox & Ffytche, 2014).

Charles Bonnet–like visual hallucinations can occur in late paraphrenia. In this setting, the visual hallucinations are accompanied by auditory hallucinations in 50 per cent, and visual impairment is also a feature in 42 per cent. As distinct from Charles Bonnet syndrome, as currently construed, only 1 in 18 patients had insight into the unreality of the experience. Four of 8 patients (50 per cent) who had structural MRI were shown to have structural midbrain abnormalities (Howard & Levy, 1994).

A variant of Charles Bonnet syndrome has been described by Oliver Sacks (2013, pp. 2318–19); in this variant, the patients present with hallucinations of musical notation. One of Sacks' subjects described her experience as follows:

> I started to see music lines, spaces, notes, clefs – in fact written music on everything I looked at, but only where the blindness exists. I ignored it for a while, but then I was visiting the Seattle Art Museum one day and I saw the lines of the explanatory notes as music. I knew I was really having some kind of hallucination. . . . I had been playing the piano and really concentrating on music prior to the musical hallucinations. . . . [I]t was right before my cataract was removed, and I had to concentrate hard to see the notes. Occasionally I'll see crossword puzzle squares . . . but the music does not go away.

The music was often unreadable and unplayable, as one of the subjects reported that 'it was inordinately complicated, with four or six staves, impossibly complex chords with six or more notes on a single stem, and horizontal rows of multiple flats and sharps' (p. 2319). In one subject, restoration of vision following cataract operation led to lessening of the hallucinations of musical notes. Another subject, a Sanskrit scholar, reported that

> the music covers a whole page and sometimes is written very ornately rather than the crude hand that occurred before, now almost like a hand of the 18th century. I have come closer to copying some of them, but I am still not sure of the accuracy of what I might write since very often the images disappear before I can verify them. Another oddity: the illusions have occurred with the Devanagari script used [in] Sanskrit. Despite the exotic nature of the script the result is still western music.   (p. 2319)

Sacks compares these visual experiences to hallucinations of texts which are usually not letters at all but lines, dots, dashes and curves and only bearing a passing resemblance to letters. The perceived musical notations, too, unconstrained by actual visual stimuli, since they are occurring in the context of visual loss are merely a 'crude simulacrum' and pseudoscores. As Sacks concludes, 'We see in hallucinations of musical notation not only notes, staves and clefts, but all the ancillary instructional notations, along with their spatial layout in the case of scores – minus the organizing principles of grammar and meaning' (p. 2322).

6.6 Conclusion

Charles Bonnet syndrome exemplifies the nature of visual hallucinations and illustrates the role of ocular pathology and anomalies in the visual pathways in the causation of visual hallucinations. Finally, Charles Bonnet syndrome forces us to reconsider how form and content are currently regarded in psychopathology. It is probable that both form and content have an underlying neural substrate.

Chapter

7

Musical Hallucinosis

7.1 Introduction

In Chapter 6, I discussed Charles Bonnet syndrome, a variant of visual hallucinatory experience that occurs often in the context of visual loss. In this chapter, I turn to musical hallucinosis, a condition in which the predominant feature is the perception of music in the absence of external stimulation. It often occurs in the context of hearing loss, but not exclusively so. This means that it has been considered by some authors as the auditory equivalent of Charles Bonnet syndrome.

Musical hallucinosis allows us to examine the neural basis of a discrete abnormal phenomenon, namely musical hallucination, and to further the goals of what Ffytche (2008) has termed *neurophenomenology*, that is, at least to attempt to identify not simply the focus of music perception but also the mechanisms and structures involved and thereby in the abnormal perception of music. Penfield and Perot (1963) showed that either spontaneously or in response to electrical stimulation, patients with a history of epilepsy requiring surgical treatment often heard music, sometimes an orchestral piece and at other times singing, piano music or a choir. Several times in their series it was reported as a radio theme song that was perceived. The localization for the production of music was put in the superior temporal convolution either on the lateral or superior surface. Examples included a 32-year-old woman with seizures starting at age 31 years, who following electrical stimulation heard 'It is a White Christmas' sung by a choir and a 28-year-old woman who began to have seizures from the age of 6 years. Stimulation of the superior and medial aspects of first temporal convolution, where the convolution lay against the insular, induced the hearing of music which the patient was able to hum and which was recognized by the theatre nurse as 'Rolling Together Again'.

This approach, the aim of localizing aberrant phenomenon or deficits, grew in the wake of Broca's (1824–1880) identification of the relationship between lesions in the left hemisphere and impairment of speech (Broca, 1861). Even though this approach has been fruitful in neurology in determining the basis of motor aphasia, sensory aphasia, dyscalculia and so on, it has not been particularly explored in psychiatry, partly because in psychiatry analysis and investigations concentrate at the level of categories of disorders such as schizophrenia rather than at the basic level of underlying and primary psychopathological abnormalities such as hallucinations or delusions.

Berrios (1990) makes the point that musical hallucinations are at the crossroads of ontological, neurological and psychiatric disorders. He also makes the important point that the concept 'music' includes harmonics, rhythm and timbres and hence that a proper understanding of musical hallucinations must be underpinned by an understanding of the neural mechanisms of the fundamental aspects of music. Berrios traces the history of recognition of musical hallucinations to Baillarger (1891) and Griesinger (1882) and identifies Regis (1881) as an important figure whose view was that musical hallucinations arise from positive and negative changes in the sensory pathways. The positive changes are the hearing of noise or tinnitus that crystallizes to musical hallucinations, and the negative change is deafness. This was a theory bearing the hallmarks of notions of release mechanisms as the basis of musical hallucinations in the context of deafness, an explanation that I would now term *deafferentation*. In order words, the hallucinatory experience arose when there was loss of external stimulation due to deafness and the central nervous system was released from the control or constraint of sensory inputs, resulting in the generation of novel and abnormal perceptions.

7.2 Case Reports

The case examples are drawn from the paper by Hammeke, McQuillen and Cohen (1983).

1. A 75-year-old, right-handed, retired female school teacher complained of annoying musical hallucinations. The first occurred four months earlier, shortly after discontinuing an antibiotic medication for a sinus infection. She was awakened during the night by the 'music', which lasted one hour. The music was loud and vivid, prompting her to search her living quarters for the source. A similar experience occurred the following night and throughout the subsequent day. During the following three weeks, the episodes increased in frequency until they were a constant experience except during periods of sleep, active conversation or mental operation. She described the experience to include both familiar and unfamiliar ('nonsense') melodies. Familiar melodies were ballads and religious hymns learned in childhood. Often the melodies were played by a single instrument (for example, guitar or chimes) and sung by a baritone voice; occasionally they were sung by a choir with orchestral accompaniment. The melodies were repetitive (line or verse) and present in both ears. Intensity increased when she was mentally inactive and ambient noise levels were low. She reported an ability to replace an ongoing musical passage with another, or alter its speed, via subvocalization of the desired song or speed. In addition, she reported a gradual progressive hearing loss over several years. ... Audiometric testing revealed moderate, bilateral sensorineural hearing loss (51 dB AD, 56 dB AS). (pp. 570–1)

2. An 80-year-old, right-handed nun and retired schoolteacher reported a three-year history of auditory hallucinations. She had been deaf in the right ear since a mastoidectomy some forty years earlier. She had been troubled by recurrent ringing and buzzing in her left ear when in the summer of 1972, she was exposed to an 'extremely intense noise (traffic)'. Several hours later she became aware of an intense noise in her head 'like a boiler factory'. This was followed by the perception of someone singing 'Jingle Bells'. Since that time she described a constant experience of repetitive sounds. At times the sounds were simply formed ('rumbling noises'). At other times words or phrases, that she had mostly read or been told, were repeated. In the first year after onset, melodies were common. In subsequent years voices repeatedly calling a name she went by as a child, or repetition of a brief religious prayer (for example, 'Lord have mercy') became more frequent. The intensity of hallucinations was greatest during periods of silence and when her hearing aid was turned down. ... Audiometric testing showed profound right ear (100 dB) and moderate left ear (50 dB) sensorineural hearing loss. (p. 571)

7.3 Explanatory Hypotheses

In order to fully grasp the underlying mechanisms of abnormal musical perception, there is a need for a more refined understanding of the brain basis for normal musical listening. Stewart et al. (2006) define musical listening as not merely the perception of music but also including *musical cognitions*, a term which refers to the ordering of incoming musical information according to rule-based structures and musical recognition. In addition to this is the elicitation of an emotional response to musical perception.

The auditory pathways actively process music, as they do other auditory sensations, relaying the information in an ascending manner to the auditory cortex situated in the superior temporal plane within the Sylvian fissure. Music is comprised of pitch, timbre and rhythm. Pitch is described as a percept, as opposed to a physical attribute of sound stimulation, and the exact relationship between the stimulus and the percept is still under debate (Stewart et al., 2006). Melody, which is a pattern of pitch over time; chords, which are the simultaneous presentation of more than one pitch at a time; and harmony, which is the simultaneous presentation of more than one melody at a time are associated with bilateral activation of the anterior and posterosuperior temporal lobes with a right hemisphere lateralization. It is interesting to note that the perceptual features of music, such as pitch, share with other sounds such as speech, an overlap in the activation of temporal structures.

Timbre, another fundamental aspect of musical perception that allows us to distinguish between different instruments, for example, is associated with different physical properties of the music stimulus, including aspects of the spectral or temporal structures. It has been shown to be associated with bilateral changes in activity in the posterosuperior temporal lobes (Stewart et al., 2006). Finally, the temporal structures of music, namely rhythm and meter, are associated with changes in the lateral cerebellum and basal ganglia during the reproduction of a rhythm. This suggests that our perception of rhythm might depend upon the motor mechanisms required for its production (Stevens & Price, 2015). Music perception involves emotional responses, and these are associated with changes in brain regions known to be involved in pleasurable activities such as the ventral striatum, amygdala, and orbitofrontal cortex.

There is considerable evidence for specialization of the musical brain, and this includes differences in the brains of musicians in auditory, somatosensory, superior parietal and cerebellar areas. Even the most minimal of musical training appears to be associated with brain reorganization. And musicians with absolute pitch also seem to have differences in brain organization from those without this attribute.

On the basis of these considerations, Stewart et al. (2006) argue that

> [w]hat emerges ... is the principle that different components of music (pitch, melody, rhythm, timbre and emotion) are underpinned by different psychological mechanisms and neural substrates. This principle is most clearly evident in the case of pitch and melody: the evidence suggests a scheme in which the perception of pitch and simple patterns of pitch is supported by mechanisms in the auditory cortices, whilst cognitive analysis of patterns within the pitch and time-domains require more distributed networks including the frontal cortices. (p. 2537)

In the light of these proposals, they put forward an explanatory hypothesis about the development of musical hallucinations in the context of deafness.

Particularly with regard to musical hallucinations associated with deafness, Stewart et al. (2006) make the point that the phenomenology of musical hallucinations, especially the fact that the perceptions are of complex patterned sequences that are in line with the previous musical listening experience of the subject, suggests that there is amplification of normal imagery that is usually suppressed by inputs from the external sensory world that decrease in the context of deafness. The proposition is that the decreased signal-to-noise ratio in auditory transmission in the deaf leads to inappropriate activation of cortical networks usually involved in perception and imagery and that the networks involved are also those involved during musical perception and imagery in the absence of deafness.

The association of deafness with abnormal perceptions of music rather than other kinds of auditory percepts such as speech requires some explanation. Kumar et al. (2014) suggest that musical perception occurs because of the statistical properties of music compared to speech, namely that music is more predictable and repetitive relative to speech. Thus, for example, hearing one or a few notes of music is sufficient to predict the upcoming notes either by mathematic rules or by retrieval from memory. In this context, repetitiveness refers to the fundamental aspect of music in which a given segment of music is repeated over time and is linked to the capacity of music to influence emotions and to give aesthetic value to a piece of music. It is also a critical distinguishing aspect of music compared to speech. Kumar et al. (2014) refer to their model of music hallucination as the *predictive coding theory*. They argue that

> [i]n this framework, each level of the cortical hierarchy tries to predict the representation of sensory objects in the level below by sending top-down predictions. Aspects of the representation that are inconsistent with the prediction (the prediction error) are then passed back to the higher level. Prediction errors are then used to update the representations at the higher level. In this framework, all bottom-up (ascending) connections communicate prediction error, and top-down (descending) connections convey predictions. This message passing changes hierarchical representations such that prediction error is minimized at all levels. . . . In summary, it is the adaptive reduction of sensory precision (estimated signal-to-noise ratio) that permits the emergence of hallucinatory predictions or percepts that are inferred with a relatively high degree of precision or confidence. (pp. 93–5)

In short, under this model, hallucinations arise because the sensory inputs are attenuated by deafness, and thus the perception is unconstrained by the precision and intensity of the sensory stimulus. Spontaneous and autonomous but abnormal perceptions, namely hallucinations, are the result of this process without the necessary checks usually brought to bear by the force of external reality.

In his analysis of six subjects with musical hallucinosis in the context of deafness, Griffiths (2000) undertook both structural and functional neuroimaging and, based on his findings, proposed a model that suggests that spontaneous activity in a module usually involved in the normal perception of pattern in segmented sounds and the perception of music is realized in a distributed network distinct from the primary auditory cortices, including the posterior temporal lobes, the right basal ganglia, the cerebellum and the inferior frontal cortices.

Musical hallucinosis also occurs significantly in association with epilepsy. Coebergh et al. (2019), in their review of the subject, distinguished four subgroups of epilepsy-related musical hallucinations comprising auras/ictal, interictal and postictal phenomena and phenomena related to brain stimulation. They concluded that musical hallucinations lie on a continuum from auditory hallucinations including verbal hallucinations and tinnitus to musical hallucinations. Their proposed mechanism is an adaptation of Kumar's predictive coding theory described earlier. There are points of departure; particularly of note is the opinion that verbal hallucinations lie in a continuum with musical hallucinations and making the case for an all-embracing theory of an auditory network that explains all auditory hallucinations. In some respects, the adaptation of Kumar's predictive coding theory can be used to explain the role of psychoactive substances in the causation of musical hallucinations. It is well recognized that benzodiazepines, opiates and dopaminergic and anticholinergic drugs may be associated with the development of musical hallucinations. In the same vein, anticholinesterases are known to be capable of diminishing or stopping musical hallucinations. The proposal is that these agents are able either to disrupt or to normalize the physiological activity in the musical hallucination network. The exact or potential mechanisms of these effects are yet to be established, but on empirical grounds, the broad proposals seem plausible.

7.4 Clinical Aspects

Musical hallucinations occur in 3.6 per cent of patients referred for audiometric testing, and the significant associations are with female sex and left-sided hearing impairments (Teunisse & Rikkert, 2012). There is also an association with being more than 60 years of age and social isolation (Cope & Baguley, 2009). In a multidisciplinary assessment of consecutive patients presenting with tinnitus, hearing loss and musical hallucinations, of the identified 16 patients, 68.75 per cent were severely or profoundly deaf, and neuroimaging showed that 43.75 per cent had small foci of gliosis or ischaemia and 25 per cent presented with mild attentional impairment. Depression was prevalent in that 68.75 per cent had recognizable depression. This association with depression was confirmed in the review of cases by Pasquini and Cole (1997). The authors conclude that patients presenting with musical hallucinations ought to be assessed by a multidisciplinary team of specialists (Cope & Baguley, 2009).

In the sample of 31 of 46 patients (67 per cent) reported by Berrios (1990) as presenting with musical hallucinations in the context of deafness, there was a preponderance of females. The onset of musical hallucinations was gradual, and musical hallucinations were the sole symptom in 40 per cent of the sample. The musical hallucinations occurred bilaterally in 31 of 46 patients. The music heard was in the majority singing, followed by instrumental music. Insight was preserved in 31 of 46 patients. Other hallucinations included tinnitus, verbal hallucinations and, in a minority (3 of 46 patients), there were visual hallucinations. There was no brain pathology in 28 of the 46 patients. The main neurological abnormalities were temporal lobe tumour, epilepsy, cerebrovascular accident, neurosyphilis, subarachnoid haematoma, localized atrophy, Behçet's syndrome, acquired traumatic brain injury and onset following electroconvulsive treatment.

In an extensive investigation using the Mayo Medical Records Linkage System (Golden & Josephs, 2015), 393 subjects presenting with musical hallucinations were identified. Once again, there was demonstrable over-representation of females (65.4 per cent), and 26.7 per cent had documented hearing impairment. In the group of patients with an underlying neurological disease (25 per cent), the female preponderance was still present (71 per cent), and documented hearing loss was present in 32.7 per cent. The most common neurological diagnosis was neurodegenerative disorder (67.3 per cent), followed by seizures

(16.3 per cent) and encephalitis (9.2 per cent). With regards to degenerative diseases, dementia of the Lewy body type was the most common (60.9 per cent), followed by Parkinson's disease and Parkinson's disease dementia. In 34 per cent of the group with neurological disorder, there was co-morbid psychiatric disorder, principally depression, anxiety, psychosis and bipolar disorder. In the psychiatric group, the mean age was 48.1 years, and 70.3 per cent were female. There was documented evidence of hearing loss in 11.6 per cent. The majority of subjects had depression, followed by bipolar disorder, schizoaffective disorder, anxiety and delirium.

Structural lesions associated with musical hallucinations were present in the following sites: temporal cortex, frontotemporal cortex, temporoparietal cortex, pons and cerebellum, and the lesions included tumours, postoperative lesions, mesial temporal sclerosis, infarcts, encephalomalacia, arteriovenous malformations, arachnoid cysts and subdural fluid. The relevant tumours were meningiomas, oligodendrogliomas, gliomas and pilocytic astrocytoma. There was no significant difference between left- and right-sided lesions. Alcohol and steroid withdrawal were most often associated with the onset of musical hallucinations. However, withdrawal of psychoactive agents such as stimulants, opiates, antidepressants and benzodiazepine was less often but nonetheless still associated with the onset of musical hallucinations. Withdrawal of lisinopril, pramipexole, ramelteon, carbidopa/levodopa and clarithromycin was also associated with musical hallucinations.

In addition to the possible causes of musical hallucinations just described, musical hallucinations have been reported in multiple sclerosis (Husain et al., 2014), post-thyroidectomy hypoparathyroidism associated with symmetrical calcification of basal ganglia (Wodarz, Becker & Deckert, 1995), following infarction of the right cerebral artery with damage to the right Heschl's gyrus (Augustin et al., 2001) and following hypertensive haemorrhage at the right pontine tegmentum (Murata, Naritomi & Sawada, 1994). There are reports of musical hallucinations in *Listeria* rhomboencephalitis (Douen & Bourque, 1997), neurological Lyme disease (Stricker & Winger, 2003) and thalamo-cortical auditory radiation infarct (Woo et al., 2014). Musical hallucinations have also been reported following cochlear implantation, developing in the context of activation and attenuated following deactivation (Low et al., 2013; Joe et al., 2015).

The treatment of musical hallucinations is of interest insofar as the varying treatments refer back to the possible underlying neurochemistry of musical hallucinations (see Section 7.3). Successful treatment with gabapentin has been reported (Holroyd & Sabeen, 2008), and antiepileptics, antidepressants, acetylcholinesterases such as donepezil and antipsychotic drugs such as quetiapine have all been shown to be effective (David & Fernandez, 2000; Ukai et al., 2007; Zilles, Zerr, & Wedekind, 2012; Blom et al., 2015; Coebergh et al., 2015). Even though there are reports of improvement of musical hallucinations in response to antidepressants, tricyclic antidepressants are also known to cause musical hallucinations (Terao, 1995), and mirtazapine has been described as causally relevant (Lee & Stewart, 2018). There is a report of steroid-induced musical hallucinations in which switching from bethamethasone to prednisolone alleviated the musical hallucination. Reintroduction of prednisolone did not cause recurrence, but reintroduction of betamethasone provoked a recurrence (Kanemura, Tanimukai & Tsuneto, 2010). Ceftazidime, a third-generation cephalosporin, has been reported as causing musical hallucinations which responded to olanzapine (Song & Jung, 2019).

The subjective characteristics of the experienced musical hallucinations were investigated in an online survey of people who reported hallucinatory experiences (Moseley et al., 2018).

The results of this investigation must be treated with some caution given the problems of bias associated with the method of study. In this study, an attempt was made to distinguish between musical hallucinations, earworms and musical imagery. Of the 255 participants, 17.3 per cent reported musical hallucinations, 40.4 per cent reported earworms, 27.1 per cent reported musical imagery and 15.3 per cent were classified as mixed experiences. The relationship to musical expertise was complex: musicians were less likely to experience solely musical hallucinations but more likely to report mixed experiences. Classical music was the most frequently reported style of music in musical hallucinations, whereas rock music was frequently reported in musical imagery and pop music for earworms. Musical hallucinations were less repetitive compared to earworms. Melody and harmonies were perceived and often involved instrumental music without voices. Musical hallucinations were likely to be mistaken for an external percept; for example, a participant said, 'There is usually a moment where I am not entirely sure if it is external or internal, but the quality of sound and the apparent feeling of "proximity" is strange when it is a hallucination. In other words, it might sound soft as if it should be coming from far away, and yet it does not sound as though it is coming through any barriers like walls … it is almost as if it is coming through earphones, close to me than the outside world, but not exactly "in my head"' (Moseley et al., 2018, p. 90). The participants reported being less able to hum along with musical hallucinations and also being less able to hum the music after the experience. In addition, participants report being less able to move along to the musical hallucinations compared to musical imagery and earworms. There did not seem to be any association between musical hallucinations, musical imagery or earworms and aspects of inner speech. In summary, in this investigation of the phenomenology of musical hallucinations, musical hallucinations were less likely to be experienced by musicians, less frequent in occurrence, less familiar and less likely to include lyrics. Furthermore, musical hallucinations were less likely to be reflective of the subject's own feelings, less easy to hum along with, less controllable and less likely to be accompanied by bodily movements. They were more likely to be mistaken for an external stimulus but likely to be experienced as one's own creation.

In the study by Berrios (1990), the subjects reported religious hymns, 'Away in the Manger' and other Christmas carols and popular songs. In one case (case 5), there was a report of the musical hallucination breaking up into short phrases (like a scratched record). This phenomenon has been reported previously as a potential trajectory of musical hallucinations from initial complexity to short musical fragments, especially in musical hallucinations in association with a neurodegenerative disease (Golden & Josephs, 2015). The music is reported as disintegrating over time into increasingly shorter melodies and tunes and sometimes terminating in repetitive single notes. This has been likened to the telescoping that occurs in phantom limb sensation, in which the sensation of the distal part of the phantom retracts over time into the stump.

In the study by Golden and Josephs (2015), there were interesting qualitative differences in the actual experience of musical hallucinations determined by the nature of the originating lesion. In patients with hearing impairment, songs tended to date back to childhood and seemed to represent over-learned material as the music was commonly religious, patriotic or cultural songs. Where the musical hallucination occurred in the context of structural neurological disease, especially epilepsy, the music was modern, taking the form of country or rock music. In psychiatric disorders, the musical tended to be mood congruent and was either sad or frightening depending on the mood of the subject at the time of the experience.

The actual musical examples given are varied for the different conditions and are probably determined by culture and age such that there is not much to be gained by itemizing them. The main message is that in deafness, musical memory probably determines the music that is perceived, and this makes sense in light of the explanatory model, the predictive coding model, that random noise is structured by a predictive model that relies on previously heard and/or learnt music. The differences in the kinds of music perceived between the different kinds of musical hallucinations may simply reflect a cohort effect in which the most elderly subjects typified by deaf subjects perceive hymns, carols or patriotic music, whereas the musical hallucinations associated with neurological disease occur in a correspondingly younger cohort who perceive country music or rock music, manifesting music that was prevalent in their youth.

7.5 Conclusion

Musical hallucinations, like Charles Bonnet syndrome, are examples of elemental phenomena that allow for an understanding of the underlying neural mechanisms of the hallucinatory experience. The association of musical hallucinations with deafferentation once again points to the role of release mechanisms in hallucinatory experience. Specifically, musical hallucinations demonstrate that when there is reduced stimulus input from the peripheral auditory system, the predictions generated by the higher neurological structures become unconstrained by reality, and the minimal sensory stimuli become transformed into hallucinatory experience.

8 Ekbom Syndrome

8.1 Introduction

Ekbom syndrome, or delusional infestation, is a condition that sits between disorders of thinking, namely delusions, and disorders of perception, namely hallucinations. It is defined

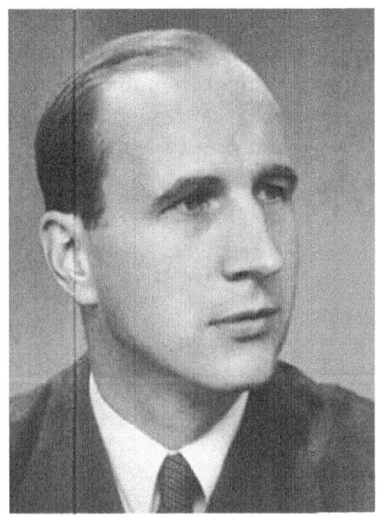

by Skott (1978, p. 11) as 'a persistent condition in which the patient believes that small animals such as insects, lice, vermin or maggots are living and thriving on or within the skin. In spite of all negative evidence to the contrary, the patient has a firm conviction that she/he is infested. This belief, if unshakeable, is best characterized as a primary delusion. It is an isolated phenomenon without relation to other psychotic symptoms.' Skott makes the point that this condition has had a variety of names dating back to Thirbierge in 1894, who termed it *acarophobia*, and in the English language literature, terms include *acaraphobia, dermatophobia, parasitophobia, delusion of parasitosis, delusion of dermal parasitosis* and *delusions of infestation*. The condition is named after Karl-Axel Ekbom (1907–1977), a Swedish neurologist who has the unusual distinction of having two psychiatric phenomena named after him – restless

Karl-Axel Ekbom 1907–1977

leg syndrome and delusional infestation. In his original description, delusional infestation was termed *Der praesenile Dermatozoenwahn* (Karroum, Konofal & Arnulf, 2009). The condition was named after Ekbom at the suggestion of Wilson and Miller (1946).

The best popular literature description is by Philip K. Dick (2011) in his novel, *A Scanner Darkly*.

> Once a guy stood all day shaking bugs from his hair. The doctor told him there were no bugs in his hair. After he had taken a shower for eight hours, standing under hot water hour and hour suffering the pain of the bugs, he got out and dried himself, and he still had bugs in his hair; in fact, he had bugs all over him. A month later he had bugs in his lungs.
>
> Having nothing else to do or think about, he began to work out theoretically the life cycle of the bugs, and, with the aid of the *Britannica*, try to determine specifically which bugs they were. They now filled his house. He read about many different kinds and finally noticed bugs outdoors, so he concluded they were aphids.

In Ekbom's original description, he explores the degree to which the condition is fundamentally an illusion, that is, a false interpretation of a real sensory experience, or a hallucination, a false perception without an object. He first examined what the evidence was for thinking that the beliefs were based on real perceptions. Firstly, the symptoms are described in a compelling, detailed and vivid manner; secondly, the symptoms are limited, typically circumscribed and localized; thirdly, many patients merely describe the skin sensations without strenuously attributing them to animals; fourthly, patients scratch themselves, and the sensations are stereotyped and unchanging for prolonged periods; sixthly, many patients conclude that the sensations still must have a cause, even if they are not the result of an infestation (in other words, the sensations are the inexplicable residue left after analysis), and finally, the patients appear to be able to distinguish between their sensory experiences and their interpretation of them. Nonetheless, Ekbom unsatisfactorily concludes that there is no conclusive evidence to assist in determining a distinction between an illusion and a hallucination, but his preference was that the symptoms were real sensory perceptions and not hallucinations (Ekbom, 1938).

The intricacies of Ekbom's thinking and argument show how perilous this conceptual terrain is. Hallucinations are best construed as like real perceptions except that there is an absence of an object. In other words, the actual perceptual experience has all the hallmarks of a true perception with regards to the character of objectivity, vividness, location in external space and the inability of the subject of experience to control or alter the experience – in essence, the experience is received with a sense of passivity. These characteristics of objectivity and placement of the experience in objective external space are easy to demonstrate in the visual and auditory domains but less so for olfaction (see Chapter 10): the objects of visual and auditory perception are located in a public, objective space wherein consensual judgement as to their existence can be easily reached by verification. These matters are far more difficult to establish for tactile and somatic experiences, where the perception is firstly private and secondly in objective but intimate space, making it impossible to establish consensual validation or verification of the veridical nature of the experience. Berrios (1982, p. 286) puts it this way: 'warmth, pressure, and vibration seem in ordinary circumstances to be related to external agencies and therefore are open to external verification. ... But sensations such as aches, pains, itches, twitches, tickles etc., depend essentially upon being "felt" and their reality therefore is not logically connected to external agencies; hence the subject's report is in normal circumstances accepted unchallenged.' Fundamentally, it is difficult to distinguish between hallucinations and illusions insofar as tactile experiences are concerned.

It is also important to distinguish between passive and active touch (see Berrios [1982] for a detailed discussion). Passive touch would include sensations such as pressure, pain, tickling and so on, whereas active touch requires movement and produces experiences such as roughness or smoothness, what we might term as *textures*. Hence, passive skin sensations such as formication (skin sensation of crawling like an ant), pinching, rubbing and crawling are common abnormalities of tactile sensation. Abnormalities of active touch are said to be rare.

Skott (1978), in her exemplary investigation, concluded that this condition resulted from a primary delusion. This view is now the dominant view, at least in the English-language literature. Although Skott does not explicitly make the point that her conclusion implies that the sensory experiences were real in nature – since to qualify as a primary delusion, the subject would have to ground their erroneous judgement upon real sensory experience – there is no disputing that the beliefs demonstrate all the characteristics of delusions. The question is, however, whether the delusions are primary or secondary. To count as secondary delusions, there would have to be present prior abnormalities such as hallucinations, but in my view it is not possible in many cases to distinguish whether the abnormal beliefs are primary or secondary. It is notable that Freudenmann and Lepping (2009a) argue that since in all cases disturbed reasoning and judgement is present whereas tactile symptoms are reported in only 82 per cent of cases, it makes sense to regard the condition as characterized by a disorder of thought.

As to the question of nomenclature, Freudenmann and Lepping (2009a) suggest that *delusional infestation* is preferable to *delusional parasitosis* as the range of probable pathogens identified has broadened beyond the select and circumscribed notion of specific parasites to any kind of pathogen, including imaginary ones for that matter. Indeed, as they argue, since 2002, an increasing number of people have been presenting with the belief that they are infested by fibres and threads that cause skin problems and unspecified neuropsychiatric symptoms. Apparently, the distinguishing diagnostic criteria are spontaneously appearing ulcerative skin lesions that contain unusual filaments lying under, embedded in or projecting from the skin. The characteristic filaments are microscopic, visually resembling textile fibres, and are white, black or a more vibrant colour such as red or blue (Middelveen, Fesler & Stricker, 2018). Brian Fair (2010) has traced the origins of this condition to Mary Leitao, who witnessed a fibre spontaneously sprout from a skin rash on her two-year-old son's face. This condition was named *Morgellons* by Mary Leitao, after a medieval French skin disease. Fair makes the point that this contested condition intersected with an already known and well-described condition, namely delusional infestation, and because of near-identical features mapped unto the pre-existing condition. Morgellons is often talked of as illustrating a contested medical condition becoming mainstream through the influence of the internet (Fair, 2010).

To return to delusional infestation, Freudenmann and Lepping (2009b) propose minimal criteria for delusional infestation, including (1) the conviction of being infested by pathogens without any medical or microbiological evidence for this and (2) abnormal sensations in the skin explained by the patients as being due to the first criterion.

Skott (1978) had previously argued that delusions of infestations ought not to be regarded as a diagnostic entity in its own right but merely as a non-specific symptom that can arise in almost any type of illness. But there are others, for example, Alistair Munro (1978a, 1978b), who make the case for recognizing delusional parasitosis as a unique condition that specifically responds to pimozide.

8.2 Case Reports

The following extracts are from Ekbom's classic paper (Ekbom, 1938; see also Yorston et al., 2003):

1. Ada K. (Admission no. 51/1937) 54 years of age, cleaner, divorced (husband joiner), two children. . . . At [the] age of 40 she developed syphilis (rash over her whole body) and received treatment for two years. At 42 [she was] run over by a car, unconscious for three hours. . . . One year ago there was sudden swelling of the face and an itching and burning rash all over the body consisting of Pfening-sized, red, round raised 'knots'. These knots disappeared after

half to one day, but no new ones came up, and it took several months for the rash to disappear. At the same time as the disappearance of the rash (or a bit later), the patient developed itching in the upper part of the back, at the neck, around the ears and at the hairline. The itching is at its worst during the daytime, but does occur sometimes at night too. Ada is of the opinion that the itching sensation is caused by the bites of little animals which run around on her skin. To alleviate the itching and kill the bugs, she has burned her skin with matches, a method that she used in the past for gnat bites. After the burning the itching disappears for a while. In this way she has got through dozens of boxes of matches. She cannot see the animals 'before they are burned', but after she can see them as black and colourful objects of various shapes. When she puts the match against her skin it crackles and there is an unpleasant smell, which she sees as clear evidence of the existence of the insects. She combs her hair several times daily with a fine comb. After rinsing the comb she can see the animals 'swimming around like fish in water'. She worried that the little animals might fall into food during cooking. More recently, it became obvious she could neither do her work nor keep her household in order because her time was mainly taken with burning and combing. … When you look at her, the skin lesions are striking, she inflicted them on herself by burning with matches. They are, as one can see, at the forehead, temples, neck and shoulders as well as in the left antecubital fossa. The wounds are hemp-seed to pea sized, irregularly contoured, superficial and covered with black brown crusts. The skin between the wounds is scarred and reddened in places. No excoriations or scabies tracks. Her hair is very short along the hairline and looks like it has been cut by a machine. There are tufts of short hair (2–10–20 cm [sic] at the centre of these shorn areas with numerous burns visible. (pp. 235–6)

2. Hilma J. 55 years old. Waitress. Divorced (husband: engineer). … At 53 she developed an itchy rash on the dorsum of the left hand and on her back. This time she did not visit a doctor; instead she bought ammonia with which she scrubbed herself. After 8–10 days the rash disappeared. One night, a few months later she developed a terrible itch over the whole of her head, and since then the itch has continued, sometimes a little better, sometime worse. The itch is particularly noticeable at night, but to some extent is present during the day as well. It has disturbed her sleep. She became nervous and anxious, which she was not before. She has the feeling that something is crawling in her hair (both on her head and on the mons pubis, but not in the axillae). Sometimes when she was hot and sweaty, she had uncomfortable sensations on her back 'like thistles on my body'. She believes that the itch is caused by scabies which she 'forced up' to her head when she scrubbed herself with ammonia. At night she feels the animals running down from her hair to her face and breasts. She has seen the scabies mites as well. They are pinhead-sized, quite long and browny black. She catches them by pulling her hair through her fingers. 'It feels the same as when you touch a louse' she says with a look of disgust. She seems to imagine that the animals stay mainly in her left ear, where she had one or two abrasions, and that they crawl from there into her hair. At her workplace she hangs up her coat some distance from those of her work colleagues so as not to infect them. She fears losing her post, because of her frequent scratching and the possibility of it coming out that she has scabies. She took drastic measures against the insects. She washes and combs her hair all the time. She spent considerable sums of money on hair tonics and lotions. She always has ointment in the left ear and in her pubic area. The hair tonic eases the itch. She got the prescription from the dermatology out-patient clinic, from which she demanded several other scabies cures. The doctors often told her that she didn't have scabies but she did not give in. 'If my head itches simply bathing my body cannot help.' She was also told that scabies doesn't affect the head but she didn't believe it. Finally the dermatologists got fed up with her, refused to write further prescriptions and sent her to the psychiatric clinic. … During a period of observation of several months her condition remained more or less unchanged. Now and then she

presents herself, often bringing along a sample of the 'bugs' in a piece of paper. The samples contain grains of sand, particles of dirt, etc. On 24.8.37 (five months after I saw her for the first time) she complained bitterly about the itch which had become rather worse. (pp. 237–9)

3. Elin N. 52 years old. Widow for 5 years (husband: butler). . . . Two years ago Elin developed a stabbing sensation in the genitals (no discharge). She believed she had got 'the infestation that you get when you hang about at night with menfolk'. She had heard talk of such infestations, but did not know what they were called. She believed, she had been infected by a 'loose woman' who rented a room from her. One day as she was making the bed for the lodger she saw an 'animal' on the sheet which looked like a white flea. It didn't move. Elin didn't dare go to the doctor, for fear of being thought a wanton old woman. Instead she washed her genitals with paraffin, alcohol and Sabadill vinegar. It burned terribly but after one week the complaint disappeared. Two to three months later she developed a stabbing sensation on her trunk, limbs and on her face. There is a momentary prick, a feeling like a needle stick or the bite of a small animal. Then she feels nothing but after a while it stabs again somewhere else. The stabbing is felt during the day as well as at night and it wakes her out of her sleep. She has also had other sensations: heat on her face and a feeling that something is running under the skin of her forehead. She has had no itching at all, but on her face, arms and breasts pinhead sized papules developed. She kept scratching these papules, because she believed they were caused by the 'louse' which had attached itself firmly into her skin. When she feels a 'bite', she quickly grabs at the place she's been bitten to catch the 'little animal'. One day she caught two in one go. She saw them clearly. They were white in colour and they do not move. The smallest are like a grain of sand, the biggest like a 'small flea'. They are not ordinary bugs. These, the patient frequently had in her flat and she knows what they look like. She showed the 'little animals' to her daughter, who on one occasion thought she saw a proboscis at one end of the 'animal'. The daughter is now of the opinion however, that everything was imagined, and she will not acknowledge her remark about the proboscis. The patient rubs her body with brandy which helps for a day or two. She was worried she might pass it on to her children or the tenants and therefore took great pains to shake out the sheets. At first she kept the illness a secret, but when she started to scratch her face her daughter found out and advised her to go to a doctor. The doctor said there were no bugs, but Elin was not satisfied with this and went to other doctors to be absolutely certain. (pp. 239–40)

Jay Traver (1951), in an article describing her own experiences, provides perhaps the most vivid and illustrative account of delusional infestation written without due cognizance of the full meaning and implications of her account. She wrote

The writer and two other members of her immediate family, all of us adult females, have been the past several years the unwilling hosts to the mite, Dermatophagoides scheremetewskyi Bogdanow. Since the published reports on this mite as a parasite of humans are not numerous, it seems desirable to present an account of the activities of the mite from first hand information. . . . Small itching papules on the scalp were noted as early as 1934. This condition persisted without much change in spite of sporadic efforts to control it, until the spring and early summer of 1943. At this time, the sensations as of some arthropod crawling, scratching and biting became very pronounced, and occurred over wide areas of the scalp. The idea that Pediculosis humanus capitus might be the causative agent was not borne out since at no time was it possible to 'comb out' a louse nor to locate nits on the hairs. Further, the infestation did not yield to treatment known to be effective against pediculosis. The itching and crawling sensations were most pronounced between 10 pm and the early hours of the morning.

By the middle of August, 1943, the annoyance had become excessive and more strenuous efforts were made to clear up the infestation and to locate the causative agent. Three areas of the scalp were principally involved, a space as large as the palm of the hand above and behind each ear, and an even larger area on the top of the head in the frontal region. The sensations as of something biting, scratching, and crawling from place to place were now almost continuous, becoming apparent as early as 10 am and continuing all day and far into the night, increasing in intensity from 11 pm onward. Sound sleep was quite impossible. The principal areas involved were also painful and swollen, and as was discovered later, the epidermis over each of them was extremely thickened. On the suggestion of a druggist, a soap containing 1% mercuric iodide was employed as a shampoo. This seemed to irritate the mites, which became very active after the use of this soap. Many of them began to move down out of the scalp, and some of the thickened epidermis began to slough off.

Those that continued down into the body soon became embedded in itching red papules reminiscent of trombiculid infestations. Treated with strong Sulphur ointment, they apparently did no further damage. They could be found on the shoulders, under the arms, beneath the breasts, on chest and both upper and lower back, occasionally around the umbilicus. The sensations of crawling and biting which were felt on legs and feet, in the latter case often on but seldom between the toes, indicated that some of the mites had migrated to the lower extremities.

Others of the mites, however, moved down on to the face, invading eyes, ears and nostrils. It was the mites in these locations that did most damage. Both eyes became so badly swollen that it was impossible to move the eyeballs; to look to right or left it was necessary to move the entire head. . . . The movements of a mite that had entered under the eyelid could be felt as it crawled slowly about, then began to 'dig in' at which moment the eye suddenly became more swollen than before. An almost continuous flow of lachrymal secretion seemed to attract the mites and made vision difficult. At no time, however, was there evidence of the formation of pus in the affected eyes.

Invasion of the nostrils produced quite distressing symptoms. . . . Early invasions of the ears seemed confined to the region of the pinna, in the folds of which the mites burrowed, producing itching red papules. . . . Even this summer (1950) live mites have been taken from all three members of the family. . . . The mites succeeded in establishing themselves temporarily on one wrist, between the third and fourth finger of one hand, just below one ear, on the ventral surface of one knee, and just below the hairline above the left temple. Applications of 2 to 5% aqueous solution of gentian to each of these affected areas except the one above the temple, repeatedly daily for a week or ten days, finally cleared up each of these sites of infestation, some of which were reminiscent of the behavior of sarcoptes scabiei. The network of red lines and itching swellings above the left temple seems also to have been brought under control, largely through the use of Sulphur ointment and Lysol. . . . Inasmuch as it has never been possible to locate a mite in the sloughed off epidermis or in the small incrustations which form over infested areas, it seems probable that the burrows are actually in the dermis. Further evidence for this belief is the fact that live mites have been captured from the deeper regions underlying such incrustation when the latter had been removed. . . . One of the most annoying runways occupied by the mites, the entire length of the right eyebrow, with extensions to and from the adjacent hairline burrow does not show any indication of its presence save a slight swelling. . . .

A dermatologist, recommended by a local physician, was apparently convinced without more than a very casual examination, that the patient's symptoms were largely imaginary, those that did exist having been caused by an ill-advised attempt on the part of the patient to rid herself of something that was not there. . . .

Capturing the mite. This was a tedious process, and the number of mites actually captured is surprisingly low. This does not mean, to me at least, that there were not many more mites present at any given time, which could not be captured by any method employed. . . . A few months after the acute symptoms subsided, however, I captured two very small

Hymenoptera which had been felt crawling on the scalp. They have been identified . . . as members of the Trichogrammatidae. . . . A rather amazing number of other arthropods have likewise been captured from the scalp. . . . Among these were several Hymenoptera of a considerably larger size than the Trichogrammatidae, an oribatid mite; what appears to be the cast skin of a small spider; an apparent jassid; and of course, many small gnats and Diptera, among these the psychodids and ceratogorids. Pollen of various sorts was also found commonly. Perhaps a study of the flora and fauna of the human scalp in summer might be interesting. (pp. 1–7)

8.3 Explanatory Hypotheses

As Reilly (1988, p. 44) remarked, 'The skin is by far the largest organ of the body. . . . [I]n both a concrete and symbolic sense the skin serves as a boundary separating the inner person from the outer world, self from non-self.' This has implication for the extent to which there is considerable subjective awareness of the cutaneous sensations and potentially explains the imputation of erroneous beliefs to ordinary sensations or the derivation of abnormal perceptions from normal sensations. It is also true that the skin shares embryonic origins with the brain, both deriving from the ectoderm. Whether this embryonic link is the basis of the degree to which the appearance of, lesions on and sensations from the skin are prone to being associated with psychiatric illness or not is unknown. It may simply be that the role of the skin and the face, too, in projecting health, sexual attractiveness and cleanliness is itself sufficient to explain the propensity for the skin's relevance to mental wellbeing. Also, the subjective experience of dermal sensations fuels metaphorical language, for example, 'it makes my skin crawl', 'I had goose bumps', and so on, signalling the degree to which dermal sensations are apt to be used in metaphor as a lexicon for feelings and emotions.

There is as yet no overarching satisfactory explanatory model for Ekbom syndrome (Freudenmann & Lepping, 2009a). This is probably also understandable given the fact that even the underlying psychopathology is yet to be fully elucidated, namely whether Ekbom syndrome is fundamentally an ideational or perceptual disorder. This means that the kinds of potential theoretical explanations that are available for Charles Bonnet syndrome and musical hallucinations, as described in Chapters 6 and 7, are not available to assist our understanding of Ekbom syndrome. Nonetheless, there is the beginning of an explanatory model, namely that delusional infestation is the result of misinterpretation of normal or aberrant dermal sensations in the context of errors of probabilistic reasoning in which the improbable is preferred over the probable (Wolf et al., 2014). Another way of thinking of this is that there is abnormal activation of the itch pathway coupled with abnormal processing and interpretation (Lai et al., 2018). The hypothesis is that abnormalities of a fronto-striato-thalamo-parietal network could explain the symptoms of delusional infestation. The potential connection with Charles Bonnet syndrome and musical hallucinations is the fact that prior to the onset of delusional infestation, some patients had demonstrable visual loss and/or hearing loss. This coupled with social isolation and loneliness may lead to reduced sensory deprivation, hence underpinning the onset of delusional infestation (Skott, 1978).

Huber et al. (2008) had previously shown that striatal lesions, principally in the putamen secondary to organic disease, were associated with delusional infestation and concluded that the striatum is involved in visuotactile perception. Wolf et al. (2013, 2014) have demonstrated widespread changes in both grey and white matter affecting prefrontal, temporal, insular, cingulate and striatal regions and pointing to disruption in prefrontal control of somatosensory representation. They show that patients with delusional infestation, irrespective of cause, have lower grey matter volume in frontal, temporal, parietal, insular, thalamic and striatal regions compared to controls. Further, only patients with organic rather than psychiatric delusional infestation cases showed increases in white matter volume. These findings confirm to some extent the hypothesized explanatory model for delusional infestation but also suggest that there may be differential neural pathways for organic as opposed to psychiatric delusional infestation.

Huber et al. (2018) reported that delusional infestation is associated with lower grey matter volume in thalamic, striatal (putamen), insular and medial prefrontal brain regions in contrast to patients with what they term non-somatic delusional disorders and control subjects. These differences were reported to be consistent at regional and network levels and suggest content-specific neural signatures in delusional disorders, once again signalling that there may be a neural basis for the content of erroneous beliefs. This proposition is significant and important precisely because it undermines the current position that only form matters in psychopathology and that content is at most a random event associated with the time that the erroneous belief crystallizes rather than that the content of abnormal beliefs actually have fundamental importance for our understanding of the neurobiology of psychopathological phenomena. Hirjak et al. (2017) concluded from their structural magnetic resonance imaging (MRI) investigation of delusional infestation cases compared with controls that there was greater cortical thickness in the right orbitofrontal cortex and smaller surface area in the left inferior temporal gyrus, the percuneus, the pars orbitalis of the right frontal gyrus and the lingual gyrus. Lower gyrification was found in the left postcentral, bilateral pre-central, right middle temporal, inferior parietal and superior parietal gyri. Their interpretation is that the regions with atrophy were the part of the neural circuits associated with perception, visuospatial control and self-awareness.

More specifically, abnormal skin sensations, as well as heightened threat processing within the amygdala and increased salience of skin representations within the insula and in concert with compromised prefrontal capacity for self-regulation and appraisal, may be at play in delusional infestation, and there is some empirical evidence to support this proposition (Eccles et al., 2015).

These are all early findings underpinning the need for further studies to give clarity and better understanding of the neural mechanisms at both structural and functional levels that are relevant in delusional infestation. In addition to the possibility of the role of changes in grey and white matter in the pathophysiology of delusional infestation, there are unrelated but yet complementary propositions implicating neurochemical anomalies in delusional infestation involving the dopamine transporter protein in the aetiology of delusional infestation (Huber et al., 2007). One hypothesis draws attention to the fact that conditions that are liable to cause decreased striatal dopamine transporter are liable to cause delusional infestation. Dopamine transporter is a key regulator of dopamine reuptake in the human brain. Case reports of delusional infestation in association with the use of substances such as cocaine, pemoline, methylphenidate and other amphetamine derivatives, substances that are known to inhibit dopamine transporter protein, are further support for this hypothesis. Furthermore, it is known that there is decreased dopamine transporter binding in such conditions as Parkinson's disease, Huntington's chorea, hyperuricaemia and so on, and these conditions also have been associated with delusional infestation. Where the foregoing is relevant for an understanding of delusional infestation secondary to drug use or to organic brain disease, in the primary delusional infestation cases, it is hypothesized that there is an aggravated age-related decline of striatal dopamine transporter. In this regard, it is notable that physiological decrease is 5 to 8 per cent per decade, but it is hypothesized that in primary delusional infestation, there is a marked decrease for reasons yet to be established.

Finally, the report by Ponson, Andersson and El-Hage (2015) on the neural basis of the role of aripiprazole in delusional infestation demonstrated, from functional MRI, that the supplementary motor area was involved both in the underlying pathological mechanism for delusional infestation and in the mechanism for the successful role of aripiprazole in treating a patient with delusional infestation. In another study with a similar design, Narumoto et al. (2006) showed that risperidone acted to increase regional cerebral blood flow (rCBF) in bilateral frontal and left temporoparietal regions, the right parietal operculum and bilateral basal ganglia, in contrast to pre-treatment images showing global decrease in rCBF in delusional infestation. This was done using a single-photon-emission computed tomography. The demonstrable changes were accompanied by dramatic clinical therapeutic response.

In summary, a well-described explanatory model for delusional infestation is yet to be proposed. Nonetheless, there are now tentative explanations drawing on clinical findings and experimental results.

8.4 Clinical Aspects

8.4.1 Epidemiology

The age- and sex-adjusted incidence of delusional infestation is reported from a population-based cohort study as 1.9 (confidence interval [CI] 1.5–2.4) per 100,000 person-years (Bailey et al., 2014). The mean age at diagnosis was 61.4 years. The incidence is reported to have increased over the four decades 1976–2010 from 1.6 per to 2.6 per 100,000 person-years. The incidence increased from 0.2 per 100,000 person-years for the age cohort 0–19 years to 16.2 per 100,000 person-years for males aged 80 years and above. Importantly in this study, the incidence in females aged 80 years and above was less than that in males and was reported as 7.2 per 100,000 person-years. The authors conclude that delusional infestation is a rare condition. The same group (Kohorst et al., 2018) reported on the prevalence of delusional infestation: the age- and sex-adjusted prevalence was 27.3 per 100,000 person-years. This increased significantly with age. The prevalence increased significantly with age for the sexes: 118 per 100,000 person-years for females aged 80 years and above and 150 per 100,000 person-years for males aged 80 years and above. This difference between the sexes was not statistically significantly. However, it is worthy of note that prior to these rigorous systematic investigations, it had always been reported that there was a marked preponderance of male to female cases – 1:2.5–3.5 (Skott, 1978; Freudenmann & Lepping, 2009b) – but these reports derive from selected samples, usually from clinics, and may only be true for patients aged over 45 years.

In another study, this time examining the incidence of diseases primarily affecting the skin derived from a population-based epidemiological investigation, it was confirmed that delusional infestation and other conditions such as non-melanoma skin cancer, lentigo maligna, herpes zoster, venous stasis syndrome, venous ulcer and burning mouth syndrome were more likely to be diagnosed in people aged over 65 years (Westermeyer et al., 1989). Indeed, the authors state that delusional infestation was typically diagnosed in persons aged over 80 years.

Lepping, Baker and Freudenmann (2010) used a different approach to estimate the prevalence of delusional infestation. They sent out questionnaires to dermatologists in the

United Kingdom and inquired into their experiences of new and ongoing cases of delusional infestation. In total, 103 British dermatologists reported 182 cases seen over three years and 54 current cases. The three-year prevalence was reported as 4.99 per million, and the point prevalence was reported as 1.48 per million. The authors concluded that delusional infestation was not that rare in dermatological practice in the United Kingdom. This stands in contrast to the earlier report by Woodruff et al. (1997) indicating that delusional hypochondriasis was uncommonly referred to liaison psychiatrists from dermatology clinics.

An examination of skin diseases in psychiatric patients showed that psychiatric patients significantly had more skin diseases compared to an age- and sex-matched control sample of individuals without psychiatric disorders (Moftah et al., 2013). The parasitic infestations were mostly pediculosis capitis and scabies. Psychogenic skin conditions occurred in 8.4 per cent of this sample of psychiatric patients, of which 50 per cent were delusional infestation cases.

The mean age of onset is reported as 57 years (Trabert, 1995; Freudenmann & Lepping, 2009b). Social isolation appears to be associated with delusional infestation, but it is unclear whether this is a risk factor the development of the condition or a result of the condition (Freudenmann & Lepping, 2009a).

8.4.2 Clinical Features

Skott (1978), in her comprehensive study including review of earlier cases, drew a picture of the typical case as follows:

> A single woman about 60 years of age with no previous history of mental illness. Apart from her present delusions of infestation she appears to be in excellent health. . . . She has always kept herself and her home scrupulously clean and dreads dirt and filth. In spite of all her cleanliness, she insists that she has now become the victim of bugs or lice. She is agitated, slightly depressed and apprehensive, which is quite understandable considering all the help she has sought in vain. She brings a small box containing either sand, breadcrumbs, skin debris, ants, or flies as evidence in order to impress on the investigator the importance of her case.

This description, although it is a caricature, gives a good sense of how cases tend to present. About half the patients presented to dermatologists with pruritus, and a third complained of being overwhelmed or greatly worried. Freudenmann and Lepping (2009a) have systematized these presenting complaints. They describe the nature of the imaginary pathogens reported by patients as including vermin, insects, parasites and 'small animals'. Often the nature of the infestation is surmised from an itch that is ascribed to mites, scabies, lice, worms, bugs, fleas, flies, ticks or spiders. Sometimes microscopic pathogens such as bacteria or viruses are identified as the cause of the patient's problem. In the Mogellons phenomenon, inanimate materials such as filaments, threads, fibres and pigments may be identified as responsible for the sensory experience.

The most common sources of the imagined infestation are other human beings, plants. animals, pets and parts of the home. The identified affected sites on the body include the skin of the hands, arms, feet, lower legs, scalp, upper back and breast and genitals (Freudenmann & Lepping, 2009a). Bodily orifices including the nose, ears, mouth, anus, urethra and gastrointestinal tract have all been identified as locations of infestation.

There are a number of behaviours associated with delusional infestation. These include attempts to remove the identified pathogen or object by digging into the skin, producing excoriations and lacerations. Sometimes patients will self-mutilate using tweezers, knives or other sharp instruments. This can include scarification of the cornea or urethra and may result in severe blood loss (Hinkle, 2010, 2011). Furthermore, the patients may treat the skin with various substances, including home remedies such as tea tree oil and cedar oil or pesticides in the home as well as on their bodies. Some patients discard or destroy their belongings, whereas others physically leave their homes. It is clear that delusional infestation has considerable impact on the lives of patients. A rare but potentially dangerous behaviour involves excessive water drinking as a means of bowel cleansing, leading to water intoxication manifest as loss of consciousness and tonic-clonic seizures (Lai et al., 2016).

Patients move from one doctor to another because they are disappointed by their responses. They see family doctors, dermatologists, entomologists, parasitologists and experts in tropical medicine. They rarely present to psychiatrists. There is also the well-recognized 'matchbox sign' in which patients bring a specimen of the presumed pathogen in order to persuade the clinician of the veracity of their claim. Formal studies of the specimens that patients bring to clinicians have revealed skin flakes, mucus, hair, debris, synthetic or textile material, nails, plant or vegetable matter, insects, insect larvae and non-pathogenic worms (Hylwa et al., 2011; Garcia-Mingo et al., 2019). In Morgellons phenomenon, the specimens included superficial skin or cellulose from cotton fibres and other materials, including polyamide, probably nylon; cellulose nitrate containing bismuth, probably from nail varnish; and polyethylene, probably from plastic container lids (Pearson et al., 2012). Freudenmann et al. (2010) have argued that the matchbox sign be re-designated the *specimen sign* because patients bring the specimens in different kinds of containers, including plastic bags, adhesive tape, paper envelopes, glass jars, tissue paper, plastic boxes, specimen or urine pots, microscopic slides, Petri glasses, pill bottles, and so on. Examination of skin biopsies shows dermatitis, excoriation, ulceration, erosion and non-specific inflammation (Hylwa et al., 2011).

Delusional infestation often presents as folie à deux (Yang, Beck & Koo, 2019) and is reported to occur in 8 to 49 per cent of cases, including as folie à deux, *folie à trois, folie à cinq* and *folie à famille* (Freudenmann & Lepping, 2009b). In the study by Skott (1978), 14 patients (25 per cent) were involved in folie à deux, 13 of whom were independently identified in the dermatology clinic, and the author estimated that there were another seven to nine people involved in the folie à deux outside the study sample. It is notable that even with married couples, the spouses saw different doctors, and in the case of a sibling pair, they consulted, independently, seven years apart. Skott concluded that the term *folie à deux* should be used with caution, in these cases, and her preferred term was *folie partagee* (shared illness). The special situation of mothers either presenting with delusional infestation by proxy (Hussain et al., 2018; Fisher, 2019), in which the child is the patient presented to dermatologists, or where the mother's abnormal beliefs are transmitted to children in *folie à famille* (Ahmed et al., 2015) need consideration as these situations have implications for child protection and management.

What is little recognized is that delusional infestation by proxy can present to veterinary surgeons. The patients present mainly with dogs and cats and an alleged infestation with anthropods and worms. Of 724 cases, 252 (34 per cent) claimed to also be affected and showed their cutaneous lesions to the veterinary surgeon. The presence of cutaneous lesions was not always confirmed. The presence of delusional infestation by proxy and also in the pet owner has been termed *double delusional infestation* (Lepping, Rishniw & Freudenmann, 2015).

Smulevich, Lvov and Romanov (2016) described hypochondriasis circumscripta as a condition in which patients present with intradermal dysaesthesia, idiopathic tactile illusions, body fantasies such as experiencing ducts or tunnels under the skin and the urge to extract objects or particles from their skin. The authors claim that this condition is distinguishable from delusional infestation, but it is difficult to see the difference that is being claimed.

The clinical outcome of delusional infestation is described as episodic, periodic or continuous (chronic; Skott, 1978). The duration of untreated illness is associated with poor response to treatment (Romanov et al., 2018). However, compared to the period before the introduction of antipsychotic drugs, full remission rates have risen from 33.9 to 51.9 per cent (Trabert, 1995). Patients report being disabled by their condition and attribute their disability to the delusional infestation (Foster et al., 2012). In another study, patients reported high levels of anxiety and depression, severe levels of concern about their appearance and poor quality of life (Shah, Taylor & Bewley, 2017).

8.4.3 Aetiology

Delusional infestation has been reported in association with a number of conditions, including cardiovascular disease, diabetes mellitus, vitamin B_{12} deficiency, chronic lymphatic leukaemia, polycythaemia rubra vera and dementia (Skott, 1978). There are reports of delusional infestation associated with peritoneal dialysis (Duarte, Choi & Li, 2011) and renal failure complicated by metabolic syndrome, hypertensive cardiomyopathy and cerebrovascular disease (Carpiniello, Pinna & Tuveri, 2011). In addition, delusional infestation can occur in thalamic pain arising from left thalamic haemorrhage (Hanihara et al., 2009) and post-herpetic neuralgia and electroencephalographic abnormalities in the left anterior parietal lobe (Harper & Moss, 1992). Multisystem atrophy involving extrapyramidal, cerebellar, pyramidal and autonomic dysfunction delusional infestation has been reported as the initial symptom in this condition (Kumbier & Kornhuber, 2002). There is a report of brain cysticercosis causing delusional infestation (Ramirez-Bermudez, Espinola-Nadurille & Loza-Taylor, 2010). These varied reports only go to show that cases of delusional infestation ought to be carefully and thoroughly investigated to rule out any underlying disease.

Delusional infestation in Parkinson's disease seems to be an adverse consequence of treatment including the use of pergolide, amantadine, trihexyphenidyl, rasagiline, modafinil, methylphenidate, carbidopa, ropinirole (Davis et al., 2017) and pramipexole (Romero Sandoval, Festa Neto & Nico, 2018). Development of delusional infestation in the context of treatment occurs with the use of psychotropic agents such as phenelzine (Aizenberg, Schwartz & Zemishlany, 1991), atomoxetine prescribed for attention-deficit/hyperactivity disorder (Howes & Sharp, 2018), the anticonvulsant topiramate prescribed for epilepsy (Fleury, Wayte & Kiley, 2008) and the antibiotic ciproflaxin (Steinert & Studemund, 2006). Delusional infestation has been reported in chronic hepatitis C treatment with pergolated interferon alpha-2b and ribavirin (Robaeys et al., 2007).

The role of drug misuse in the aetiology of delusional infestation is well recognized. In a prospective study of delusional infestation, 33 per cent of patients tested positive for recreational drug use, mostly cannabis, and there was a history of drug use in 22 per cent of a retrospective sample of 86 patients (Marshall et al., 2017). The role of cocaine in delusional infestation is also important to note (Brewer et al., 2008), as are the roles of prescribed opiates and psycho-stimulants (Zhu et al., 2018).

Finally, it is well established that there are cases of primary delusional infestation. I described earlier the physical illnesses that have been reported in the literature in association with secondary delusional infestation. I now turn briefly to confirm what is already well established, namely the fact that delusional infestation also occurs in the context of schizophrenia, affective disorder and mental retardation (Skott, 1978; Morris, 1991, Freudenmann & Lepping, 2009a).

8.5 Conclusion

Delusional infestation is on the borderline of abnormalities of belief and abnormalities of perception. Thus, the provenance of the phenomenon is disputable. It illustrates the precariousness of identifying what is a normal tactile experience and distinguishing it from an aberrant experience. Furthermore, the ascription of abnormal beliefs to explain an illusory experience draws our attention to the relationship between beliefs, judgement and subjective experience.

Vulvodynia and Penoscrotodynia

9.1 Introduction

The conditions described in this chapter are distinct from those in the preceding chapters in this section on disorders of perception in that both vulvodynia and penoscrotodynia are disorders of sensation rather than of perception. The distinction that I seek to draw is that between *sensation* and *perception*. Sensation is the first stage in receiving information from outside the self. The sensory system includes the visual, auditory, tactile, olfactory, gustatory, kinaesthetic and proprioceptive pathways. These pathways deal with the receipt, transformation and transmission of raw and disparate sensory data from peripheral receptors to the central nervous system (CNS). The transformation of raw sensory stimuli into sensory information is then decoded into meaningful perception involving active processes that are influenced by attention, affect, cultural expectations, context, prior experiences, memory and prior concepts (Oyebode, 2018). What is important is to recognize that such a distinction exists between the awareness of primary sensations and the awareness of perceptions.

In the preceding chapters I dealt with abnormal visual perceptions in Charles Bonnet syndrome, abnormal auditory perceptions in musical hallucinations, and abnormal tactile perception in delusional infestation. To emphasize this point, in Charles Bonnet syndrome, the abnormal subjective experience is not merely of elementary sensations such as light and colours but of perceived objects. And in musical hallucinations, it is not mere sensations such as noises or elementary noises but music. This is also true for delusional infestation, where the subjective experience is not simply sensations in or on the skin but experience of worms, insects or parasites moving.

In this chapter, the focus is on awareness of abnormal sensations in the genital areas, namely vulvodynia in females and penoscrotodynia in males. Both conditions rarely present to psychiatrists. The term *vulvodynia* refers to vulvar pain occurring in the absence of an underlying recognizable disease (Moyal-Barracco & Lynch, 2004). Skene (1889, p. 94) described 'excessive sensitivity' and 'hyperaesthesia' of the vulva in his classic text, *Treatise of the Diseases of Women*, published in 1889. In this classical description, Skene writes

> This disease as the name implies is characterized by a supersensitiveness of the vulva. Pruritus is absent, and on examination of the parts affected no redness or other external manifestation of the disease is visible. When however, the examining finger comes into contact with the hyperaesthetic part, the patient complains of pain, which is sometimes so great as to cause her to cry out. Indeed, the sensitiveness is occasionally so exaggerated as to keep the patient from consulting her physician until it becomes absolutely intolerable.

103

Sexual intercourse is equally painful, and becomes in aggravated cases impossible. This condition must not be confounded with vaginismus, or with other conditions of increased sensitiveness of the vulva due to inflammatory conditions.

It is now recognized that the condition is a syndrome of unexplained vulvar pain, sexual dysfunction and psychological disability (Paavonen, 1995). It is distinct from vulvar pruritus and until recently was subdivided into dysaesthetic vulvodynia and vestibulitis, and some authorities included cyclic vulvovaginits, vulvar papillomatosis and vulvar dermatoses as subsets (Paavonen, 1995). However, more recently, given the absence of inflammatory pathogenesis in vestibulitis, vulvodynia has become the preferred term irrespective of whether the vulvar pain is spontaneous or caused by physical provocation. The term is used to describe chronic burning and/or pain in the vulva (Lotery, McClure & Galask, 2004). Originally, several terms were used to describe vulvodynia, including *non-pathogenic vaginitis, psychosomatic vulvovaginitis* and *burning vulva syndrome.*

Penoscrotodynia is regarded as the male equivalent of vulvodynia. Indeed, it has been argued that the definition and classification should be modelled on that which has been suggested for vulvodynia. Markos (2011) described penoscrotodynia as a condition in which there is a genital skin-burning sensation in otherwise normal skin and in which there is absence of any pathology or where there is no clearly identifiable aetiology. Furthermore, penoscrotodynia may be a generalized condition of pain or burning sensation affecting most of the genital skin, or it may be localized to the scrotum, penis or glans exclusively. In addition, the pain or burning sensation may be spontaneous or provoked. There is the suggestion of a classification of severity where (1) severe is defined as a condition that interferes with the daily normality of life or sexual relationships, (2) moderate is defined as a condition that the patient describes as troublesome but not to the extent of interfering with daily living or sexual relationships and (3) mild is defined as a condition in which the patient perceives the problem as sporadic, non-severe or both but does not interfere with daily living or sexual relationships.

Aside from the idiopathic variety of penoscrotodynia, generally referred to as *dysaesthetic penoscrotodynia*, there are a number of other conditions, namely alcohol-induced penodynia, caffeine-induced genital skin pain, red scrotum syndrome and restless genital syndrome, that are said to be included within the ambit of the term *penoscrotodynia* (Markos, 2011).

9.2 Vulvodynia

9.2.1 Case Report

A 40-year-old woman, gravida 2, parity 1, abortion 1, presented with a 5-month history of vulvar burning. She denied a history of nocturia, dysuria and unrinary frequency. There was no history of physical or sexual abuse. Pelvic examination did not reveal any erythema, ulceration or hypopigmentation of the posterior fourchette. Internal examination revealed no tenderness of the levator ani muscles, no vaginismus and no pain associated with the bladder. Urinalyses, urine, vaginal and cervical cultures and smear were negative. Vaginal culture did not grow any enteric organisms and no yeasts were detected on KOH examination. A biopsy of this area was normal. . . . We learnt from her history that she had had a divorce 7 months earlier and her symptoms started then. We thought that her disease might be attributable to psychiatric trauma and she was referred to a psychiatrist. She was diagnosed as having somatoform disorder and depression. She continued selective serotonergic reuptake inhibitors and her symptoms improved rapidly. (Gumus et al., 2008, p. 156)

9.2.2 Explanatory Hypotheses

There is as yet no overarching explanatory hypothesis underpinning our understanding of vulvodynia. There are reports of increased intraepithelial and papillary innervation in vulvodynia (Tympanidis, Terenghi & Dowd, 2003) and of significantly increased vanilloid receptor (VR1) and VR1-positive fine epidermal fibres in vulvodynia tissues compared to controls (Tympanidis et al., 2004). These findings suggest that nociceptors are expressed in response to inflammation in people with vulvodynia and that these increased receptors and fibres play a role in the symptoms of vulvodynia. Indeed, there is evidence not merely for increased innervation but also for increased vestibular mast cells, subepithelial heparanase activity and intraepithelial hyper-innervation. Heparanase is degranulated from mast cells and is capable of degrading vestibular stroma and epithelial basement membrane, thus permitting stromal proliferation and intraepithelial extension of nerve cells. This intrusion is likely to have a bearing on the hyper-innervation seen in vulvodynia and may account for the pain disturbance experienced (Bornstein et al., 2008). The presence of mast cells in the vulva of women with vulvodynia also raises the possibility of an altered immune inflammatory response to environmentally induced allergic reactions, and there is indirect evidence for this: women with vulvodynia are more likely to have self-reported hives before vulvodynia, a history of allergic reactions to insect bites and a history of seasonal allergic responses (Harlow, He & Nguyen, 2009).

Furthermore, women with vulvodynia, whether generalized vulvar dysaesthesia or localized vestibulodynia, showed greater pain sensitivity to pressure in both the vulvar and peripheral body regions such as the thumb, deltoid and shin. This suggests a central component to the mechanism mediating vulvodynia (Giesecke et al., 2004). It is possible that these findings are due to alterations in neuroplasticity at a central level following chronic ongoing local irritation in susceptible individuals with vulvodynia, resulting in more widespread mechanical hyperalgesia (Giesecke et al., 2004). The possibility that central factors are involved in vulvodynia is supported by findings that demonstrated augmented brain responses in the insula, dorsal midcingulate, posterior cingulate and thalamus to pressure stimuli remote from the vulva, namely in thumb pressure-evoked pain (Hampson et al., 2013). Altered sensory adaptation, a measure of central sensitization that is linked to dysfunction in CNS inhibitory pathways mediated by gamma-aminobutyric acid (GABA) has been shown to be impaired in a subset of patients with vulvodynia, further indicating that CNS mechanisms may have a role in vulvodynia (Zhang et al., 2011).

The finding that vulvodynia is associated with the presence of other chronic pain conditions such as interstitial cystitis, irritable bowel syndrome and fibromyalgia demonstrates the centrality of pain perception to the pathophysiology of vulvodynia. Indeed, patients with vulvodynia are two to three times more likely to have one or more co-morbid chronic pain conditions. This fact emphasizes the likelihood of a shared basic pathophysiology (Reed et al., 2014).

In addition to the investigations of pain in vulvodynia, there are also electromyographic studies of the pelvic floor demonstrating significantly differences between women with vulvodynia and normal controls. The contractile amplitudes involving the tonic, phasic and endurance contractions were significantly less in the vulvodynia group (Glazer et al., 1998; Jantos, 2008). The full implications of these findings are yet to be understood.

9.2.3 Clinical Aspects

The prevalence of vulvodynia is reported as 7 to 8.3 per cent, and this prevalence remained stable through to age 70 years, declining thereafter. Among sexually active women, the prevalence was similar at all ages (Reed et al., 2012; Harlow et al., 2014). The lifetime prevalence is estimated as 16 per cent (Vieira-Baptista et al., 2014). The incidence rate is reported as 4.2 cases per 100 person-years and is higher at age 20 years (7.6 cases per 100 person-years) compared to women at age 60 years (3.3 cases per 100 person-years). The rate is also increased in Hispanic women (Harlow et al., 2014), in married women and in those with a past history of chronic pain or specific co-morbid pain disorders (Reed et al., 2014). A history of pain after intercourse is also known to be predictive of vulvodynia, and remission was commoner in women without a history of pain after intercourse (Reed et al., 2008). Women with vulvodynia were seven to eight times more likely to have a history of pain with their first tampon use (Harlow & Stewart, 2003). The onset of symptoms was often associated with a specific event, for example, yeast infection, sexual intercourse, surgery, menopause, childbirth and first insertion of tampon (Bachmann et al., 2006). The total duration of symptoms was 7.1 years and 2.7 years before diagnosis (Bachmann et al., 2006).

There is a demonstrable association with fibromyalgia, bladder pain syndrome and irritable bowel syndrome, and there is a considerable impact on quality of life and on sexual life (Arnold et al., 2006; Ponte et al., 2009; Reed et al., 2012; Vieira-Baptista et al., 2014). There are reported associations with candidiasis, genital herpes, urinary tract infection and papillomavirus infection (Turner & Marinoff, 1988; Vieira-Baptista et al., 2014). The use of oral contraceptives (Harlow, Vitonis & Stewart, 2008; Vieira-Baptista et al., 2014), premenstrual tension, hysterectomy and scoliosis have all been found to be associated with vulvodynia (Vieira-Baptista et al., 2014).

In an investigation of 300 patients, Sadownik (2000) reported the mean age as 38 years and the mean duration of vulvodynia symptoms as 38 months. The symptoms were constant in 67 per cent, intermittent in 26 per cent and cyclic in 4 per cent. Patients used the term *constant* to refer to the fact that the symptoms were present during sexual intercourse but necessarily also present outside of sexual activity. The symptoms were reported to involve the vagina (77 per cent), labia minora (54 per cent), labia majora (40 per cent), anus (12 per cent), pelvis (8 per cent), back (4 per cent) and legs (2 per cent). The symptoms included dyspareunia during penetration, associated with ejaculation and after intercourse. There were also complaints of vulvar burning, vulvar itching, abnormal vaginal discharge and sexual concerns such as loss of interest, loss of sexual arousal and problems with orgasm. There were reported limitations to sexual intercourse, sexual foreplay, clothing choice and sitting.

In relation to the localization of pain and the relationship of the pain to provocation, Edwards (2004) reported that only a minority of patients (6.7 per cent) reported discrete pain localized to the vestibule and provoked by intercourse, and 8.3 per cent reported unprovoked pain that was generalized. The majority did not fit into a formally recognized pattern, including experiencing both provoked and unprovoked pain but limited to the vestibule and also extending beyond the vestibule. In conclusion, Edwards makes the point the current distinction drawn between site of the pain and whether the pain is provoked or not does not reflect empirical findings.

There is evidence that adult-onset vulvodynia is more likely to occur in women exposed to childhood physical and/or sexual abuse, and the likelihood is particularly strong where the abuse was by a primary family member (Harlow & Stewart, 2005). But this finding is not universal (Edwards et al., 1997). In addition, antecedent mood or anxiety disorder predisposes to vulvodynia, and unsurprisingly, vulvodynia also predisposes to new-onset depression and anxiety (Wylie, Hallam-Jones & Harrington, 2004; Khandker et al., 2011; Iglesias-Rios, Harlow & Reed, 2015). And morning awakening cortisol level has been reported to be blunted in women with vulvodynia, confirming that these patients are under chronic stress (Ehrström, Kornfeld & Rylander, 2009). However, the findings in relation to psychological functioning have to be taken with caution because Reed et al. (2000) reported that there is no difference between women with vulvodynia and control individuals in terms of demographic characteristics, sexual relationships, sexual behaviours, current and past depression, somatic sensitivity and history of sexual or physical abuse.

The subjective experience of vulvodynia has been investigated by Ayling and Ussher (2008), who reported a number of themes, including (1) feelings of being an inadequate sexual partner, (2) feelings of being an inadequate woman, and rarely (3) feelings of being an adequate woman/sexual partner. In the inadequate sexual partner theme, the women expressed feeling worthless, useless and broken, and these feelings flowed from the sense of not being able to satisfy the perceived sexual needs of their partner. In the inadequate woman theme, the women expressed feeling that they were not real women, and this feeling was linked to their identity as women and this was itself associated with the ability to attract and to keep a man. It is clear that vulvodynia has deep effects not merely on sexual activity but also on the sense of self.

In terms of outcome, 22.2 per cent of women in a two-year follow-up study reported full resolution of their symptoms (Reed et al., 2008). In another study, 33 per cent of women reported 75 per cent diminution in pain, and 21 per cent reported a decrease in pain levels of between 50 and 75 per cent. When women who had taken antidepressants or anticonvulsants were analyzed, more than 50 per cent reported significant improvement, but this was equally true for those who had not taken any medication (Reed, Haefner & Cantor, 2003). In a report on the use of electromyography-assisted pelvic floor rehabilitation, 88.4 per cent reported having no vulvar pain following treatment, with a further 11.6 per cent reporting marked improvement (Glazer, 2000). However, the truth is that the treatment options and likelihood of benefit are still under investigation.

9.3 Penoscrotodynia

9.3.1 Case Reports

There are very few case reports of penoscrotodynia. I have included cases of red scrotum syndrome and restless genital syndrome to illustrate this condition.

1. A 60-year-old man presented with burning sensations of scrotal skin for at least 12 months. Topical treatment with corticosteroids so far had not improved his complaints. On examination we found an erythematous scrotal skin without any scaling or scratch marks. The border to the adjacent skin was sharp. He was otherwise healthy. A diagnostic biopsy

was taken that was unremarkable besides superficial telangiectasia. The diagnosis of RSS [red scrotum syndrome] was made. We started treatment with doxycycline p.o. and tacrolimus 0.1% ointment twice daily with a complete remission of his burning sensations. The redness also improved markedly within 10 days. After 4 weeks treatment was stopped because of complete remission. (Wollina, 2011, p. 39)

2. A 74-year old married man with three children. He was referred to our outpatient department by his general physician. His medical history revealed a laparoscopic radical prostatectomy due to local prostatic carcinoma at the age of 73 years. After surgery, continence remained normal with no problem of micturition, ejaculation disappeared but with intact sensations of orgasm, and previously existing erectile difficulties became complete. Seven months after prostatectomy, Mr. A began to feel increased 'very unpleasant' sexual urge in his genitals as if he is on the edge of getting an orgasm in the absence of conscious thoughts or fantasies about sex. These genital sensations are experienced as a sort of 'restlessness' in the genital area. These sensations were very disturbing and unwanted, making the patient feel upset, irritable, restless, and desperate. Although Mr. A and his wife accepted the loss of erectile function and abstained from sexual activity since prostatectomy, he attempted to masturbate simply to get rid of the genital sensations. However, after masturbation attempts, the unwanted genital sensations typically re-occurred within 15 minutes against his will. The genital sensations got worse when sitting and diminished during walking or lying down. Since the onset of the genital sensations was recorded, there was increased urgency to void, but only in small amounts. Mr. A did not report restless legs. Since his prostatectomy he has developed complete erectile dysfunction and anejaculation. Prior to his prostatectomy, intercourse frequency was once a week with an estimated intravaginal latency time of about 10 minutes. However, since the onset of the genital feelings, a sensation of orgasm occurs 20–60 seconds after start of masturbation. The weird sensations are described as a type of tingling and are located above the pubic bone and along the penis or testes. The sensations are triggered by touch of the glans penis along his clothes (allodynia), sitting, and after defaecation. His medical history does not reveal prior child abuse, mood or anxiety disorder, obsessive compulsive disorder, or traumatic sexual experiences. ... Routine laboratory assessments in our hospital ... were normal, and EEG and MRI scan of the brain showed no abnormalities. Ultrasound examination and an MRI scan of the pelvis showed a varicocele at the inguinal canal bilaterally, but mainly on the left side, and around the spermatic cords. Sensory testing of the genital region elicited a considerable number of points of static mechanical hyperaesthesia bilaterally of the pubic bone, and above the penis in the pudendal dermatome. ... Manual examination of the ramus inferior of the pubic bone and, particularly along the dorsal nerve of the penis, elicited the sensations of an imminent ejaculation and sensation of restless at the previous[ly] mentioned trigger points. (Waldinger et al., 2011, p. 327)

9.3.2   Explanatory Hypotheses and Clinical Aspects

There is as yet, as with vulvodynia, no overarching understanding of the pathogenesis of penoscrotodynia. This is even more acutely so for penoscrotodynia precisely because it remains a term covering a number of disparate conditions (see earlier).

The prevalence of this condition is unknown. It is noted to be associated with alcohol use in a subset of patients (Markos, 2011). This is thought to be an allergic reaction to ethanol that is demonstrable on oral provocation testing and that occurs as a dose-dependent, non-IgE-mediated pathogenic mechanism but nonetheless presents as a hypersensitivity reaction to ethanol (Ehlers et al., 2002). It is also possible to hypothesize that ethanol works by potentiating the response of vanilloid receptor 1 to heat, and hence, in ethanol-induced penoscrotodynia, ethanol acts to make the patient sensitized to heat at a temperature lower than body temperature leading to a burning sensation (Trevisani, 2002; Markos, 2011). Furthermore, caffeine has been reported as a potential inducer of penoscrotodynia (Markos, 2008). The mechanism for this effect is unknown.

Red scrotum disease is another condition that is recognized as being liable to cause penoscrotodynia. It is conceived of as a neurovascular disorder that is characterized by burning sensation and hyperaemia of the anterior half of the scrotum that may extend to the posterior scrotum or the base of the penis and may be a phenotypic expression of localized primary erythromelalgia (Fisher, 1997; Prevost & English, 2007; Markos, 2011). But it is worth keeping in mind that it may result in misuse of topical steroids (Narang et al., 2013).

Another condition of interest is restless genital syndrome, which presents with unprovoked sexual arousal/orgasm of uncertain cause, usually primarily reported in women but also known to occur in men (Oaklander et al., 2020). The full range of symptoms includes involuntary feeling of stimulation of the clitoris which is prolonged; feeling of arousal that is unabated by sexual orgasm and genital stimulation unaccompanied by the subjective feeling of sexual desire (Mosiołek et al., 2016). In women, it can occur between the ages of 10 and 70 years. In 80 per cent of patients, daily out of context sexual arousal occurred in episodes that usually included orgasm but may also include lesser, longer-lasting non-orgasmic arousal. Most of the female patients had symptoms attributable to sacral neuropathy, including perineal or buttock pain. The authors of this series of cases suggest unprovoked firing of C-fibres in the regional special sensory neurons that subserve sexual arousal may be responsible (Oaklander et al., 2020). There are other possible causes including pelvic venous congestion and drugs such as trazodone and phytoestrogens (Mosiołek et al., 2016). In addition, there are reports of associated restless leg syndrome, overactive bladder syndrome and urethral hypersensitivity and intolerance of tight clothes and underwear. As in the male case described earlier, there is often static mechanical hyperaesthesia demonstrable by finer touch investigation on various trigger points in the dermatome of the pudendal nerve. Three of the 23 women reported in one study showed sensory stimulation–induced uninhibited orgasm during physical examination (Waldinger et al., 2009). In summary, there are similarities in the presentation of vulvodynia, penoscrotodynia, persistent genital arousal disorder and restless genital syndrome to at least consider whether a shared common underlying abnormality exists. Markos and Dinsmore (2013) make the case for an underlying neurovascular dysfunction.

Finally, the role of psychological and psychiatric disorders cannot be ignored. Anyasodor et al. (2015, 2016) investigated dysaesthetic penoscrotodynia and reported on a case series of consecutive patients over a period of 18 months from two hospitals. They described 10 men with a mean age at referral of 49.6 years and a mean duration of symptoms of 34.2 months (range 4–96 months). All the patients had evidence of psychopathology. Four patients had a prior diagnosis of mood and anxiety disorders, including bipolar disorder. One had a family history of bipolar disorder in a sibling and also death by suicide in his mother. The others all had evidence of anxiety and/or depression based on their scores on the Hospital Anxiety and Depression Scale, the Generalized Anxiety Disorder scale, and the Patient Health Questionnaire. The authors concluded that invariably all patients with penoscrotodynia have demonstrable psychopathology and that treatment of the psychiatric disorders alleviated the physical symptoms. They argued that penoscrotodynia be regarded as a somatoform disorder and make the case for regarding vulvodynia also as a functional somatic symptom disorder.

9.4 Conclusion

Vulvodynia and penoscrotodynia are both conditions that are rarely seen by psychiatrists but nonetheless illustrate the distinction between sensations and perceptions. In the former, the abnormal sensations are not treated as any more than the rare sensations that they are, whereas in the perceptual disorders, the rare sensations have already been transformed into perceptions. This distinction probably underlies the fact that vulvodynia and penoscrotodynia are rarely referred to psychiatrists despite both being conditions that challenge and that have no understandable cause.

Chapter 10

Olfactory Reference Syndrome

10.1 Introduction

Olfactory reference syndrome was codified as a condition worthy of attention by Pryse-Phillips in his seminal paper published in 1971 (Pryse-Phillips, 1971). He described 36 patients presenting with the belief that smells emanated from their bodies without the intervention of any external agency, what Pryse-Phillips termed *intrinsic hallucinations*. This belief was accompanied by a 'contrite' reaction manifest as a deep sense of shame, embarrassment and self-abasement and sensitivity to the reaction of people around them. There were also behavioural responses to this belief, including excessive washing, excessive changing of clothing and social withdrawal. This condition was distinguished from olfactory hallucinations in the context of schizophrenia, mood disorder and epilepsy.

Pryse-Phillips makes the point that olfactory reference syndrome has been previously described in the literature and given different names, including *délire à bâse olfactive, parosmia,* and *bromidrosiphobia* (Potts, 1891; Tilley, 1895; Bullen, 1899; Sutton, 1919). What is significant is that in describing olfactory reference syndrome, Pryse-Phillips was focusing on olfactory hallucinations as the presenting complaint in the absence of other primary psychiatric or neurological conditions. Current definitions of olfactory reference syndrome now concentrate on the following criteria: (1) a persistent false belief that one emits a malodorous smell (this belief may encompass a range of insights); (2) the belief causes clinically significant distress and is time consuming or results in significant impairment in social, occupational or other important areas of functioning; and (3) the belief is not accounted for by another mental disorder or a general medical condition (Begum & McKenna, 2011). In other words, the role of hallucinatory experience has been de-emphasized in the definition of olfactory reference syndrome, even though a significant number of the reported patients make the claim that they can smell the odour.

To make the point even more clearly, olfactory reference syndrome is distinct from the other conditions in this section precisely because the role and importance of either the abnormality of sensation or of perception in its conceptualization are markedly diminished. It is the belief that one smells and not the actual sensing of the smell that is critical here. In addition, the role of values for the first time enters into the experience and characterization of a psychopathological phenomenon. I mean by this the fact that in olfactory reference syndrome, the smell is believed to be 'bad'. The odour that the patient believes that he or she emits is not described as a neutral smell, nor is it assigned a positive value. It is invariably a 'bad' odour, a smell that is foul and that is liable to influence how the patient is socially perceived by others. In essence, there is social disvalue attendant on the possibility that the patient has a negatively evaluated odour associated with him or her. This sense of social disvalue comprises feelings of low self-esteem, lowered self-confidence and a preoccupation with social rejection and exclusion. This direct linkage between bodily odour and social rejection speaks to the fundamental role of odour in social affiliation. This is quite distinct from how the other disorders of perception described in this section influence the patients who experience them. Visual, auditory and tactile perceptions themselves rarely have a direct effect on the social standing of the individual patient. The objects that are abnormally perceived do not have an intrinsic value that is distinct from the distress that they may cause, whereas in olfactory reference syndrome the particular odour is itself labelled as 'bad', and the distress that it causes is because it is believed by the patient to affect his or her social standing.

There is a notable similarity between olfactory reference syndrome and the Japanese concept of *taijin-kyofu-sho*, which involves notions akin to social anxiety, and in severe form, *jiko-shu-kyofu*, where the patient believes that he or she offends others by giving off a smell (see Section 10.3 for a fuller description).

10.2 Case Reports

Case 1

Patient 9. Male, married, aged 39 years, machinist. Complaint: 'I think I smell; body odour or something like that.' Background: Two paternal uncles had had treatment for depression, as had his younger brother. His eldest son had asthma, and the second son was 'very sensitive'. A sister had had mental hospital treatment. His early development was normal, and his health was very good. He became a sergeant in the army after the war, and later earned a high wage as a night worker in a factory. He said he had always had many friends, but was a sensitive, retiring, and temperamental man, and 'fanatically clean'. History: When aged 11 years he had to wear clothes which had been contaminated by smoke from a fire in the house and at school he was laughed at and teased because of the resulting smell. From that time on, only ceasing when he was away in the army, he had feared that a sweaty, body-odour smell emanated from him and had been certain that others could smell it, as he was aware of remarks – 'old smelly' or 'stinker' – which were continually made around him; and he had seen people making gestures of disdain. He agreed that neither he nor his family smelt anything, and produced many ingenious reasons for this, such as that it only came on when he sweated excessively at work. He moved jobs repeatedly on this account, had no social life (except at home where he seldom worried about the smell), and washed frequently and changed his clothes each day. On examination, the secondary delusions, ideas of reference, ruminations, and mild tension were the only features detected. The situations producing his smell could be ranked as a hierarchy so that, for instance, hot crowded buses brought on the worry about the smell badly, while talking to a stranger over the garden wall produced little anxiety about a smell.   (Pryse-Phillips, 1971, p. 492)

Case 2

Mr. A. was a 17-year old male who described a persistent preoccupation, which had begun about 6 months previously, with the idea that he smelled of urine. Each time he urinated, for example, he worried that he had wet his underwear, and that consequently people would think that he smelled of urine. He stated that these thoughts occurred most of his waking time. As a result of the thoughts he would repeatedly check his underwear for urine stains, would change his clothing excessively often, and would use more deodorant than usual. In addition, shame and embarrassment about the perceived odour gradually led him to avoid more and more social interactions, and he even began to miss days at school. He became increasingly demoralized and at the time of presentation exhibited a number of symptoms of depression. . . . On close questioning, the patient said that he was 95% certain that he did in fact smell of urine, although on occasion he felt that his preoccupations about odour were excessive and unreasonable. There was no history of classic obsessions or compulsions or of definite hallucinations or delusions. There was no history of substance abuse or an underlying general medical condition.   (Stein et al., 1998, pp. 96–7)

Case 3

A 75-year-old African American woman, widow, unemployed, and domiciled with a past medical history of hypertension, osteoarthritis, and asthma. The patient was brought to the Emergency Room by Emergency Medical Services on account of an attempted suicide due to a 3-year history of 'bad odour coming from my vagina'. The patient reported that the foul smell from her vagina was making her body 'rotten'. She reported that 'the smell came back recently and it is stronger'. Although she has been having odour for the last three years, it has recently gotten worse, the culmination of which resulted in her attempted suicide this time. She reported that she has seen several gynaecologists who have treated her to no avail and later advised her to see a psychiatrist. She stated that there is a 'devil' in her body that does not let go and she said 'I need help'. The patient had significant impairment in social functioning evidenced by a reported avoidance of social events, she could no longer go out to the store for her basic needs; according to the patient's son, she has also stopped going out to get groceries or to the church. She reported that she has been unable to have any romantic relationships because of her 'odour'. The patient stays at home all day, showers several times daily, and has tried many vaginal products and creams all in vain. At the time of initial evaluation, the patient appeared paranoid, reporting that people stayed away from her because of her smell. She also endorsed ideas of reference claiming that people around her cover their noses, stand next to the windows, or look at her in 'a certain way' and then talk about how much she 'stinks' to each other. She endorses profound feelings of hopelessness, helplessness, and guilt and was tearful during the interview.   (Jegede et al., 2018, p. 2)

10.3 Explanatory Hypotheses

There is as yet no overarching explanatory hypothesis for olfactory reference syndrome. Indeed, our understanding of the relationship between olfaction and the brain is in its infancy. We know that our experience of a smell or odour does not refer to any specific molecular feature of the odorant, that there is a large variety of perceptual experiences of odours commensurate with variety of odorants and, finally, that our perception of a smell is holistic in nature such that complex admixtures such as the smell of coffee appear as a single percept in the same manner that a single odorant molecule does (Mackay-Sim & Royet, 2006). For our purposes, in a chapter on olfactory reference syndrome, the most singular fact is that one of the most salient aspects of an odour is its pleasantness. Aversive odorants activate the left orbito-frontal cortex and amygdala bilaterally. Emotionally valenced olfactory, auditory and visual stimuli all activate left orbito-frontal cortex, temporal pole and superior frontal gyrus, whereas the left amygdala seems to be specifically activated by highly emotionally charged olfactory stimuli. In addition, there is the role of the insula, serving as an internal alarm system alerting individuals to potentially distressing interoceptive sensory stimuli and imbuing them with negative emotional significance, and this has been shown to be true for the inhalation of disgusting odours (Mackay-Sim & Royet, 2006).

It is recognized that both the insula and basal ganglia are involved in the perception of disgust, and as discussed earlier, the insula and orbito-frontal cortex are involved in the processing of olfaction and highly charged emotions. There is evidence that abnormalities of disgust processing are present in some but not all patients with obsessive-compulsive disorder and of differential deficits in recognition of facial expressions of disgust in schizophrenia (Heining & Phillips, 2006). This overlap between the brain systems mediating emotion and olfactory processing suggests that there is merit in studying the brain mechanisms in psychiatric disorders and especially in conditions such as olfactory reference syndrome.

Finally, it is well established that smell plays a role in mating, parenting, social affiliation and prey-predator relationships in other mammals, and hence it is reasonable to assume that it has a role too in social functioning in human beings (Malaspina, Corcoran & Goudsmit, 2006). There are two distinct but intricately interwoven olfaction systems: the first detects a finite number of pheromones, which are species-specific olfactory signals conveying information relevant to social status and potential sexual reproduction, and the second is able to detect a broad array of odours that are important not only for establishing social status and sexual reproduction but also for the recognition of food and danger. Well-understood influences of odours on endocrine function include induction of menstrual synchrony, dampening of female cycle length irregularities by males, beard growth acceleration by exposure to females, hastening of puberty in females who reside with unrelated males and the augmentation of male testosterone and sexual behaviour by exposure to vaginal secretions (Malloy, Miller & Kane, 2015).

These findings all point to the immense importance of odour perception in human beings and the significant role that odours play in determining social behaviour including sexual behaviour. While there is as yet no comprehensive or even schematic understanding of the underlying pathological mechanisms in olfactory reference syndrome, it is safe to assume that mechanisms exist particularly as this syndrome fortuitously brings to our attention the links between odour perception and the fear of social exclusion, social rejection and abandonment. For the present, what we have is a model that attempts to integrate the social and cultural context in which olfactory reference syndrome emerges with the individual vulnerabilities of the patient. There are obvious problems and questions about this approach, but for the moment, it will have to do.

In Pryse-Phillips's seminal paper, he argued for a role for 'sensitivity reaction' as the context in which olfactory reference syndrome emerges. He based this proposition on Kretshmer's classical 'sensitive Beziehungswahn' a concept best enunciated as follows:

> The Sensitive ... sees the whole world as though it were coloured by the same reaction as, in reality, only torments him inwardly. He has a feeling that his whole humiliation has become notorious, that everyone knows about his painful experience, that people in the street turn round and look at him when he passes, grin, and make signs. He detects veiled allusions to himself in harmless conversation, even in the newspapers. [These reactions] ... have certain starting typical points particularly

calculated to give rise to humiliating feelings of inferiority, chief of which are provided by sex complexes ... less frequently ... inferiority feelings of non-sexual kind lead to the formation of sensitive ideas of reference.   (Quoted in Pryse-Phillips, 1971, p. 501)

Pryse-Phillips makes the point '[s]uch a formulation fits exactly the clinical picture of the olfactory reference syndrome if the bad smell is taken as the key experience, a humiliating and shameful attribute' (Pryse-Phillips, 1971, p. 501).

A more precise understanding of the relationship between self-perception and the evolution of olfactory reference syndrome is available if the similarities of the Japanese concept of *taijin-kyofu-sho* are examined. *Taijin-kyofu-sho* was first defined by Morita and is defined as an obsession that the patient would displease or embarrass others by symptoms such as blushing, a defect in appearance, staring inappropriately or emitting foul odours (Suzuki et al., 2004). Latterly, Kasahara et al. (1972) have conceptualized it as a continuum ranging from a highly prevalent but transient adolescent social anxiety to delusions. *Jiko-shu -kyofu* is regarded in the Japanese nosological system as a subtype of *taijin-kyofu-sho* and is recognized as a culture-bound phobia of a self-emanating odour which is indistinguishable from olfactory reference syndrome (Suzuki et al., 2004).

Sasaki, Wada and Tanno (2013) propose that there is a conceptual relationship between (1) erythrophobia, which is the fear of blushing, (2) the fear of eye-to-eye confrontation (*jiko-shisen-kyofu*), (3) olfactory reference syndrome, (4) delusions of soliloquy, (5) delusions of sleep talking and (6) thought broadcasting. The point that Sasaki et al. want to make is that these six symptoms have an underlying central abnormality that they term *egorrhoea*, the leaking out of body odour, for example, and the concomitant belief that whatever it is that leaks out is offensive to others. This conceptualization is problematic for many reasons but principally because it focuses on six disparate symptoms which, on the face of it, are distinct but ignores other phenomena that also illustrate a disturbance of ego boundary, which after all is what the notion of egorrhoea is a novel term for. But where Sasaki et al. are helpful to our understanding of olfactory reference syndrome is in their analysis of how culture determines and structures the relationship between internal feelings and the external expression of these feelings. They argue that in East Asian culture there is great cultural value in maintaining group harmony, and this determines the desire to be sensitive to how an individual's behaviour impacts others around him or her, accentuating the wish to ensure that one regulates one's own behaviour to maximize other people's welfare and thereby maintain social harmony. This position is in contrast to the Western perspective that focuses on oneself and how other people's behaviour influences one's own feelings. In this regard, the sensitivity is one's own internal state, and there is less attunement to the demonstrable feelings of others. It then becomes understandable that the individual with *taijin-kyofu-sho* and its many variants comes to believe that their own inner feelings and behaviours induce others to look at them with contempt and conversely that the individual who looks at the patient with contempt believes that the patient should feel ashamed. There is also the associated belief that one's feelings are transparent, what Sasaki et al. term the 'illusion of transparency'. The emphasis here is that this relational dynamic, as described earlier, which is comprehensible in the light of culture, may provide an understanding of what lies at the root of olfactory reference syndrome, namely the belief that odour is leaking from oneself and that the social consequence is contempt from others and social rejection for the patient.

There is evidence that individuals with reported preoccupation of subjective oral odour were also more likely to report bodily odour and in the context of social anxiety more likely to have olfactory reference syndrome. The findings from this study must be taken with caution as the participants were community-based female university students attending a health science course. There is also some evidence from a relatively small study that individuals with olfactory reference syndrome have demonstrable impairments in processing speed, executive functioning, recognition memory bias for olfactory reference syndrome–related words and olfaction functioning including odour detection and discrimination and, finally, in emotional processing (Sofko et al., 2020). How far these impairments are specific to olfactory reference syndrome rather than to psychotic disorders in general is moot.

10.4 Clinical Aspects

In Pryse-Phillips (1971) seminal paper, the age of onset of olfactory reference syndrome was 25.4 years. The majority of patients were male (78 per cent), and most patients were single (75 per cent). A considerable percentage of patients (50 per cent) had prior referrals to other physicians aside from psychiatrists, including general surgeons, neurologists, dermatologists and ear, nose and throat specialists. Pryse-Phillips reported that in 75 per cent of cases there was evidence for true olfactory hallucinations, and there was a loss of insight in 60 per cent. Finally, there was evidence of suicidal ideation and actions in 43 per cent of cases. Significantly, Pryse-Phillips made the distinction between intrinsic and extrinsic olfactory hallucinations and remarked that in olfactory reference syndrome, as opposed to schizophrenia, for example, the olfactory hallucinations were deemed to come from the patient's own body (i.e., the olfactory hallucination was intrinsic), whereas in schizophrenia where olfactory hallucinations were present, they were described as coming from the external environment (i.e., the olfactory hallucinations were extrinsic in nature). Furthermore, in olfactory reference syndrome, the hallucination was associated with marked contrite reaction because the hallucinations were thought by the patient to be offensive to others.

This characterization needs to be modified in light of more recent findings. In a systematic study of 20 patients by Phillips and Menard (2011), the mean age of the patients was 33 years, and most were female. This preponderance of females is different from the earlier report by Pryse-Phillips. The odour was reported as emanating from the mouth in 75 per cent of cases, followed by the armpits (60 per cent) and the genitals (35 per cent). A minority of patients reported emanating both a bodily odour and a non-bodily odour such as the smell of ammonia, an 'oily' fishy smell, vegetable soup odour or the smell of stale food and cigarettes. Eighty-five per cent of patients reported that they could smell the odour, and 95 per cent believed that others too could smell the odour. Practically all patients believed that people took undue notice of them because of the supposed smell and claimed that other people behaved in ways that indicated that the patient smelt badly.

Practically all patients in this study carried out repetitive behaviours in response to their preoccupation with bodily odour. These included smelling themselves to check for the odour (80 per cent), excessive showering to remove the odour (68.4 per cent) and excessive changing of clothing in order to remove the offending clothing (50 per cent). Other behaviours include drinking fluids, talking softly to minimize bad breath and checking their breath by blowing into their nose. In addition, practically all patients tried to mask the odour with the use of perfumes, powder, deodorants, chewing gum or mints.

There is a considerable effect upon social functioning. Periods of social avoidance are reported by 75 per cent and avoidance of occupational, educational and role activities. Many of the patients (44 per cent) had sought treatment from non-psychiatric healthcare professionals, and treatment had included tonsillectomy, nasal sprays, electrolysis of the armpits and prescription mouthwash.

In a systematic review of 84 case reports, Begum and McKenna (2011) reported that in the vast majority of cases, the age of onset was before age 20, and the mean duration of illness was 8 years with a wide range (6 months–48 years). There was a preponderance of males (62 per cent), and a family history of psychiatric disorder was available in 18 of 84 cases. There was associated low mood in 39 per cent of cases, and taking a broad definition of anxiety, this was present in 42 per cent of cases. In 49 per cent of cases, there was an identifiable precipitating event, including unrelated stress about the time of the onset (17 per cent) and smell-related events in 85 per cent of cases. The type of smell-related events described included 'sister told him his feet smelled', 'teased by classmates about leaking wind', 'wife said that he stank in order to humiliate him during a phase of frequent quarrelling', and so on (p. 456). The smell emanated from a wider source than in the study by Phillips and Menard (2011) and included from the feet, underarms or groin, sweat, urine, flatus, faeces, bad breath and anal, genital or sexual odours. Other smells included garbage, dirty socks, gases, burning fish, medicines, old cheese or rotten eggs. All the patients believed that the smells emanated from their bodies. In 59 per cent of cases the patient could not smell the odour, and in only 22 per cent was there an unreserved belief that they could smell the odour. In 57 per cent the belief was described as fixed and firmly held, whereas in 43 per cent there was evidence that the belief was held with less than full conviction. Nonetheless, ideas of reference were present in 74 per cent, and this was demonstrable as misinterpretation of the comments, gestures and actions of others as indicating that the patient had a bad smell.

Begum and McKenna (2011) concluded that this was a condition with an age of onset before 20 years and that was associated with low mood and anxiety. The condition appeared to be grounded in abnormality of personality traits such as avoidant, dependent and obsessional personality traits. The long-term outcome is described as chronic by Phillips and Menard (2011), but Begum and McKenna found that two-thirds showed improvement or full recovery. Nonetheless, they concede that their findings may reflect selection bias from the published literature.

Many of the findings of earlier studies were confirmed by the large internet-based survey of 253 subjects reported by Greenberg et al. (2016). In essence, the mean age of onset was confirmed as 21 years, and 54 per cent reported a chronic course. The most severe symptoms appeared to be associated with being female and having poor insight and higher levels of impairment of occupation, leisure and relationship.

The role of hyper-vigilance to the body language and facial cues of others is underlined in the personal account reported by Martin et al. (2018, p. 509). The patient reported that

[o]ne symptom ... that became characteristic of my behaviour was an acute sensitivity to the body language and facial cues of people around me. The tiniest gestures such as the twitch of a nose were perceived as confirmation that I was emitting a bad smell.

Furthermore, the patient commented on the effects of olfactory reference syndrome on his functioning as follows:

I became withdrawn and hated being physically close to anybody in case they detected the malodour that I was certain emitted from my body. I rationalised the fact that I couldn't detect the odour myself by assuming that I had become desensitized by constant exposure to it. My bathing, scrubbing and cleaning rituals became progressively more elaborate, but nothing seemed to make any difference. After trying countless hygiene products with no success, I became convinced that the problem was due to an underlying metabolic disorder, and made the hesitant decision to seek medical advice. (p. 509)

There is continuing discussion about the nosological status of olfactory reference syndrome. Veale and Matsunaga (2014) and others (Lochner & Stein, 2003; Singh, 2006; Lochner & Stein, 2014) point to the similarity of the behavioural aspects of olfactory reference syndrome and obsessive-compulsive disorder, and Skimming and Miller (2019) suggest that there are overlapping neuro-circuitry systems between olfactory reference syndrome and obsessive-compulsive disorder. This issue is yet to be resolved. Olfactory reference syndrome, alongside other conditions such as body dysmorphic disorder and hypochondriasis, cuts across categorical boundaries in the current systems. In many respects, if these conditions are regarded merely as symptoms rather as syndromes, then the variety of presentation cutting across categories (as they do in fact) will become subsumed under the relevant categories as necessary. The disadvantage of this approach is that conditions that may benefit from thematic unity and theoretical unification may end up in disparate categories, hence undermining the advancement of knowledge.

In general, olfactory hallucinations occur in many medical conditions. Pryse-Phillips (1971) showed that a third of olfactory hallucinations were attributable to depression, a quarter to schizophrenia, a quarter to olfactory reference syndrome and 8 per cent to epilepsy (see also Meats, 1988). However, in addition to the established linked between olfactory hallucinations and epilepsy, olfactory reference syndrome itself has been reported in temporal lobe epilepsy with right focus (Devinsky, Khan & Alper, 1998) and in a right-sided arteriovenous malformation underlying a psychomotor seizure (Toone, 1978). The authors highlight the already established relationship between right-sided lesions and the development of delusional disorders. Olfactory reference syndrome independent of drug treatment has been reported in Parkinson disease (Moroy, Bellivier & Fénelon, 2012). Olfactory reference syndrome also has been reported in hyperhidrosis (Gama-Marques, Jesus & Brissos, 2014).

The risk of suicide is highlighted in the papers by Jegede et al. (2018) and Lodhi (2020). In the one case, a 75-year-old African American woman was admitted following a suicide attempt. The suicidal act was a direct response to the worsening 'bad smell' that she reported emanated from her vagina and that had a rotten odour that was getting stronger and unresponsive to treatment from gynaecologists (Jegede et al., 2018). In the other case, a 51-year-old woman presented to the emergency room with the complaint of vaginal odour that was unresponsive to the use of deodorants, household cleaning products and bleach used as a douche. In desperation, she presented threatening to end her life by suicide if she did not receive appropriate assistance (Lodhi, 2020).

Another notable feature of olfactory reference syndrome is the propensity for the patients to present across medical specialties, including gynaecology, dermatology and oral medicine. Patients also present to dentists, and a report from Nigeria described a series of patients identified by the fact that there was no objective evidence of halitosis despite the subjective complaint of oral malodour. The characteristics features were as described earlier (Uguru et al., 2011).

10.5 Conclusion

Olfactory reference syndrome is important because it focuses attention on olfaction and the role of values in perception. Unlike other hallucinatory disturbances, the abnormal perception is deemed unpleasant and has implications for the social standing of the individual. The hallucination is regarded as intrinsic in nature; that is, it emanates from the person and thus is intimately connected to the social value of the individual. Furthermore, there is the difficulty in distinguishing between perception and abnormal belief.

Chapter 11

Cross-Modal Perceptual Syndrome (Synaesthesia)

11.1 Introduction

In the preceding chapters, I focused on the psychopathology of perception or of sensation. These pathologies often, if not invariably, are recognized as indicating underlying disorders or diseases. I now turn to synaesthesia, a condition that is not usually thought of as a disorder or disease but rather as a variant of normal experience. Put simply, it is the merging of the senses, in which a stimulus in one sensory modality both evokes a normal perception, as expected, in the same modality and an anomalous perception in another modality. In other words, there is cross-modal perception.

This definition is best illustrated with an example. Cytowic et al. (2009, p. 14) give the example of Deni Simon.

> When I listen to music, I see the shapes on an externalized area about 12 inches in front of my face and about one foot high onto which the music is visually projected. Sounds are most easily likened to oscilloscope configurations – lines moving in colour, often metallic with height, width, and most importantly, depth. My favourite music has lines extended horizontally beyond the 'screen' area.

In this example, we see that music, an auditory phenomenon, is heard, as expected, as music but is also perceived as colourful visual phenomena.

Even though synaesthesia is not an example of psychopathology, it is of interest and importance to psychiatrists for at least five reasons. Firstly, it is a perceptual anomaly that deserves further investigation by psychiatrists as it may illustrate the manner in which sensory stimuli are transformed into perceptions and thereby assist in illuminating the underlying cognitive processes of aberrant perceptions such as hallucinations and visual distortions.

Secondly, synaesthesia may demonstrate the underlying physiological underpinnings of perceptions and thus shed light on the pathophysiology of hallucinations and other abnormalities of perception, including the structural anomalies responsible for these abnormalities. Thirdly, as I describe later, it is a phenomenon which demonstrates the possibility of potential differences in the subjective experience of things, the so-called qualia, and the degree to which these differences are so embedded in reality that it takes considerable self-awareness to recognize that the experiences are not shared by others. Here it is plain that it is a potential model for the problem of insight in psychiatry. In other words, if an experience is so veridical in its subjective manifestation and hence profoundly compelling, insight into its anomaly is likely to be compromised.

Fourthly, as I describe later and as exemplified in the example of synaesthesia cited earlier, the experience of synaesthesia illustrates very well the problem of the nature of space in psychiatry. Part of the definition of a true perception and of a true hallucination is the notion that the experiences occur in 'objective' space. This criterion is problematical because many patients with auditory hallucinations have difficulty describing the spatial location of their hallucinations. This problem also occurs in synaesthesia, and it raises the possibility of fine distinctions between objective space and subjective space. This issue will be further discussed later in this chapter.

Finally, functional hallucination and reflex hallucination have much in common with synaesthesia. Functional hallucination is the provocation of a hallucinatory experience by a normal stimulus in which both the resulting perception and the hallucinated perception are in the same modality (Oyebode, 2018). Reflex hallucination is described as a hallucination that occurs in response to a sensory stimulus in one modality producing both a true perception in the same modality and a hallucination in another perceptual modality (Oyebode, 2018). In other words, with the exception that functional and reflex hallucinations are encountered in a psychiatric context and often occur alongside other psychopathological phenomena, they share many features with synaesthesia, and thus, investigation of synaesthesia may assist greater understanding of these phenomena.

Francis Galton (1822–1911) is credited with the first formal description of synaesthesia (Galton, 1883), but George Sachs (1786–?) submitted a thesis in 1812 in which he described his own and his sister's synaesthetic experiences (Sachs, 1812), and Eugene Bleuler (1857–1939), who is best known for his work on schizophrenia, had earlier published on synaesthesia jointly with Karl Lehmann in 1881 (Bleuler & Lehmann, 1881). Synaesthesia has been reported in well-known figures such as Vladimir Nabokov (1899–1977); his son Dmitri Nabokov and his wife Vera Nabokov as well (Cytowic et al., 2009); in Richard Feynman, the famous physicist (Ward, 2009); and in Olivier Messiaen (1908–1992; Bernard, 1986) and Alexander Scriabin (1872–1915; Myers, 1914), both musical composers.

Dmitri Nabokov writes of his own experience as follows:

In music the association is not simply with the written name of the note but with its sound as well. And this goes further, into territory that requires a musical ear. The key in which a particular composition is written, played or sung gives the piece an overall colouring. For example, Schubert's *'Doppelgänger'*, when performed in E-flat minor, has a deep yellowish shade, while, if it is done in E minor, the hue approaches white. I have begun with samples from music because it is a domain to which I have devoted much of my life. Coloration, however, extends in my case to numbers, to the ensemble of an occurrence, to an individual, or to a train of thought. It can go further. I am not a religious person in the sense that I do not endorse a liturgy or pray in formulae. Nonetheless, for a number of years, when there is something I devoutly wished – say, the well-being of a loved one – my yearning tended to be integral with the sense of a profound cavity, with the violet number 4 in its depths. The more distinct the image, the more likely I considered the fulfillment of my wish. And, in more general sense, the more intently I have wished that that loved one should recover. (Cytowic et al., 2009, pp. 249–50)

This example shows how complex the experience of synaesthesia is and demonstrates that there are manifold ways in which it can be expressed. Importantly, it points to the need for classification and enumeration of types and to the requirement to determine whether the varying types are variants of the same underlying process or not.

11.2 Classification and Types

To reiterate, synaesthesia is a conscious experience that is involuntary but yet routinely experienced by a small proportion of people. Grossenbacher and Lovelace (2001) describe two interrelated components, namely the *inducer*, which is the inducing event, and the *concurrent*, which is the synaesthetically induced sensory attribute(s). For example, in Grossenbacher and Lovelace's example, one synaesthete describes the sound of her crying baby as having an unpleasant yellow colour. In this example, the sound of her baby's cry is the inducer, and the yellow colour is the concurrent. The relationship between inducer and concurrent is systematic such that each specific inducer is correlatively accompanied by the same concurrent and is stable over time. This description of the relationship between an inducer and a concurrent allows for a classification in which, for example, sound induces colour, to be termed *sound-colour synaesthesia*.

Several different types of synaesthesias have been described (Cytowic et al., 2009), including

1. Grapheme–colour
2. Time unit–colour
3. Musical sound–colour
4. General sound–colour
5. Phonemes–colour
6. Musical notes–colour
7. Smells–colour
8. Pain–colour
9. Vision–taste
10. Touch–taste
11. Taste–touch

See Cytowic (1997) for an exhaustive list.

There is consensus that in grapheme–colour synaesthesia (viewing black digits or letters induces colour experiences termed *photisms*), the induced photism, which is the concurrent, is either projected onto external space, that is, in external objective space (*projectors*), or is experienced in the mind's eye, that is, in inner subjective space (*associators*). Projectors are in the minority (11 per cent) of a sample of grapheme–colour synaesthetes (Dixon, Smilek & Merikle, 2004).

Another account of the phenomenology of grapheme–colour synaesthesia is that by Ramachandran and Hubbard (2001). These authors make a distinction between the nature of the inducer versus that of the concurrent as described earlier. In this account, the distinction is between a higher- or lower-order inducer. A higher-order inducer acts via the meaning of the inducer; that is, it is conceptual in nature or acts as a lower-order inducer, acting via the actual perceptual form of the inducer. Higher-order synaesthetes are reported, for example, to have the same colour photism to the digit '4', the Roman numeral 'IV' and four dots, whereas in lower-order synaesthesia, the digit '4' and the Roman numeral 'IV' induce different photisms. Another way of thinking of this distinction is that proposed by Grossenbacher and Lovelace (2001), which is described as synaesthetic perception versus synaesthetic conception.

However, perhaps the most common type of synaesthesia, even if not the most studied, is number forms or spatial sequence synaesthesia. According to Cytowic et al. (2009), this is the coupling of colour, perspective, and spatial configurations with concepts involving sequence or ordinality. Numbers or other ordered sequences such as days of the week or months of the year are seen to lie on a path that twists or zigzags, looping around or encircling the body, and executing a variety of angles, bends and curves. Synaesthetes who experience number form synaesthesia are surprised that not everyone sees numbers and that other people find the spatial configurations exceptional.

Here is an example drawn from Galton's original study of synaesthesia (Galton, 1881, pp. 97–8):

> George Bidder, Esq., observed that he had possessed the faculty of mental visualization . . . so long as he could remember. He imagined the mental pictures to be survivals of some early associations in childhood, which however, in most cases it is impossible to trace. In the mental picture or diagram that numerals appear to him to assume, the first twelve numbers are placed as if on a clock face, and probably the idea was originally derived from that source. In his diagram there was an angle at 10, and again at 12. He could only account for this by supposing it to be the result of a struggle between the decimal and duodecimal systems of notation. He explained that not only numbers, but almost all subjects of thought and memory, present themselves to his mind in a visualized form – For example, the months of the year are arranged in a circle. The days of the week in a line from right to left. The dates and events of history have also a definite local arrangement.

To summarize, synaesthetic experiences are automatic and involuntary, are spatially extended in some individuals or experienced in inner subjective space in others. They are consistent over time.

11.3 Case Reports

Case 1

> The subject of this note, whom for convenience we shall call A, is about 30 years of age. . . . A has had synaesthesia as long as he can remember. He does not think it has undergone any change. The colours are particularly apt to appear when he is at a concert, but he often actively suppresses them. Words and numbers evoke no colour and no spatial schemes. Voices, on the other hand, are coloured; Madame Clara Butt's, for example, being violet, and male voices (definite instances given by A) being pink, red, or brown, according to their depth and timbre. Similarly, the tones of the violoncello are brown to pink, of the bassoon brown to yellow, and of the horn to rose. The tones of the trombone are still redder, while the tones of the violin are pink to blue, and those of the fife are light blue verging towards green. Green, says, A, occurs very rarely among the sounds of nature, the notes of certain birds 'shading from blue through peacock colour to green'.   (Myers, 1911, p. 232)

Case 2

> During his recent visit to England, the well-known Russian composer, Alexander Scriabin, kindly allowed me to carry out an examination of his coloured hearing. . . . Colours form for Scriabin so important a part of the total effect of sounds that he desired his *Prometheus* to be performed to the accompaniment of concealed lamps which shall flood the concert-hall with a light of ever changing colour; the music of his *Mystery*, when completed, will be presented with a similar play of colours, and with odours. Scriabin's

attention was first seriously drawn to his coloured hearing owing to an experience at a concert in Paris, where, sitting next to his fellow-countryman and composer Rimsky Korsakov, he remarked that the piece to which they were listening (in D major) seemed to him yellow; whereupon his neighbour replied that to him too, the colour seemed golden. Scriabin has since compared with his compatriot and with other musicians the colour effects of other keys, especially B, C major and F# major, and believes a general agreement to exist in this respect. He admits, however, that whereas to him the key of F# major appears violet, to Rimsky Korsakov it appears green; but this deviation he attributes to an accidental association with the colour of leaves and grass arising from the frequent use of this key for pastoral music. (Myers, 1914, pp. 112–13)

Case 3

The following report concerns itself with the synaesthesia of the author. He was first cognizant of the phenomenon during the year 1918. Whether it had been present before that year he is unable to say. During that year he was physically run down and nervously unstable. Whether he became subject to these secondary sensations because of his physical condition he is unable to assert. . . . Localisation–Colours are projected in the direction of the sound, if the sound comes from without. In inner speech, as when the letter *a* is inwardly pronounced, the colour is located somewhere within the head; and so rapidly does the colour follow upon the sound that it is located, I am almost sure, just against that part of the palate and mouth used in pronouncing a vowel. Thus, the white photism for the vowel *e* (me) is localized against the roof of the mouth, and the photism for *e* (met) is localized down in the throat. Taste photisms are localized in the mouth, and odour photisms in the nose. Temperature photisms are localized on that part of the body experiencing the sensation. Pain photisms are localized on the part of the body experiencing the pain. The photisms for all sensations are localized on the part of the body concerned in the primary sensation. (Ginsberg, 1923, pp. 582–8)

11.4 Explanatory Hypotheses

Ramachandran and Hubbard (2001) showed in an elegant investigation that grapheme–colour synaesthesia is a perceptual phenomenon. In this study, synaesthetically induced colours led to perceptual grouping even though the inducing graphemes did not. Other important findings include the fact that only Arabic numerals induced photisms, whereas Roman numerals did not, and that graphemes presented at higher than 4 Hz failed to induce photisms. This study put paid to the notion that grapheme–colour synaesthesia was down to memory-dependent association. The authors speculated on whether synaesthesia was due to cross-wiring in specific areas of the brain, caused perhaps by excessive proliferation (or defective pruning) of neuronal connections between adjacent brain maps, for example, between area V4 and the number area in the fusiform gyrus. Ramachandran and Hubbard go further in speculating about the possibility that understanding the neural basis of synaesthesia may very well assist our understanding of the anatomical basis of metaphor. They define metaphor as the linking of one conceptual map, for example, taste, to another, for example, tactile sensation. And they also point out how systematic shifts exist between one sensory domain and another in the use of adjectives, exemplified by terms such as *loud colours* and *bitter cold.*

Furthermore, Ramachandran and Hubbard (2001) speculate that this capacity for an overlap between disparate but contiguous brain maps that underlies synaesthesia may also underlie exceptional creative abilities. It has been widely reported that many outstanding musicians such as Rimsky-Korsakov, Duke Ellington, Franz Liszt, Olivier Messiaen and Scriabin (see earlier) were synaesthetes (Pearce, 2007).

To summarize, Ramachandran and Hubbard's hypothesis suggests that synaesthesia results from aberrant connections between contiguous brain areas. In other words, the connections are horizontal in nature. A distinct hypothesis is that by Grossenbacher and Lovelace (2001). They propose a normative mechanism, namely that synaesthesia is mediated by neural mechanisms that exist in normal adult human brains. In their hypothesis, there is disinhibition of feedback mechanisms that would normally constrain the activation of the pathways that are involved in the genesis of the concurrent in the inducer–concurrent relationship already highlighted earlier. To put this another way, where the aberrant connections hypothesis emphasizes horizontal connections, this disinhibition of feedback hypothesis emphasizes top-down connections.

Smilek et al. (2001) advance further the proposal by Grossenbacher and Lovelace just described. This is a complex and sophisticated explanation that relies on a systematic understanding of the pathways and processes underpinning recognition of colour and form as well as the semantic meaning of a grapheme. Colour is processed in the primary visual cortex (areas V1 and V2), and the resulting information is conveyed to the colour-specific areas of the fusiform gyrus. Form activates the shape-processing areas of the primary visual cortex as well as the extrastriate areas in the lingual and fusiform gyri. Then anterior fusiform areas determine the meaning of the form. In the hypothesis of Smilek and colleagues, it is here that the synaesthetes' processing of graphemes (digits) departs from normal colour and form perception. Activation of the meaning of the form activates colour processing in area V4 via feedback connections, and it is this, the re-entrant phenomenon, that influences the perception of the external presented grapheme (digit), lending it photism. There is independent evidence that the meaning of the grapheme ultimately determines the synaesthetic photism (Myles et al., 2003) and that syllable stress, as part of other linguistic determinants (Ward, Simner & Auyeung, 2005), determines the photism associated with graphemes (Simner, Glover & Mowat, 2006). This is further independent evidence for the importance of meaning in synaesthetic photism.

These hypotheses have arisen in the context of cognitive psychological investigations and hence only speculate about the possible neuronal architecture of synaesthesia. There is evidence confirming – on the basis of tensor diffusion imaging to determine the connectivity of white matter tracts and structural magnetic resonance imaging to determine volumes of specific brain regions – that differences exist that may explain the phenomena experienced by the investigated synaesthete (Hänggi et al., 2008). A subject E.S., a multiple synaesthete with musical interval–taste and musical tone–colour synaesthesia was shown to have hyperconnectivity in bilateral perisylvian-insular regions and also bilateral structural differences in auditory areas, namely the planum temporale and Herschl's gyrus, insular cortex and occipital regions. It is worthy of note that trans-magnetic stimulation over the parieto-occipital cortex disrupted grapheme–colour synaesthesia, demonstrating the importance of this region for the binding of graphemes and colour to different spatial reference frames (Muggleton et al., 2007).

The ability of chemical agents such as lysergic acid diethylamide, mescaline, psilocybin, ketamine, ayahuaca and so on to elicit transient experiences of synaesthesia in subjects who do not have developmental synaesthesia suggests that serotonergic mechanisms may underlie synaesthesia, as the agents just listed mainly act through serotonergic pathways (Luke & Terhune, 2013). However, it is important to note that the current consensus is that chemically induced synaesthesia does not qualify as genuine synaesthesia since it does not appear to be automatic, consistent or specific.

As described earlier, one of the distinct differences between synaesthetes is that between *projectors* and *associators*. There are distinctions, too, between projectors in grapheme–colour synaesthesia who project colour onto the surface of a page and those who experience colour in externalized near space termed *space-projectors*. Furthermore, associators can also be distinguished from those who see colour in internal subjective space and those who simply know the colour (Ward et al., 2007). These distinctions are of great interest to psychopathologists. Usually, hallucinatory experiences are defined by their similarity or identity with normal perceptions (with the proviso that there is no sensory stimulus), and one of the yardstick is the degree to which the hallucinatory experience is in external objective space, an experience which is thought to be identical to normal perception.

What Ward et al. (2007) show is that in synaesthesia, the perception, namely the grapheme–colour photism, can be projected onto the actual grapheme, or be projected in near space, or be seen as an imagery in inner subjective space, or not be seen at all but simply be known. In psychopathology, much is made of whether the perception is in external objective space or in internal subjective space – this distinction determining whether an experience is a true hallucination or a pseudo-hallucination. Another possibility is that spatial frames of reference that support normal imagery, normal perception, synaesthetic imagery and perception all exist in the brain and that the differences between subjects reflects the spatial frame of reference evoked during synaesthesia (Ward et al., 2007). A possibility that has not been considered but is relevant especially for hallucinatory experiences is that in normal perception, the perception has an object in the external world onto which the perception is projected. In a hallucination, given the absence of a real external object, descriptions of where the false perception is complicated and the subject's descriptions are hampered by the unusualness of the situation as much as by the spatial frame of reference that the brain uses to designate the position of objects in the external world.

Time–space synaesthesia refers to the experience of time units such as days of the week, years, and months occupying specific spatial locations. Individuals report that time units are arranged in ovals, oblongs, circles and towers and that these can be projected in front of them or appear in their mind's eye. This phenomenon is reported as being highly prevalent (76 per cent) in grapheme–colour synaesthesia and is also closely linked to letter–space and number–space associations, all three frequently occurring with colour synaesthesia (Smilek et al., 2007). It is the role of time units in directing attention and responding to attentional cues in time–space synaesthesia, acting independently of the subject's intentions and rapidly to spatial locations, that is important. This turns our interest to the role of attention in verbal hallucinations, for instance, and hallucinations in general. It is well recognized by clinicians that patients cock their ears to given spatial locations, for example, to better hear a hallucinatory voice. The role of attention in rendering hallucinatory perceptions more salient and the degree to which attentional resources are directed towards hallucinatory experiences and the implications of that for other cognitive tasks are yet to be fully explored.

It is clear that synaesthesia is not a homogeneous phenomenon. Most of the research literature is on individuals with grapheme–colour synaesthesia. In order to have a comprehensive understanding of synaesthesia, there is a need for more work on a wider range of phenomena. For example, vision–touch synaesthesia is a phenomenon in which visual perception of touch elicits conscious tactile experiences in the perceiver. Blakemore et al. (2005) investigated an individual, a female subject C, and demonstrated that in addition to the areas activated in a control group when studied while observing a person being touched on the face or neck, the subject had activation bilaterally in the anterior insular cortex and increased activation in the left premotor cortex, confirming an overactive mirror system for touch. The authors favoured an explanation emphasizing the importance of thresholds in distinguishing between grasping that an observation of another person's face or neck being touched was that, an observation, and the fact that in C the threshold was crossed in such a way that C consciously experienced her own face or neck being touched. And there is evidence of enhanced colour sensitivity in synaesthetes who experience photisms and enhanced tactile sensitivity in synaesthetes who experience touch, suggesting a hypersensitive concurrent perceptual system, at least, in some synaesthetes (Banissy, Walsh & Ward, 2009). This explanation adds to the other possible explanatory mechanisms described earlier and is further advanced by reports of *shared pain*, a condition in which an individual experiences pain on observing another person in pain – a phenomenon that has been reported in amputees who experience synaesthetic pain in their phantom limb (Fitzgibbon & Giummarra, 2010). These phenomena are termed *mirror–sensory synaesthesia* (Fitzgibbon, Enticott & Rich, 2012). For a fuller discussion of these conditions, see Banissy et al., 2009).

11.5 General Aspects

Francis Galton (1881) estimated that one man in 20 and one woman in 15 experienced visualized numerals. There have been several reports since then providing estimates between 1:200 and 1:2000 (Baron-Cohen, Burt & Smith-Laittan, 1996; Ramachandran & Hubbard, 2001), but perhaps the most thorough is that by Julia Simner et al. (2006), in which they report on (1) 500 participants, opportunistically recruited from universities in Edinburgh and Glasgow, and (2) 1190 participants recruited from visitors to the London Science Museum in June–August 2004. In the university study, a prevalence of 4.4 per cent was found (female-male ratio 1.1:1). In the museum sample, a prevalence of 1.1 per cent was found (female-male ratio 0.9:1). In the university sample, day–colour synaesthesia was prevalent in 2.8 per cent of respondents, making it the commonest type of synaesthesia, and it constituted at least one form of synaesthesia in 46 per cent of subjects. The finding of similar prevalence between males and females was in sharp contrast to previous reports of a significantly high prevalence in females versus males, in some reports as high as 6:1.

Baron-Cohen et al. (1996) suggested that the increased prevalence in females indicated that synaesthesia is likely to be inherited as an X-linked trait, but the finding of an absence of female bias (as described earlier) calls this possibility into question. Familial patterns of synaesthesia have been investigated in order to determine individual differences and general characteristics of synaesthesia within families (Barnett et al., 2008). In this study, 95 per cent of subjects reported experiencing synaesthesia throughout their lifetime, and 5 per cent reported the onset as being in very early childhood. The majority reported grapheme–colour synaesthesia alone or with other forms of synaesthesia such as music–colour synaesthesia or number forms synaesthesia. Forty-two per cent of the total sample reported that numbers, days or months are spatially arranged (spatial sequence synaesthesia). Forty-two per cent reported at least one other first-degree relative with synaesthesia. Most families had only one type of synaesthesia, namely grapheme–colour synaesthesia, but the exact inducer and the concurrent photisms were not consistent within families. Twenty-seven per cent of families had different types of synaesthesia, for example, grapheme–colour synaesthesia and taste–shape synaesthesia.

In a study of 615 children in British primary schools aged six to seven years, the prevalence of was 1.3 per cent, with a female-male ratio of 1.6:1. This was an estimate for the prevalence of grapheme–colour synaesthesia. These children had, on average, 10.5 stable grapheme–colour associations at six to seven years of age, and at age seven to eight years of age, they had 16.9 stable associations, demonstrating that this form of synaesthesia evolves over time following environmental exposure to linguistic units (Simner et al., 2009). There are anecdotal reports of synaesthesia ceasing at puberty and the contrary claim that the onset is associated with puberty (Cytowic et al., 2009).

Synaesthetes often discover by accident that their experiences are unique. Cytowic et al. (2009) quote a number of examples in their book, *Wednesday Is Indigo Blue*.

> As seven-year old, for example, synaesthetic artist Carol Steen once said to a schoolmate, 'The latter "A" is the most beautiful pink I've ever seen'. Thinking she must be crazy, Carol's schoolmate gave her a withering look. After that, Carol never mentioned her colours to anyone until she was 20, when, as she and her family were sitting around the dinner table one evening, she told them that the number 5 was yellow – whereupon her father startled her by insisting, 'No, it's yellow ochre!' and then refused to say anything more about it.

This aspect of synaesthesia – the fact that the subjective experience of the world differs from that of the majority of people but is yet veridical and compelling – has echoes of the manner in which patients with unusual experiences and beliefs in the psychoses find them compelling and hence are described as without insight. It is not that synaesthesia is a model for psychosis but rather that subjective experiences that are imbued with a sense of reality are by definition woven into the fabric of reality, and it is difficult, if not impossible, to stand outside them with a critical eye.

There are reports of an association between synaesthesia and prodigious memory. This is best illustrated by Solomon Shereshevskii, who was studied by Aleksander Luria in the 1920s. It is reported that for him, sound elicited touch, taste and visual perception so that, for instance, 'a 2000 hertz tone at 113 decibels looked something like fireworks tinged with a pink-red hue, felt rough and unpleasant, and had the taste of briny pickle' (Ward, 2009). Ward describes one of Shereshevskii's most extraordinary feats as follows:

> In June 1936 he was presented with the most difficult material that he had ever been asked to memorise during a performance. It consisted of a long list of meaningless repeating syllables that were read aloud to him – 'ma, va, na, sa, na, va, na, ma, va. sa, na, ma, va, na' and so on. Most people find it difficult to remember words if they sound similar, even if the words have meaning and the list is short. ... At the start of his attempt to learn the list, Shereshevskii spontaneously relied on his synaesthesia. He saw an extremely thin greyish-yellow line that was related to the fact that all vowels were A. He then saw 'lumps, splashes, blurs, bunches', all of different colours, weights, and thicknesses, appear on the line that corresponded to the different consonants. The coloured line would switch direction as the reader paused to begin another section of the list. This spontaneous use of a spatial map to represent a sequence is highly characteristic of synaesthesia. ... However, as soon as he realised that the list would continue like this he felt a sinking feeling that it would take him too long to recall it if he had to decode each synaesthetic splash and lump. As such, he switched to a mnemonic technique. He grouped the meaningless syllables into the closest

meaningful words that he could think of, relying on his knowledge of Russian, Yiddish, Polish and Latvian. . . . Shereshevskii reproduced the list flawlessly. He did so again, without prior warning some four and eight years later. (pp. 115–16)

This relationship between synaesthesia and enhanced memory has been confirmed in empirical studies. Rothen, Meier and Ward (2012) show that synaesthetes have an enhanced memory in comparison to matched controls and that this tends to be visual rather than verbal memory. The suggestion is that the features of synaesthesia lead to richer encoding and retrieval of information but that there may very well be wider cognitive systems at play in this demonstrable advantage of synaesthesia for memory functions.

Finally, there is work to suggest that synaesthesia is associated with creativity. There are anecdotal reports of synaesthesia in individual artists such as Liszt, Nabokov and Hockney. There is a higher prevalence of grapheme–colour synaesthesia in art students (7 per cent) versus a control sample (2 per cent; Rothen & Meier, 2010). But it is noteworthy that there is no demonstrable association between synaesthesia and psychometric measures of creativity despite the fact that synaesthetes were more likely to engage in creative arts and to show preference for creative activity depending upon the nature of their synaesthesia (Ward, Thompson-Lake & Ely, 2008).

11.6 Conclusion

Synaesthesia is a naturally occurring anomaly that is not regarded as pathological. Its importance resides, for psychiatrists, principally in the fact that it illustrates the possible nature of the neural mechanisms underlying hallucinatory experiences and also the nature of the relationship between veridicality and insight in the psychoses.

Depersonalization

12.1 Introduction

The nature of the self is essential to an understanding of the conditions described in this section. For Jaspers (1997), the self has four formal characteristics, namely (1) the feeling of activity, that is, an awareness of being active; (2) awareness of unity; (3) awareness of identity; and (4) awareness of being distinct from an outer world and all that is not self. The awareness of activity depends upon kinaesthetic information from our joints and muscles and proprioceptive information regarding the position of bodies in space. In addition to these two sensory modalities, the other senses, including vision, hearing and touch, also contribute to our knowledge of being active. Thus, sensory data play a significant role in the definition of the body schema, in the manner in which our body exists in space and how it is engaged in particular activities. It is plain from the preceding that the awareness of activity is derived from our being embodied such that it is difficult to imagine a sense of activity of the self without corporeality. I discuss embodiment and the abnormalities of the body in the next section.

Depersonalization is a condition that undercuts this link between a sense of self and feelings of activity. Jaspers (1997) gives an example from Kurt Schneider.

> I feel nameless, impersonal; my gaze is fixed like a corpse; my mind has become vague and general; like a nothing or the absolute; I am floating; I am as if I were not . . . I am only an automaton, a machine; It is not I who senses, speaks, eats, suffers, sleeps; I exist no longer; I do not exist, I am dead; I feel I am absolutely nothing . . . I am not alive, I cannot move; I have no mind, and no feelings; I have never existed, people only thought I did. . . . The worst thing is that I do not exist. . . . I am so non-existent I can neither wash nor drink.
>
> (Jaspers, 1997, p. 122)

This example is of a severe case, so severe that it merges with Côtard syndrome, a condition that will be discussed in Chapter 16. Nonetheless, it well exemplifies the degree to which depersonalization can influence the experience of the body in action and how this experience, the defective awareness of one's activity, may influence the sense of self.

In addition to the four formal characteristics that Jaspers introduced, Scharfetter (1981, 2003) added a fifth – awareness of vitality. This can be defined as 'being present as a living being and existing [and being] actually present in a given situation' (p. 274). He gives self-accounts illustrating abnormalities of self-vitality as follows:

> I am not alive anymore; I do not exist at all; That is the core question: do I really exist? Am I alive? I am afraid that I will lose all life; My ego does not exist any longer . . . I do not feel/sense myself as living; I am dying, my heart stopped beating; I have to breathe forcedly

and repeatedly to reassure myself that I am alive; I have to see my blood, to inflict pain on myself, so that I know I am still alive; I am rotting; I am destroyed – the world is destroyed; I am totally dried up, tomorrow everything is dead; My face, my cheeks are of plastic, not living. (p. 274)

It is evident, given the foregoing, that there is an overlap between awareness of activity and awareness of vitality. The former derives from the sense of self that is constituted in activity, and the other seems to be far much more foundational, deriving from the visceral and intuitive awareness of being alive. It is possible to speculate that this sense of vitality derives from interoception, sensing from the automatic, autonomic workings of the body, for example, spontaneous breathing, heartbeat and the unaccounted but present gestures and mannerisms that make up the background rhythm of living, that we are indeed alive.

Paul Schilder (1950, pp. 138–9) describes depersonalisation as follows:

In a case of depersonalisation the individual feels completely changed from what he was previously. This change is present in the ego as well as in the outside world and the individual does not recognize himself as a personality. His actions appear to him as automatic. He observes his actions and behaviour from the point of view of a spectator. The outside world is foreign and new to him and is not as real as before. . . . The patient sees his face in the mirror changed, rigid, and distorted. His own voice seems strange and unfamiliar to him, and he shudders at the sound of it as if it were not himself speaking. [He] . . . feels that his movements are interrupted. His body feels as if it were dead and he has the sensation that a dynamo is hissing in his head. The body feels too light, just as if it could fly.

Ackner (1954a) drew attention to the problems with defining depersonalization. He noted previous emphasis on abnormalities of sense perception, primary emotional disturbance, specific anomalies of action, memory or peculiarities in self-monitoring and concluded that descriptions of depersonalization have more or less agreed on the territory of the disorder but had hitherto failed to agree as to what the boundaries of the condition are. Ackner put forward what he regarded as the most salient phenomena of depersonalization.

The most prominent feature in states of depersonalisation appears to be the statement by the patient of a subjective awareness of a feeling of change. This feeling of change can extend both to the outer and inner world, and the two aspects may be associated together or occur separately. . . . In addition, therefore, to the mere subjective awareness of a feeling of change, must be added a further necessary quality of experience, namely that of unreality or strangeness. . . . The outer world seems strange and has 'lost its character of reality'. . . . The quality of unpleasantness . . . emerges as a further important feature of depersonalisation. . . . Another important feature, in addition to the above, is a particular type of affective state, often characterized by a complaint of lack of capacity for emotional response, variable in degree and extent. (pp. 844–5)

Ackner (1954b) concluded that the term *depersonalization* included

[t]hose complaints of a change in the relationship of the patient to the world, his body or his psychic functioning which are formulated in terms which indicate to the patient, they have the quality of unreality, strangeness, foreignness, etc., and which, whilst not accepted by the patient as within his normal range of experience, are yet not expressed in frankly delusional terms. (p. 856)

Ackner (1954a) also contended that other features such as difficulty in thinking and concentration, impairment of memory, difficulty in time appreciation, poor imagery and subjective sensory abnormalities were all associated with depersonalization but were not an integral part of the condition but were ancillary features. To summarize, the leading features are (1) a subjective feeling of internal and/or external change, (2) experience of strangeness or unreality, (3) accompanied by a highly unpleasant or distressing emotion, (4) in the context of retention of insight and (5) a loss of affective response.

Sierra and Berrios (2001) showed that the phenomenology of depersonalization has remained stable for more than 100 years and that there was an invariant core of features including visual de-realization, altered body experience, emotional numbing, loss of agency feelings and changes in the subjective experience of memory.

An aspect of the subjective experience of depersonalization that needs to be emphasized is that which is often described as the 'as if' quality to the experience. Ackner (1954a) describes Miss W.D., aged 54, suffering from an involutional illness in which feelings of change occurred in the setting of depression, who made the following comments:

> It's *as if* I am living in a world of horror all on my own [emphasis mine], I feel cut off. I'm a sort of horror people would not want to be near. . . . Trees seem to be stark and staring and ugly, not attractive anymore. I used to see people nice and attractive, now those that are nice look ugly. Even fair people look dark to me now. The rooms seem different and people's faces seem behind a sort of smoke. . . . My body does not seem to have any shape or form. There's a hollowness, like a 'sack tied up in the middle' sensation. *I know* [emphasis in original] my head has shrunk, I think my leg must have shrunk, in fact everything has shrunk. My feet seem to lose themselves at times, and I feel as though I have no neck. I've got a terrible appetite and yet I feel empty all the time. . . . Now that I'm wicked, I'm just horrid. *I know* [emphasis in original] I look horrible and I feel that other people don't want to look at me for the same reason. (p. 850)

There is an important distinction being made by the patient between experiences that have an 'as if' quality and those which have a compelling veridical quality and are described with the word *know*. In general, the term *depersonalization* refers to anomalous experiences that are difficult to describe such that the subject of the experience is forced to use analogical terms in an attempt to make the experience comprehensible both to themselves and to the interviewer. Several other linguistic terms are employed to communicate to the clinician this aspect of depersonalization. Often patients use the terms *seem*, *think*, *feel* and *would* as a means of signalling the tentative quality of their descriptions and their analogical comparisons.

Other terms are used in the literature to broaden the scope of the experiences of depersonaliaation. These include *de-realization*, *de-affectualization* and *de-somatization*. De-realization refers to the subjective distortion of perception, including alterations in the size of objects and their shapes. Objects may become twisted, their colours dimmed, and faces may become unfamiliar or frightening. One patient of Mayer-Gross (1935) said: 'The world looks perfectly still, like a postcard. It is standing still; there is no point in it. A bus moves without purpose. It does not feel real. Everything in vision is dead; branches of trees are swaying without purpose' (see also Slater & Roth, 1970a). De-affectualization refers to the attenuation of emotional experience such as loss of affection, pleasure, fear or disgust. Some patients describe an absolute inability to feel and subjectively experience emotions

(Sierra, 2009). De-affectualization can include loss of empathy, and Sierra (2009, p. 32) gives an example.

> I just cannot feel anything when somebody else is suffering or in pain. My best friend was diagnosed with cancer a few months ago. We were all telling him how sorry we felt, but I just did not feel a thing, and had to pretend and say all the right words. . . . It was the same thing when my mother died.

De-somatization refers to the manner in which some patients experience their bodies. Slater and Roth (1970a) describe patients who experience their heads as numb or large or the body below the neck as dead or lifeless. Often patients use descriptions such as 'made of marble' and 'filled with cotton wool' to convey their experiences. The limbs may feel heavy and swollen, or the hands may feel unreal or unfamiliar or in some cases fill the patient with a sense of dread. Sierra (2009) makes the point that de-somatization is composed of (1) feelings of lack of ownership of one's body, (2) feelings of loss of agency over one's actions, (3) feelings of disembodiment and (4) somatosensory distortions.

12.2 Case Reports

These illustrative case examples are all drawn from Ackner (1954b).

1. Miss E.H. 30. According to the patient she had always felt apart from people and somewhat separate from events. 'I was never quite in things', she said. Severe depersonalisation symptoms had however only been present for a year prior to admission and followed the termination of an unfortunate love affair. These symptoms were present without relief and were associated with intermittent free-floating anxiety and depressive spells. She described her feelings as follows: 'The part of me that is there talking is like part of a machine, then it breaks down and I can't cope with others. ... In essence this is a feeling of unreality and sometimes I lie in bed and feel so unreal that I move just to see if I am. . . . I seem so unreal to myself, everyone else seems to have ideas and purposes, but I do not – I am not part of anything and so nothing seems real. (p. 866)

2. Mrs. N. P. 42. During the 18 months prior to admission the patient had become increasingly depressed. She was worried over her work and her marriage was unsatisfactory. She began to feel 'automatic'. Everything seemed 'detached and apart' and her brain seemed to be 'bursting up'. Two weeks before admission she had made an unsuccessful suicide attempt by walking on railway lines. Following this, the 'depression seemed to go but I felt empty and dead inside'. Superficially she was able to make a social effort and appeared brighter, 'but my brain seemed scooped up and it seemed that everything was going from me – all ideas and everything else'. ... The patient presented as a rather untidy looking woman with a somewhat expressionless face. She was tense, was somewhat aggressive in manner, answered questions slowly and appeared a little bewildered. She discussed her suicidal thoughts and ideas of hopelessness with no change of expression and little show of feeling. She was preoccupied with her feelings of change, especially with feelings related to her head and she described these repeatedly in vivid terms: 'Things look the same and my body is alright, it is the brain that is the trouble. I am conscious of myself but I'm a vacuum. When I went out recently I felt like a bag of skins with a vacuum inside. . . . There's a jammed up feeling in my head – it feels split in two if my brain was peeling off. Nothing comes into my head. There's an emptiness there. . . . I don't seem to think unless anyone says anything to me. . . . I don't respond to anything, everything seems to have gone, it started going sometime ago. Now I've

no feelings for anyone. Nothing would affect me. I can't get disturbed or upset over things though I worry and can't see any future. Things just go on and I am not part of them. I know things have happened, but I can't picture things vividly or recall them properly. (pp. 868–9)

3. Mr. E. U. 26. The patient first experienced attacks of feeling 'strange' 5 years before admission. He was at the time a Captain in charge of a Commando Unit in North Africa, and during a talk to his Unit he suddenly felt as though he was talking like an automaton. The attack lasted a few minutes, but took a few hours to disappear completely. He recalled that he was feeling tense at the time as a result of recent disputes amongst his fellow officers. Subsequently he experienced two or three attacks a week, lasting a few hours, often sudden in onset, and always preceded by a period of mounting emotional tension. Initially, he only suffered a feeling of lifelessness and automatic-like activity, but later disturbances of bodily experience appeared. He put his symptoms down to the stress of military life, but after leaving the Services and beginning a university course his symptoms further increased in duration and severity. He had increasing difficulties with his studies, became progressively more depressed and was finally admitted to hospital. ... The patient was a tall, rather awkward individual, ill at ease initially but gradually able to relax. He appeared moderately depressed but his depression cleared in the first week after admission to hospital. His attacks of depersonalisation continued however. They varied in severity but a fully developed attack had the following characteristics: There was marked loss of affective response for external events accompanied by a feeling of increased irritability and a tendency to rumination. Things looked dull, flat and lifeless. He claimed that his experience of bladder and rectal fullness seemed diminished and other sensations such as taste, tickle and pain were reduced. There was usually a singing sensation in his head. His hands and feet felt detached, as though they did not belong to him and sometimes seemed to disappear altogether. He felt clumsy in his movements and unsteady at times. His mouth seemed like 'an empty cavern' and when he chewed it sometimes felt as though he was biting powdered glass. Of himself he said 'I seem to have no personality, as if I had no background, no future and no ties at all with anyone or anything. I feel non-existent as a personality – like a vacuum.' (pp. 869–70)

12.3 Explanatory Hypotheses

In 1970, Sedman (1970) reviewed the leading theories at the time regarding depersonalization. He divided these theories into (1) an organic basis to depersonalization, (2) depersonalization as a disturbance of particular psychological functions, (3) psychoanalytical theories of depersonalization, and (4) theories that considered depersonalization as a precursor to schizophrenia. With respect to the organic basis to depersonalization, Sedman relied, to a degree, on Mayer-Gross's (1935, p. 123) opinion about the manner in which organic disease acts to cause depersonalization, described as a 'preformed functional response of the brain', much like epileptic seizures, delirium, states of semi-consciousness and catatonic states are preformed responses to organic brain insults. This description of the place of depersonalization as a symptom locates it as a release psychic phenomenon, which illustrates something of the hierarchical relationships between different brain structures in light of Hughlings Jackson's (1835–1911) conception of neurological symptoms. In this paradigm, the higher neurological structures, namely the cortex, exert control over the lower structures. Lesions of neurological structures, depending on their place within the hierarchy, produce release phenomena that are general in nature yet indicating the site of the putative lesion. In this, depersonalization can be conceived as being a non-specific symptom occurring in different kinds of diseases.

Mayer-Gross (1935) and Slater and Roth (1970) also point to the possibility that depersonalization is closely allied to anxiety and that it has been considered as a defence against anxiety, confining anxiety within tolerable limits. This view is supported by an investigation into the relationship between the clinical diagnosis of anxiety assessed by forearm blood flow, which demonstrated the lowest mean basal blood flow in patients with depersonalization, versus agitated depression, schizophrenia, phobic states and so on (Kelly & Walter, 1968). Further support came from the description of an anxious patient who experienced an attack of depersonalization while measurements of skin conductance and heart rate were being made and who surprisingly showed an alteration from what is typical for an anxious person to that of a normal person (Lader & Wing, 1966). In summary, in depersonalization there is a discrepancy between subjective anxiety and objective measures of the autonomic concomitants of anxiety.

More recent investigations into the neural underpinning of the blunting of emotional responses in depersonalization using presentation of facial expressions of emotions showed decreased response in the subcortical limbic region with increasing intensity of facial emotions compared with the control group. This was demonstrable in the right amygdala in response to increasing intensity of sadness and in the right hypothalamus with increased intensity of happiness. In addition to these findings, the participants with depersonalization showed increased inhibitory responses in the prefrontal cortex (Lemche, Anilkumar & Giampietro, 2008). There was also evidence that contradicted the established proposition of a general dampening of autonomic response in depersonalization. In a study by Lemche et al. (2008), there was a marked variability of skin conductance levels in subjects with depersonalization compared with normal control individuals and of increased rather than decreased mean skin conductance levels.

A different approach to studying basal anxiety in depersonalization was employed by Stanton et al. (2001) using basal cortisol levels and showing that in depersonalization, basal cortisol level was significantly lower than in major depression but higher than in a control health sample.

These studies point to the possibility that the severity of anxiety is integral to an understanding of the genesis of depersonalization. Sierra (2009) puts the point this way:

> Depersonalisation represents a 'hard-wired' response to deal with extreme anxiety, by combining a state of increased alertness with a profound inhibition of the emotional response system by the prefrontal cortex. According to this 'fronto-limbic' model of depersonalisation, once a threshold of anxiety is reached, the prefrontal cortex will down-regulate emotional processing on the limbic system, leading both dampened sympathetic output and reduced emotional experience. (Sierra, 2009, p. 152)

Nonetheless, there are reports that do not support this proposition and point in a different direction. Simeon, Guralnik and Hazlett (2000) report a positron-emission tomographic study of depersonalization that suggests abnormalities in visual, somatosensory and auditory processing pathways, as well as abnormalities in regions underpinning integrated body schema. Specifically, there were glucose utilization abnormalities, manifest as greater activity in portions of the sensory cortex, namely temporal, parietal and occipital lobes. The study also failed to find evidence for a primacy of temporal lobe involvement in depersonalization. Furthermore, a study of Kleine-Levine syndrome patients who also present with de-realization demonstrate marked hypoperfusion during symptomatic periods in the right dorsomedial prefrontal cortex and right parietotemporal junction, underscoring the importance and role of cross-modal regions in depersonalization (Kas et al., 2014).

The reports of demonstrable functional imaging abnormalities in regions involved in integration of sensory perception in depersonalization are matched by reported abnormalities in structure, namely lower cortical thickness in the right middle temporal region, bilateral temporal lobes, inferior temporal regions and right posterior cingulate. There was also increased cortical thickness in the right gyrus rectus and left precuneus (Sierra et al., 2014).

What is significant here is that Ackner's original view that depersonalization is the result of a relative failure of integration of an experience and not a problem of the experience itself seems pertinent once again (Ackner, 1954b). This view conceptually links depersonalization alongside other phenomena such as delusional misidentification syndromes and asomatognosia, in which there may be disruption in cortico-limbic and visual pathways resulting in failure of integration between emotions and perception (Sierra & David, 2011; see also Chapter 1).

The role of body image in aiding our understanding of depersonalization has receded in importance in recent times probably because it was originally put forward by Schilder (1936) as part of a psychoanalytical understanding of depersonalization and there is little doubt that the current influence of psychoanalysis on psychopathology is negligible. Schilder was of the view that 'patients with depersonalisation not only feel a change in perception concerning the outside world, but also have clear-cut changes concerning their own body' (p. 139). He emphasized the fact that the disturbance becomes stronger the more the perception belongs to the subject's own body, and he exemplified this view as follows: 'The patient sees his face in the mirror changed, rigid, and distorted. His own voice seems strange and unfamiliar to him, and he shudders at the sound of it as if it were not himself speaking' (p. 139).

Adler et al. (2016), in an elegant study using somatosensory event-related potentials to investigate the temporal dynamics of mirroring self-related information, exemplified by seeing touch on one's own face compared to seeing touch on a stranger's face, demonstrated that in individuals with high levels of depersonalization, determined by scores on the Cambridge Depersonalisation Scale, there was evidence of early, implicit mirroring for self-related events. This study is important because it focused on our current understanding of pre-reflective representation of body-related information, a feature that is built on sensorimotor coherence and which is driven by interaction with others and with one's own body. Singularly, this area of study on the development of the embodied self and the underlying neural mechanisms, which in principle ought to be regarded as fundamental to our understanding of depersonalization, has been little investigated. The development of a basic sense of a self-structuring body and the implications for reciprocity, social engagement and communication are outside the scope of this chapter, but it is nonetheless important to recognize the influence of self-perception of the body in social interactions.

In this regard, the relevance of the mirror neuron system, the neural correlates of self-related processes and the underpinning of how we come to understand others by mapping them onto our own bodily representations becomes significant for an understanding of depersonalization. What Adler et al. (2016) show is how these matters may be fruitfully investigated and, secondly, that there is an absence of mirroring effects for self-related stimuli in people with high levels of depersonalization, perhaps indicating that the self in these individuals is treated no differently from the body of others.

12.4 Clinical Aspects

The experience of depersonalization seems to be relatively common. A systematic review showed that between 26 and 71 per cent of individuals have experienced transient symptoms of depersonalization in a lifetime and that between 31 and 66 per cent do so following traumatic events (Hunter, Sierra & David, 2004). Examples of actual studies include that by Dixon (1963), who reported that 51 of 112 college students (46 per cent) had experienced symptoms of depersonalization over a 12-month period, and that by Sedman (1966), who reported that 35 of 50 medical students (70 per cent) had experienced symptoms of depersonalization in a lifetime. Community surveys using standardized diagnostic interviews reported 1.2 to 1.7 per cent for one-month prevalence in a UK sample and 2.4 per cent for Canada (Hunter et al., 2004).

Prevalence rates of depersonalization estimated from consecutive inpatient admissions are reported as between 1 and 16 per cent, and in clinical samples of patients with post-traumatic stress disorder, 30 per cent of war veterans and 60 per cent of those with unipolar depression are included (Hunter et al., 2004).

The age of onset is reported as between 16 and 22 years (Khanna & Ramasubbu, 1985; Simeon, Knutelska & Nelson, 2003; Baker et al., 2003). The male-female ratio is reported as 1:1 by Simeon et al. (2003), but other studies report increased prevalence in females (Myers & Grant, 1972). The onset is often sudden in nature, and the course is typically chronic and often continuous (Baker et al., 2003; Simeon et al., 2003). The mean duration was 13.9 years in the study by Baker et al. (2003).

The most frequently reported experience was 'my body felt it was not part of me'. This was followed by 'I had the feeling that I was two people. One was "going through the motions" while the other "me" was observing me' and '[M]y body seemed detached, as if my body and self were separate' (Sedman, 1966, p. 908). The least frequent experiences were 'there was no distinction between "me" and "not me". There was feeling but it was not me feeling' and '[M]y ordinary feelings of self-awareness seemed different. There seemed to be less difference between self and not-self' (Sedman, 1966, p. 908).

The features of depersonalization reported in the study by Myers and Grant (1972) are similar to those reported by Sedman (1966). These features included (1) 'I feel slightly unreal and as though I wasn't part of my surroundings, but watching from a distance; my voice sounded strange to me and did not seem to be part of me' (Myers & Grant, 1972, p. 60); (2) '[t]he feeling of not being part of my body but being outside it' (p. 60); (3) 'I don't feel the sensation of it being my hand; it is something else which is there but nothing to do with me' (p. 60); (4) 'I suddenly felt that I was really behind myself, not watching myself but detached from everything including my body to some extent' (p. 60); (5) '[m]y mother and I were walking towards each other from opposite ends of a street, and I suddenly felt an odd sense of estrangement, as if I had never seen her face in my life before' (p. 60); and (6) 'I felt disembodied . . . only my mind seemed to exist. . . . I would have to pinch myself to reassure myself that I did exist' (p. 60).

Other associated phenomena included micropsia, subjective alteration in the passage of time, difficulty in thinking and concentrating, heaviness or lightness of the body and déjà vu experiences (Sedman, 1970), and the examples given to Myers and Grant (1972) included 'I feel my big toe, thumb or any portion of my anatomy swell up to gigantic proportions'; 'I can see my body in the dark and it seems to be immensely long'; and '[g]enerally my head and lower jaw feel disproportionately large for my body and my arms and fingers thin out' (Myers & Grant, 1972, p. 60).

The experience of depersonalization occurred in clear consciousness in 13 of 35 subjects (37 per cent), and in the others, it occurred in the setting of fatigue, use of alcohol and physical illness as well as in hypnagogic states (Sedman, 1970; Myers & Grant, 1972). A number of subjects associated depersonalization with anxiety or feelings of sadness (Sedman, 1970).

It is well recognized that depersonalization can occur in a number of different medical or psychiatric settings. Ackner (1954b) described organic depersonalization as occurring in the setting of encephalitis, epilepsy, chorea, toxic and delirious states, head injury, intracranial tumours, carbon monoxide poisoning and mescaline poisoning. A case of episodic de-realization reported in association with focal cortical dysplasia of the right supramarginal gyrus, a region recognized as a hetero-modal association cortex, demonstrated the importance of the neurological site responsible for the integration of sensory input for depersonalization (Gupta, Das & Panda, 2016).

Depersonalization has been reported in vestibular disease. In an investigation of 50 patients with vestibular disease, mainly due to unilateral canal paresis, vestibular neuritis, vestibular schwannoma and benign paroxysmal positional vertigo, there was a higher prevalence of symptoms of depersonalization than in normal control individuals (Sang et al., 2006). The commonest depersonalization symptoms in patients were dizziness, sensation of shifting ground, feeling spaced out, body feeling strange and not being in control of self. Caloric stimulation in normal subjects produced the same depersonalization symptoms as the vestibular patients had reported. The authors proposed that vestibular disease caused symptoms of depersonalization/de-realization because the distorted vestibular signals create a misleading spatial reference that is mismatched with the other senses, hence giving rise to illusory or unreal perceptions. These findings have been confirmed (Jáuregui-Renaud & Ramos-Toledo, 2008), and there is a suggestion that the same is true for patients with retinal disease.

Depersonalization symptoms have been shown to emerge in normal subjects following the smoking of marijuana. The exact symptoms were not reported in the study by Mathew et al. (1993), but the Depersonalisation Inventory and Temporal Disintegration Inventory showed elevated scores at 30 minutes after smoking. In addition to these increased scores on both inventories, the subjects also had elevated anxiety, sensation of being 'high', tension, anger and confusion. Unusually, the feelings of depersonalization were not unpleasant for the subjects. Some subjects go on to develop episodes of depersonalization, so-called uncontrolled depersonalization, outside the use of marijuana, and this becomes associated with anticipatory anxiety and panic attacks (Moran, 1986).

Depersonalization occurs in anxiety disorders, including panic attacks, post-traumatic stress disorder, social anxiety and phobias. It can be a symptom of depression and of dissociative identity disorder. A full description of the relationship of depersonalization to other psychiatric disorders can be found in Sierra (2009).

The term *primary depersonalization* was applied to cases in which the depersonalization does not appear to be secondary to any other psychiatric disorder. Often it occurs in immature individuals, negotiating the tasks of adolescence with undue introspective attitude and with difficulty in establishing relationships. Davison (1964) reported seven patients and showed that the condition starts suddenly in adolescence and tends to recur over a period of years. His investigation did not reveal any structural cerebral lesion, nor was there any other psychiatric disorder present. An example is as follows:

> Miss EH., born 1923, experienced her first depersonalisation episode in 1945 and thereafter at intervals of 1–2 years. Her most recent attack in 1962 was her tenth. The episodes begin and end abruptly – 'something goes click in my head' – and, if untreated, last for three months. No physical or psychological precipitant has been discerned except that one episode in 1960 developed immediately after she recovered consciousness after having a general anaesthetic (thiopentone and nitrous oxide) for a minor operation. During each episode she feels strange and unreal – 'like in a dream' – her movements feel automatic and she has difficulty grasping what is being said to her. Although at times looking depressed and tearful, she maintains that her emotions are numb and she experiences neither pleasure nor sadness.

These cases are similar to those reported by Shorvon (1946, 1947), and it is of interest that primary depersonalization also formed the basis of Slater and Roth's (1970a) description of phobic anxiety–depersonalization syndrome in which feelings of unreality are closely associated with phobic and anxiety symptoms.

12.5 Conclusion

Depersonalization is a subjective experience that focuses on the self, indicating a disruption to the usual experience of awareness of activity and vitality and core components of the self. In addition to estrangement from the self, there can also be estrangement from the environment and detachment from one's emotions.

Chapter 13

Autoscopy and Related Syndromes

13.1 Introduction

The term *autoscopy* literally means 'seeing oneself'. It refers to a complex set of experiences involving the duplication of the self. These experiences and the underlying notion of self-duplication have a compelling influence on popular culture manifest in the writings of authors such as Fyodor Dostoyevsky (1821–1881) in *The Double*, Shusaku Endo (1923–1996) in *Scandal*, José Saramago (1922–2010) in *The Double*, Edgar Allan Poe (1809–1849) in his short story 'William Wilson' and R. L. Stevenson (1850–1894) in *Dr. Jekyll and Mr. Hyde*. This influence is extensive enough to include literary theory in such works as Karl Miller's *Doubles: Studies in Literary History* and Robert Rogers's *A Psychoanalytic Study of the Double in Literature*. Indeed, there are traces going back to the mythology of various human groups, including notions about the *fetch* in Irish mythology, *doppelgänger* in German folklore and *wraith* in Britain. The sighting of the double is usually regarded as a portent of imminent death.

In Dostoyevsky's *The Double* (Dostoevsky, 1846/2009, p. 43), the first experience of autoscopy of the protagonist of the novel, Mr. Golyadkin, is described as follows:

> With an indescribable feeling of uneasiness he started looking around. But no one was there, nothing out of the ordinary had happened and . . . meanwhile . . . he felt that someone had been standing right beside him just then, his elbows similarly propped up on the railings and – amazing to relate – had even said something to him and which concerned him.

This initial experience is an example of the 'feeling of presence'. This first experience culminated in Golyadkin's face-to-face encounter with his double.

> There was the stranger, sitting before him on his own bed, also wearing a hat and coat, faintly smiling, screwing up his eyes a little, and giving him a friendly nod. Mr. Golyadkin wanted to cry out, but he was unable to; he wanted to protest in some way, but his strength failed him. His hair stood on end and he squatted where he was, insensible with horror. And besides, he had good reason. Mr. Golyadkin had fully recognized his nocturnal friend: his nocturnal friend was none other than himself, Mr. Golyadkin in person – another Mr. Golyadkin, but identical to him in every way – in brief, in all respects what is called his double. (p. 49)

Brugger, Regard and Landis (1997) describe the phenomenology of the six main types of autoscopy. The main types include (1) autoscopic hallucination, (2) heautoscopy proper, (3) feeling of presence, (4) out-of-body experience, (5) negative heautoscopy, and (6) inner autoscopy. Autoscopic hallucination involves the pure visual experience of seeing one's own body or its upper parts as if reflected in a mirror. In other words, in autoscopic hallucination, the percept is often, but not always, a mirror image of the patient. The hallucinatory experience is in natural colours and is usually of a motionless perception, or the percept may imitate the gestures, movements or facial expressions of the patient.

Heautoscopy proper also involves visualization of the double, but in addition there may be other anomalous experiences, including a feeling of detachment, strangeness of one's body as well as feelings of lightness and, occasionally, the experience of vertigo. The double may appear transparent, grey or ghost-like. The double may imitate the patient's actions but may also act autonomously, not necessarily mirroring the patient's actions or movements. The characteristics of the double may differ from those of the patient such that it might be smaller or bigger, younger or older, and the gender may not be congruent with that of the patient. And, surprisingly, the patient may feel that he or she can see the world through the eyes of the double. Jean Lhermwitte (1951, p. 432) described it as follows:

> Sometimes the hallucinatory image appears very thin, as if it were a projection on the screen; at other times, on the contrary, it would seem to be made of jelly-like or glass-like substance, so that the patient can see everywhere around him through this ghostly illusion, which would be impossible if the image were real. This is not a constant rule, and often the phantom seems to be made of an opaque substance, not transparent to the eye.

The term *feeling of presence* describes a feeling of the physical presence of another person close to the patient who is not seen but appears to be just out of sight. The patient may, in addition, experience altered or anomalous phenomena regarding his or her body.

Out-of-body experience involves seeing one's body from an outside perspective. The core of this experience is the separation of the body from the experiencing self. Typically, the body is observed from a detached and elevated spatial position. The body is usually motionless during the observation. The surrounding environment is also seen from an elevated perspective. There is an associated strong emotional accompaniment and significance to the experience, and the emotions are more often positive, except in cases where the experience is a precursor to a seizure.

Negative heautoscopy refers to the failure to perceive one's own body in a mirror or when looked at directly. It is often accompanied by depersonalization and the loss of awareness of one's own body, sometimes termed *aschematia*. Negative heautoscopy can be unilateral, affecting the perception of only one half of the body. Finally, inner/internal heautoscopy refers to the experience of visual hallucination of one's own internal organs outside the body. Both negative and inner heautoscopy are rarely reported.

These conditions all point to severe disruption in the relationship between the self and the body. But, as Dening and Berrios (1994) say, despite the relatively extensive literature, there is significant vagueness and inconsistency in the use of the term *autoscopy* and its related terms, thereby resulting in the collection of disparate phenomena under the same rubric. And furthermore, the term *heautoscopy* is sometimes used, as earlier, following in the tradition of Menninger-Lerchenthal (1935, 1961). But this term probably adds little to a greater understanding of the phenomena under investigation.

There is the added problem that these phenomena sit within an age-old dispute within philosophy of mind and cognitive science, namely whether or not the self is separable from the body – in other words, whether autoscopy, heautoscopy proper and out-of-body experience are clinical and concrete examples of the concept of Cartesian duality, thereby confirming the dual nature of the relationship between the self and the body. This issue points at the importance of autoscopy and related phenomena for illuminating the neural underpinning of the representation of the self. This matter will be discussed in greater detail in Section 13.3. Suffice to say at this point that there may be a multiplicity of neural representations of the body that are liable to fracture in given conditions and that the phenomena that are described in this chapter shed some light on those representations.

13.2 Case Reports

13.2.1 Autoscopic Hallucination

A 31-year-old housewife presented when 27-weeks pregnant with complaints of restlessness and voices debating in her head. These symptoms had commenced one month before she conceived. . . . Some weeks after admission a new symptom was related. She had suddenly seen a vision of herself which was fleeting and caused her considerable amusement. She described it thus: 'I see myself just as I am, in clothes I'm wearing. It comes out of the blue when I least expect it and it would stagger you. It's the front view as if in a mirror. It's just a second or two. I turn away quickly whenever I see it and when I look back it's gone. It's just me and I don't do a thing.' In the following weeks as an in-patient the spectre reappeared frequently, dressed exactly as the patient, the clothing being fully coloured. It was solid and objects could not be seen through it. She felt it belonged to her and was under her complete control, though it would appear unexpectedly. No movement or action was carried out, but the apparition would stand just ahead with its face showing the patient's feelings. She never tried to approach it. The hallucination was as if she were seeing herself in a mirror, differing only in the absence of any signs of pregnancy, which were obvious in the patient at the time. The aesthetic qualities of the double gave her pleasure. 'No, it wasn't all of a bundle, not stretched out or anything like that. . . . I thought I wasn't bad looking at all, I was quite pleased.' The enthusiasm shown for this aspect of the phenomenon contrasted with the reticence displayed when other facets were discussed. The patient's explanation was that she was thinking of herself as someone else, objectifying herself. 'I am standing myself out in front of me and looking at myself. I think of "me" as "she".' The phantom double became a less compelling symptom, gradually diminishing in extent to a vision of the upper body and then of the face alone.   (McConnell, 1965, p. 67)

13.2.2 Heautoscopy Proper

A 55-year-old professional man employed by an Oxbridge college was walking across the college quadrangle when he had a sudden autoscopic experience. He saw himself directly ahead and several yards away. The image was vivid and coloured, although it did not speak to him. He stopped and the image persisted for 5–10 minutes before disappearing. During this time he also felt depersonalized and dysphoric. He then proceeded to have a full-blown panic attack. He had two similar episodes over the next few months and, fearing he was losing his sanity, consulted a psychiatrist. It emerged that he had always been an anxious man, who nevertheless had a distinguished record as an air force pilot, before leaving because of anxiety after a new plane was introduced. His present post was stressful and there were financial problems within the college which concerned him. He was currently suffering from a depressive illness with prominent anxiety symptoms.   (Dening & Berrios, 1994, p. 815)

13.2.3 Feeling of Presence

A taxi driver of 62, treated for recurrent depression, complained of the following autoscopic experience: 'Sometimes I *feel* with the special feeling of a blind man approaching a wall, or with the extra sense of a man who feels his way in a pitch-dark room, my "other self" moving about a foot in front of me or beside me. I have never seen him with my eyes, but I feel him around me and sometimes when I sit down I feel that I am resting on my own, or so to say, on my "double's" knees. After a while our two bodies merged into one again.'

(Lukianowicz, 1967, pp. 34–5)

13.2.4 Out-of-Body Experience

A 26-year-old Danish citizen, a former member of the German SS Corps. Charged with the murder of two Danish patriots, to which he pleaded guilty. Neurological diagnosis: Contusio cerebri regionis paroetalis dext. Seq. . . . On 5 February 1944 in an encounter on the Eastern Front, a shell splinter struck the left side of his head. He fell unconscious for a few minutes. After a while, he managed to walk back to the camp hospital. He was operated on four hours later. Shell splinters were removed from the *right* parietal region. As a sequela of the surgical intervention, complete, left-sided hemiplegia developed. He remembered nothing about sensory anomalies in the extremities. Within two or three months, the paralysis subsided and, according to the patient, disappeared completely by December 1944. About five months after the operation, while still in hospital on account of the moderate, left-sided hemiparesis, he had within one month five episodes of the character described below. All were identical, all began after breakfast: Suddenly, it was as if he saw himself in the bed in front of him. He felt as if he were at the other end of the room, as if he were floating in space below the ceiling in the corner facing the bed, from where he could observe his own body in the bed. The episode lasted for several minutes, ample time for the details to be impressed on his mind; he saw his own completely immobile body in the bed; the eyes closed. He noted the large [medical] dressing (which he had often seen in a mirror), the colour of the hair, the pale complexion. The experience seemed real; for the duration of the episode, he felt convinced that he was watching his own dead body. He failed to detect the respiration and was fully convinced that he had died. The vision terrified him, he was struck dumb with horror; consequently, he could not communicate with his room mates. Throughout the episode, he distinctly heard their voices coming from 'below', his own self being suspended in space. He felt positive that he had been fully conscious throughout. The vision had gone as abruptly as it had come. Afterwards, he had palpitations, and it was some time before he realized that he was still alive.

(Lunn, 1970, pp. 121–2)

13.2.5 Negative Heautoscopy

There are no convincing clinical reports of negative heautoscopy. Guy de Maupassant (1850–1893) in one of his short stories, 'The Horla', gives an account of a psychiatric patient presenting with a complaint of sense of presence and also of negative heauto-scopy. This account is often quoted to illustrate negative heautoscopy and is thought to be semi-autobiographical, as Guy de Maupassant is said, personally, to have experienced autoscopy, hallucinations, migraine and neurosyphilis (Álvaro, 2005).

> So there I was, pretending to this presence which I knew was spying on me that I was reading. All of a sudden I felt it reading over my shoulder, brushing against my ear. Leaping to my feet, I turned round so quickly that I nearly fell over. Believe it or not, though the room was bright as day, there was no sign of me in the mirror. It was empty, clear and full of light. But my reflection was not in it, despite the fact that I was standing directly in front of it. I looked at the large glass, clear now from top to bottom. I looked at it in terror.
>
> (Maupassant, 2004, pp. 241–2)

It is worth noting that negative heautoscopy is often said to be associated with depersonalization and the loss of awareness of one's own body, sometimes termed *aschematia*. An example is given by Villiers Lunn (1970).

> A 26-year-old man who five months after traumatic lesion of the right parietal region had autoscopic experiences; later there were somato-sensoric disturbances. Obviously the episodes were not combined with general impairment of consciousness. . . . For about a year prior to admission, the patient had attacks of non-characteristic headaches, most intense in the left side of the head. Whenever he stooped or moved his head violently, the headache intensified. Epileptiform episodes had occurred within the past six months; there had been vague symptoms of epigastric aura, accompanied by dyspnea; on one occasion, a right-sided Jacksonian seizure was followed by moderate, right-sided hemiparesis and hemianaesthesia lasting 24 hours. . . . Two days before admission, the patient was in bed with a severe headache when he experienced the following: Suddenly, he felt as if he were standing with folded arms, leaning over the end of the bed. He could distinctly feel the pressure across his chest. He saw his own silent, motionless body in the bed: 'I looked very pale and emaciated and I could not help thinking that I must be very ill if I look so bad.' He was extremely upset by the experience but, by a big effort of will, had managed to pull himself out of this 'split personality' state. . . . Two days before, he experienced the following: He was driving in his car to visit some friends. Suddenly, it was as if his left arm had gone leaving in its place a 'gap', almost as if his arm had been cut off at the shoulder. The sensation had been very realistic and, horrified, he had felt with his right hand to discover what had happened. He had felt much relieved when he found that everything was all right. The sensation had lasted for two hours and was equally intense throughout. Although he repeatedly convinced himself of the presence of his arm, he had to reassure himself time after time.

13.2.6 Internal Autoscopy

> In 1983 a 70-year-old Brahmin was admitted to hospital with symptoms of sadness, sleeplessness, lack of appetite, lack of interest in work and personal hygiene and markedly decreased psychomotor activity of two months duration. . . . The patient was diagnosed as suffering from M.D.P. (Depression) in accordance with ICD 9 criteria. During interview, patient reported that he could 'see' his brain as a lotus coloured pinkish mass of flesh with grooves and bulges. He further stated that it was covered by a layer of smoke. He expressed surprise over this phenomenon agreeing that it is impossible for a person to see his internal organs. He claimed he could recognize his brain, based on a vague recollection of an illustration of the brain in a textbook of Biology which he had seen as a student in seventh

standard. However, he maintained that he had never seen a real brain either human or animal, either in museums, exhibitions or at a butcher's shop. (Rao, 1992, p. 280)

13.3 Explanatory Hypotheses

The starting point is Melzack's notion of neuromatrix (Melzack, 1990; Melzack, Israel & Lacroix, 1997). This notion suggests that the basic experience of our bodies is not merely derived from a sensory pathway with inputs from sensory receptors. Rather, a network of neurons, a neuromatrix, which consists of loops that integrate the somatosensory thalamus and cortex, the limbic system and the association cortex, determines our perception of our bodies, and this perception is dynamic, fluid and constantly changing depending on our position. In this model, the neuromatrix is partly innately determined but is influenced by sensory inputs from birth onwards. This hypothesis was developed to account for the empirical fact that children with congenitally absent limbs can and do experience phantom limbs, which shows that our perception of our body is not a passive process that merely reflects inputs from the body but is continuously generated by a distributed neural network, the neuromatrix. The neuromatrix is conceived of as having stable genetic determinants and variable spatial and temporal inputs.

The profound implication of this is that there may be multiple bodily schemas, determined by the different sensory inputs, namely tactile, somatic, proprioceptive, kinaesthetic, visual and vestibular. These differing inputs, at least theoretically, are dissociable, and the anomalous bodily experiences seen in the clinic are pointers to this fact. In ordinary day-to-day experience, these differing inputs cohere to form an integrated experience of the self and body.

Olaf Blanke and Shahar Arzy (2005), in a series of studies, have worked to further our understanding of the role of the temporoparietal junction in encoding for self-location in space and also in the ascription of first-person perspective. For example, in out-of-body experience, they identify three components, namely disembodiment, which is defined as location of the experiencing self as being outside of one's body; an extracorporeal/egocentric perspective, which involves seeing the world from a distant and elevated visuospatial perspective; and autoscopy, which involves seeing one's own body from this elevated perspective. They conclude from their review of the neurological literature that in autoscopic phenomena, including autoscopic hallucination and heautoscopy proper, there is no disembodiment in autoscopic hallucination, and even where there is disembodiment such as in heautoscopy proper, the self is localized at multiple extracorporeal positions, but the visuospatial perspective is always body centred.

They show that in cases where focal brain damage is associated with the out-of-body experience, often there is involvement of either the temporal or parietal region or both and there is a suggestion that right-sided lesions predominate. This suggests that autoscopy (autoscopic hallucination and heautoscopy proper) reflects the failure of integration of proprioceptive, tactile and visual information regarding one's own body resulting in discrepant representation and ultimately leading to seeing one's own body in a position that does not coincide with the tactile/proprioceptive/kinaesthetic-experienced position. To simplify this, in autoscopy, the visual self, that is, the visual image of the self, is dissociated from the tactile/proprioceptive/kinaesthetic images, but importantly, the visuospatial perspective is retained as body centred.

Blanke and Arzy (2005) make a case for the involvement of vestibular mechanisms, particularly graviceptive functions deriving from otoliths that seem to induce sensations of floating and of elevation in out-of-body experiences. The proposition is that otolithic dysfunction may have an important causal role in out-of-body experience. The vestibular dysfunction leads to disembodiment and the elevated visuospatial perspective because of the discrepancy between personal (vestibular) space and extra-personal (visual) space.

In an in-depth study of six subjects, Blanke et al. (2004) definitively showed that brain dysfunction in the temporoparietal junction is associated with out-of-body experiences and autoscopy. All patients describing out-of-body experiences were characterized by what the authors termed a *parasomatic* body, that is, a body outside of the physical body. The visuospatial experience of this parasomatic body was experienced as immediately elevated and described as inverted by 180 degrees with respect to the extrapersonal visual space and the habitual physical body position. In addition, the parasomatic body was 2 to 3 metres above the actual physical bodies. The experiences were often described as vivid and veridical but sometimes as dreamlike. Self-recognition of the parasomatic body was immediate even when the face was not seen. In all out-of-body experiences, the actual physical body was lying prone on the ground or in bed, whereas autoscopic hallucination involved seeing the hallucinated body in an upright standing or sitting position. All patients who experienced out-of-body sensations reported vestibular sensations such as feelings of flying or floating.

In this study, complex partial epilepsy was the cause of the reported out-of-body or autoscopic hallucinatory experience in four of six patients; transitory familial hemiplegic migraine was the cause in one patient; and in the sixth patient, the experience was artificially induced by electrical stimulation of cortex distant from the primary epileptic focus. In conclusion, Blanke et al. (2004) proposed that the main forms of autoscopy (autoscopic hallucination, heautoscopy proper and out-of-body experience) result from a double disintegration in (1) personal space and (2) between personal and extrapersonal space at the temporoparietal junction. In essence, they argue that there is a requirement of an integration of our representation of our bodies with our representation of extrapersonal space for rapid and effective enactment of action within our surroundings. They speculate that ambiguous inputs from proprioceptive, tactile, visual and vestibular information underlay the anomalous experiences that are described as autoscopy. In further work, Blanke and Mohr (2005) compared patients with autoscopy with those with heautoscopy and showed right hemispheric dominance in patients with out-of-body experience and autoscopy. whereas a left hemisphere dominance was demonstrable in patients with heautoscopy. In all three forms of autoscopy, there was involvement of both the temporal and parietal lobes. These findings suggest that disembodiment from one's own body is determined by independent mechanisms that are distinct from the mechanisms involved in perspective taking (Cacioppo, 2016).

Finally, in a number of experiments, Blanke and colleagues (Lopez, Halje & Blanke, 2008; Aspell, Lenggenhager & Blanke, 2009; Lopez & Blanke, 2010; Aspell, Lenggenhager & Blanke, 2011; Ionta, Gassert & Blanke, 2011; Ionta et al., 2011) showed, using robotic technology, that it is possible to induce fundamental changes to the sense of self-location of healthy subjects. These changes were accompanied by demonstrable activity in the temporoparietal junction using functional magnetic resonance imaging. These experiments confirmed that the temporoparietal junction encodes self-location and, furthermore, that multisensory integration at the temporoparietal junction is responsible for the feeling of being an entity localized at a specific position in space and perceiving the world from this position and perspective. It is beyond the scope of this book to describe in detail these ingenious experiments (see Ionta et al. [2011] for details). An example of the experimental approach involves participants viewing a three-dimensional video image on a head-mounted display that was linked to a video camera that was placed 2 metres behind the subject, filming the participants from behind. Participants thus saw their body from an 'outside' third-person perspective. In one study using this approach, subjects viewed the video image of their body (the 'virtual body') while an experimenter stroked their back with a stick. The stroking was thus felt by the participants on their back and also seen on the back of the virtual body. The head-mounted display showed the stroking of the virtual body either in real time or not, therefore generating synchronous and asynchronous visuotactile stimulation (Blanke, 2012).

These ingenious and elegant experiments demonstrate that subjects who viewed the video image of their body while an experimenter stroked their back with a stick experienced illusory self-identification with the virtual body, and referral of touch to the virtual body was stronger during synchronous rather than asynchronous stroking. Taking account of the different approaches used to keep motor and vestibular factors constant while investigating visuotactile stimulation, the authors were able to show that a subject could experience tactile sensation located in a virtual body and, in addition, that this illusory self-identification with the virtual body includes nociceptive and physiological changes such as skin conductance response to a threat directed towards the virtual body (Blanke, 2012).

Furthermore, Blanke (2012) showed that egocentric versus allocentric mental transformations have distinct brain processes. When participants were asked to imagine shifting their position and perspective to a new position and perspective in space and make judgements about variable attributes or spatial relations of stimuli from the imagined position and perspective, these mental operations were associated with activation in the right middle temporal gyrus, supplementary motor area, left middle occipital gyrus and the left temporoparietal junction. When subjects were asked to generate egocentric mental imagery by imagining themselves at the position and perspective of virtually presented human figures, there was associated activation of the bilateral temporoparietal junction and bilateral extrastriate cortex in proximity to the extrastriate body area. Allocentric mental transformations were associated with activation of the right posterior parietal cortex.

The role of the vestibular-related areas has been studied by exposure of healthy subjects to weightlessness and caloric and galvanic stimulation with the consequence of disintegration of bodily information and altered body ownership and embodiment, thereby further clarifying the contributions of vestibular processing to these issues (Lopez et al., 2008). These hypotheses linking the temporoparietal junction to autoscopy were confirmed in a report of a patient who reported an out-of-body experience during an awake craniotomy for resection for a low-grade glioma. Stimulation of the subcortical white matter in the left temporoparietal junction repetitively induced out-of-body experiences. The patient described floating above the operating table and looking down on herself (Bos et al., 2016). In a different report, two patients with epilepsy had electrical stimulation of the right medial occipitoparietal cortex, including the right precuneus and occipitoparietal sulcus, reported seeing their own faces, facing themselves in the left visual field. This study suggests that the stimulated region may be involved in representations of one's own face (Jonas, Maillard, Frismand & Colnat-Coulbois, 2014). Nakul and Lopez (2017) make the point that out-of-body experience is very rarely induced by electrical brain stimulation, and they conclude from this that the neural underpinnings of the anchoring of the self to the body must be exceedingly robust and that in the case reported by Bos et al. (2016), the effect was produced by stimulation of subcortical tracts. Indirect confirmation for the role of the temporoparietal junction was supported by the finding in another study in a patient who had electroencephalograph recordings during a heautoscopy experience and a right parietal electrical focus (Anzellotti et al., 2011).

13.4 Clinical Aspects

Mora and Jenner (1980) described the clinical features of autoscopy, including autoscopic hallucination and heautoscopy proper, as follows: the appearance of the double occurs suddenly and without warning, although occasionally it can be preceded by a feeling of 'presence'. In epilepsy and migraine, it is usually preceded by sensory aura. The frequency of the experience is indeterminable. In some patients there are one or two episodes in a lifetime, whereas in others there are reported frequent episodes or even continuous experiences of the double. The experience can occur at any time. The double is usually situated within the visual space of the patient. There is often an emotional affinity between the patient and double. The double is reported to be just beyond reach of the arm or may be further away. The double may copy the patient's movements and facial expressions. Occasionally, the double only stares at the patient and fades away or disappears if the patient attempts to approach or touch it. The double appears grey or misty but is occasionally flesh coloured. The double may be transparent, vitreous or jelly-like. It is reported sometimes to be solid in appearance but rarely, if ever, casts a shadow. The patients report feelings of anxiety, discomfort, sadness or amazement on seeing the double. The actual physical body may be experienced as cold and lifeless, behaving like an automaton, whereas the double may seem more alive and real. Finally, the double may seem sad, cold or weary.

It is now established that the feeling of presence is not preferentially lateralized to the left side of the body, as was previously thought. Brugger (1994) showed that in the 11 cases where focal brain lesions were associated with a feeling of presence, there were 6 right-sided lesions and 5 left-sided lesions. The feeling of presence was not preferentially lateralized to the left hemispace.

In a large study of 1,000 British adults, aged 18 years or over, responding to a questionnaire about anomalous experiences, 10 per cent of respondents reported out-of-body experiences (Pechey & Halligan, 2012). Blackmore (1986) conducted a survey of patients with schizophrenia for out-of-body experience and found in the control group of patients attending a general hospital without psychiatric history that 13 per cent had previously had out-of-body experiences. In patients with epilepsy, the prevalence of out-of-body experience is 7 per cent, and this was not associated with demographic factors, medical history, or seizure characteristics (Greyson, Fountain & Derr, 2014). In patients presenting with dizziness, out-of-body experience occurred in 14 per cent compared to 5 per cent in healthy aged-matched control individuals. In this sample, out-of-body experience was associated with peripheral vestibular disorders and was predicted by depersonalization/de-realization, depression and anxiety, as well as by migraine (Lopez & Elziere, 2018). In summary, evidence suggests that out-of-body experience occurs in approximately 5 to 10 per cent of the general population.

In their survey of the published literature dating back to 1935, Dening and Berrios (1994) reported on 56 cases. The mean age was 39.5 years, and there were 38 men (67.8 per cent). Most cases (58 per cent) were associated with neurological disease, most commonly epilepsy. There was no significant association with hemispheric laterality. The commonest psychiatric disorder associated with autoscopy was depression, which was present in 18 per cent of cases. Eight cases (13 per cent) were associated with schizophrenia or organic hallucinosis. The autoscopic experiences lasted less than 30 minutes in most cases. The patients reported seeing the face of the double, the upper body, but less often the whole body. Most patients were in bed at the time of the experience or in a sitting position. The commonest affective response was dysphoria, including distress, fear, anxiety and depression. Positive affective response very rarely occurred. Thirteen patients (23 per cent) reported the doubles as talking. These were all male patients, and autoscopy occurred in the context of psychosis in these cases.

The three cases reported by Dewhurst and Todd (1956) illustrate the relationship between focal neurological lesions and autoscopy: case 1 had subarachnoid haemorrhage, case 2 had a multicystic malignant glioma of the left posterior temporoparietal region, and case 3 had sustained traumatic brain injury from shrapnel, in 1917, that destroyed his right eye, passing through the right orbit into the right temporal lobe and causing epilepsy. Bhaskaran, Kumar and Nayar (1990) reported on a case in which the double appeared in the hemianopic field in a 60-year-old man who had suffered a right occipital infarct. Computed tomographic scanning showed a mixed-density, irregular lesion with contrast enhancement and surrounding oedema in the right occipital cortex consistent with an infarct.

It is reported that autoscopic phenomena occur in 6.3 per cent of individuals with simple partial, complex partial or generalized tonic-clonic seizures. In the case series reported by Devinsky, Feldmann and Burrowes (1989), the temporal lobe was involved in 86 per cent of cases. In patients presenting with ictal lateralized autoscopic phenomena, the underlying well-defined epileptic focus is mostly contralateral to the side of the autoscopic appearance (Hoepner et al., 2012).

Rarely, autoscopy may involve multiple doubles. Brugger et al. (2006) reported a 41-year -old male patient presenting with polyopic heautoscopy in the context of a tumour in the insular region of the left temporal lobe. This case suggests that the purported breakdown in the integrative functions underlying autoscopy may rarely involve multiple mappings of the body, in the so-called neuromatrix, thereby resulting in the illusory experience of multiple doubles.

There are reports of autoscopy in multiple sclerosis (Arias et al., 2007), Huntington's disease transient (Martínez-Horta, Perez-Perez & Pagonabarraga, 2020), hyperglycaemia (Arias et al., 2007), as migraine aura (Podoll & Robinson, 1999) and post-eclamptic brain damage involving the occipital cortex and basal ganglia bilaterally (Zamboni, Budriesi & Nichelli, 2005). In Parkinson's disease, patients who experience a feeling of presence reported it as not distressing, characterized as usually brief in duration, and experienced as occurring beside or behind the patient. Most of the patients checked for a real presence, yet their insight was preserved. Finally, the feeling of presence was associated with a higher daily dose of levodopa-equivalent dose (Fénelon, Soulas & Langavant, 2011).

Autoscopy has been reported in association with psychiatric disorders. In Lukianowicz's (1967) classic paper on disturbances of body image in psychiatric disorders, they reported on three cases, one presenting with migraine, another with recurrent depression and the third with schizophrenia, and Mora and Jenner (1980) summarized the literature, confirming that autoscopy can occur in the context of schizophrenia, depression, obsessive-compulsive disorder, anxiety, somatoform disorders and fatigue and exhaustion. A questionnaire survey of patients with schizophrenia inquiring into out-of-body experiences, among other symptoms, found that even though 42 per cent of patients with schizophrenia endorsed having had out-of-body experiences, when they responded to a follow-on questionnaire, this proportion decreased to 14 per cent, which was no more than the control group. The authors concluded that there is no evidence that out-of-body experience is symptomatic of schizophrenia (see also Blackmore, 1986).

There are reports of autoscopy in the context of childbirth as part of postpartum psychosis. Craske and Sacks (1969, p. 344) reported a rare variant of double autoscopy in a 32-year-old female patient arising in the seventh week postpartum.

> On each occasion that the two images appeared they were both static, silent, opaque and blue in colour. . . . One image always appeared sitting in a chair straight ahead of the patient. It was always dressed in a blue sari which the patient recognized as her own. . . . [T]he other image, occurring simultaneously with the first image covered the patient's body . . . 'like a mask, but was separated from it by a thin layer'. It felt very light in weight, but 'although it was made of air I could feel it resting on me'.

There are single case reports suggesting an association between autoscopy and suicide. Brugger et al. (1994) reported on a 21-year-old male patient with a history of complex partial seizures with bilateral temporal lobe foci. Computed tomography showed a hypodense lesion in the mesiobasal temporal lobe that magnetic resonance imaging demonstrated as multicystic in nature. The lesion was removed and shown to be a dysembryoplastic neuroepithelial tumour. The authors write

> On the respective morning he got up with a dizzy feeling. Turning around, he saw himself lying in bed. He became angry about 'this guy who I knew was myself and who would not get up and thus risked being late at work'. He tried to wake the body in the bed first by shouting at it; then by trying to shake it and then repeatedly jumping on his alter ego in the bed. The lying body showed no reaction. Only then did the patient begin to be puzzled about his double existence and become more and more scared by the fact that he could no longer tell which of the two he really was. Several times his bodily awareness switched from the one standing upright to the one still lying in bed; when in the lying mode he felt quite awake but completely paralysed and scared by the figure of himself bending over and beating him. His only intention was to become one person again and, looking out of the window (from where he could still see his body lying in bed), he suddenly decided to jump out 'in order to stop the intolerable feeling of being divided in two'. At the same time, he hoped that 'this really desperate action would frighten the one in bed and thus urge hIm to merge with me again'. The next thing he remembers is waking up in pain in the hospital. (p. 839)

Misuse of ketamine is associated with a number of anomalous experiences, including illusory movement experiences, out-of-body experiences and out-of-body autoscopy (Wilkins, Girard & Cheyne, 2011, 2012). In the sample studied, 91 per cent reported having at least one illusory movement experience, 83 per cent reported at least one out-of-body feeling and 48 per cent reported at least one out-of-body autoscopy. The control sample consisted of individuals who had a history of drug misuse other than ketamine, including alcohol, cannabis, lysergic acid diethylamide and 3,4-methylenedioxymetamphetamine. The lifetime frequencies while under the influence of ketamine were 77 per cent for illusory movement experiences, 63 per cent for out-of-body experiences and 24 per cent for out-of-body autoscopy. This compared with the control sample as follows: 78, 52 and 30.5 per cent, respectively. This suggests that autoscopy is also associated with misuse of alcohol, cannabis and other psychotropic agents. Autoscopy also has been reported in glue sniffing (Hitomi, 2001).

13.5 Conclusion

The varying subjective experiences that make up autoscopy can only be understood in light of the concept of a neuromatrix, a network of neurons which consists of loops that integrate the somatosensory thalamus and cortex, the limbic system and the association cortex that determines our perception of our bodies, and this perception is dynamic, fluid and constantly changing depending on our position. The real importance of autoscopy is thus in highlighting the possibility of dissociation of the component parts of the body concept and bringing attention to the processes on which unity of the body concept is based.

Dissociation

Possession States and Dissociative Identity Disorder

14.1 Introduction

The nature of the self depends on at least four presuppositions, namely a subjective awareness of activity, a subjective awareness of a sense of unity of self over time, an awareness of a persisting and singular identity over time and, finally, a distinct sense of being separate from other material objects and other selves. In this chapter, I deal with two conditions, possession states and dissociative identity disorder (multiple personality disorder), both of which seem to undermine the presupposition that the sense of self is predicated upon a unified sense of self over time and a sense of a persisting and singular identity over time.

It is worthwhile to understand the roots of our notion of the self. John Locke (1632–1704), in *An Essay Concerning Human Understanding*, equated self with person and wrote 'person is a forensic term, appropriating actions and their merit, and so belongs only to the intelligent agents, capable of law' (Locke, 1817, p. 189). He goes on, saying that a person 'owns and imputes to itself past actions, just upon the same ground and for the same reason that it does the present' (p. 189). Finally, Locke says, 'What a person stands for . . . is a thinking intelligent being that has reason and reflection and can consider itself as itself, the same thinking thing in different times and places; which it does by . . . consciousness' (p. 180).

In the Lockean approach to the concept of self, reason and intelligence matter, and the capacity for continuity of identity is important. And the continuity of identity over time is itself dependent, in Locke's approach, on 'participation of the same continued life, by constantly fleeting particles of matter, in succession vitally united to the same organized body' (p. 177), even though for Locke it is consciousness that counts irrespective of how personal identity is itself preserved. To put this simply, the identity of the self is guaranteed by its vital unity to the same body over time, even though it is the capacity for memory that safeguards identity, not the mere co-location of self and body.

The conditions discussed in this chapter demonstrate that even though the self remains vitally united to a single physical body, the possibility exists for the self to experience itself as only one of a potential group of other selves inhabiting this singular body. And in some circumstances the multiple selves have different appreciations of autobiographical memory or experience disruptions of their autobiographical memories.

This empirical fact was anticipated by David Hume (1711–1776), the Scottish Enlightenment philosopher. In *A Treatise on Human Nature*, Hume argued that '[w]hat we call *mind* is nothing but a heap or collection of different perceptions, united together by certain relations, and suppos'd, tho' falsely, to be endowed with perfect simplicity and identity' (Hume, 1817, p. 207). He continued:

When I enter most intimately into what I call *myself*, I always stumble on some particular perception or other, of heat or cold, light or shade. ... I never catch *myself* at any time without a perception, and never can observe anything but the perception. When my perceptions are remov'd for any time, as by sound sleep; so long as I am insensible of *myself*, and may truly be said not to exist. (p. 252)

Finally, Hume wrote the following, accentuating his proposition not only that the self is both elusive and illusory but also that our notion of its unity and the singularity of its identity are fictitious in nature:

The mind is a kind of theatre, where several perceptions successively make their appearance.... There is properly no *simplicity* in it at one time, nor *identity*. ... There are successive perceptions only, that constitute the mind; nor have we the most distant notion of the place, where these scenes are represented, or of the materials of which it is compos'd. (Hume, 1817, p. 253)

To summarize, the self is not a thing but a complex concept that continues to elude definitive description. The formal characteristics that seem to determine its very essence are problematical and open to critical inquiry. Nonetheless, when we take an ordinary attitude, which is dependent on our subjective experience, towards the nature of the self, it seems obvious that there is a unity of experience despite there being disparate functions such as memory, perception and agency and that this unity of experience belongs to a single, recognizable identity. To emphasize this point, Immanuel Kant (1724–1804), in the *Critique of Pure Reason*, wrote

When I seek to draw a line in thought ... obviously the various manifold representations which are involved must be apprehended by me in thought one after another. But if I were always to drop out of thought the preceding representation (the first part of the line . . .) and did not reproduce them while advancing to those that follow, a complete representation would never be obtained: none of the aforementioned thoughts, not even the most elementary representations of space and time, could arise. (Kant, 1999, p. 133)

For Kant, this unity of consciousness is the precondition for all our experience of the world. What is intriguing are the possibilities which possession states and dissociative identity disorder open up for, at least the contention that, the self may be fissile in nature or at the very least that there may be situations in which the self may appear to be capable of splintering or coexisting with other centres of agency and awareness.

14.2 Possession States

It is essential, at the outset, to make clear that possession is a culturally sanctioned phenomenon and that it exists across all cultures. It is distinct from possession states and related phenomena that occur in the context of psychiatric disorders. The relationship between culturally sanctioned phenomena and the manifestation of motifs drawn from these phenomena embedded within psychiatric disorders illustrates the manner in which psychopathological objects can be parasitic upon normal cultural artefacts. This is hardly surprising given that the contents of consciousness, by definition, are derived from the social world and that this fact is as true for normal experiences as they are for psychopathology.

It is often said that the three subjects that anthropology has focused on are the concepts of totems, trance possession and witchcraft. This is not the place to offer a critique of the structure of anthropological discourse, its relationship to European imperialism and its preoccupation with what it sees as 'primitive peoples' and the 'othering' of non-European populations. But it is important to say at the outset that trance possession and its related phenomena are human phenomena and not, in my view, some characteristic behaviours that signal non-European sensibility or culture.

Erika Bourguignon (1973) sets possession trance in the context of institutionalized forms of altered states of consciousness, namely a structured and normalized pattern of behaviour that exists within a religious context. The emphasis here is that these are not pathological behaviours; rather, they are behaviours that occur in the complex interplay between religious beliefs and institutions and that are emergent in the context of cultural change. In this framework, as Bourguignon puts it,

> A person in an altered state may be thought of as 'possessed' by certain spirits or, on the other hand, his soul, or one of his souls, may be thought to be temporarily absent. Such beliefs account for the individual's behaviour as well as for his altered subjective experience of himself and of the world. If he behaves strangely, the behaviour may be attributed not to him but to a possessing spirit. If he hears or sees unusual things, these may be spirits he is seeing or hearing, or messages from spirits he is receiving. (Bourguignon, 1973, pp. 3–4)

Bourguignon reports that in her sample of 488 societies, 90 per cent had institutionalized forms of altered states of consciousness ranging from 97 per cent in aboriginal North America to 80 per cent in the circum-Mediterranean region. Thus, the capacity to experience altered states of consciousness is a biologically human one, but the utilization, institutionalization and patterning of these states depend on culture and hence are variable in their features and manifestations (Bourguignon, 1973). Next, Bourguignon makes a distinction between possession trance and trance, the former referring to altered states of consciousness that involve the experience of hallucinations or visions that are interpreted as the experiences of the soul of the person, its temporary absence or its journeys or adventures, and the latter may involve the repetition of messages of spirits to an audience, the imitation of the actions of spirits or the narration of the subject's spirit journey. Possession trance in this scheme is the impersonation of spirits, the acting out of their speech and behaviour.

Finally, Bourguignon reports that societies that predominantly had possession trance rather than trance alone or a combination of trance and possession trance are more likely to have a degree of societal complexity, by which she means a large population, and the largest local group, the presence of slavery or a recent history of slavery, social stratification, sedentary settlement pattern and a complex hierarchy of jurisdictional levels. They also tend to have marriage by bride price rather than marriage without compensation and to have extended rather than independent nuclear families. In addition, these societies are more likely to have patrilineal or matrilineal kin groups, are more likely to have duo-lateral cousin marriages and to practice the segregation of adolescent boys (Bourguignon, 1973).

The phenomenology of possession trance (spirit possession) is well described in Mischel and Mischel's (1958) report of spirit possession in Shango worshippers in Trinidad. In this description, Tanti, a woman in her forties is the individual being described.

> When the spirit begins to manifest 'on' or 'catch' Tanti, a dramatic physical transformation takes place. If in a standing position, she staggers, appears to lose her balance, begins to sway (bending her body forward and backward rhythmically), and may fall either to the ground or into the arms of bystanders. Her entire body begins to vibrate, while her arms are either rigid at her sides or stretched out above her. Her feet are planted widely apart and she may lurch back and forth from toe to heel. The vibrations increase in intensity, and somewhat resemble the convulsions of a seizure state. At the same time, she emits deep grunts and groans. Her

jaw begins to protrude, her lips pout and turn down sharply at the corners, her eyes dilate and stare fixedly ahead. . . . In the standing position her stomach and pelvis are thrust forward, her head and shoulders are thrown back, legs wide apart, hands on hips. The entire posture is quite rigid. At this point the spectators recognize that full possession by the particular power has occurred. From then on the individual who is possessed, the 'horse', becomes identified with the power, and is referred to and treated as such. (p. 250)

Mischel and Mischel report that in the Shango ceremony in Trinidad, possession may never occur in the lifetime of an individual who attends the ceremonies, or it may occur five or more times in one night. Such is the variability of the phenomenon. The same individual may be repeatedly possessed by the same power or by different powers at different times. The period of possession may last a mere 10 minutes or 5 or more hours, but on average, the state lasts less than an hour. The possession trance appears to be induced by drumming and the participants talk about 'falling with (or to) the drums'. In addition to the drumming being integral to possession trance, the atmosphere of crowd excitement, singing, the darkness, candles, circular dancing and ceremonial rituals seems to have a facilitative aspect too.

The intensity of the altered state of consciousness appears to vary. But even in cases where there seems to be profound partial or temporary loss of consciousness, the individual appears to continue to recognize those around her and may refer to them by name and make references to past experiences. Finally, recovery from possession often terminates with the person spinning rapidly and suddenly falling to the ground (Mischel & Mischel, 1958).

The features of all possession trances do not all follow this description. Among the Muria people of Central India, possession trance is induced by the pursuit of religious vertigo through dance and swinging. The ritual use of the swing is not confined to the Muria but is described in the Vedic ritual of Mahavrata (Gell, 1980). Despite the difference in the method associated with inducing possession trance, the behaviours associated with possession are similar, if not identical.

The individuals whom I observed going into trance seemed to do so in sequence of regular stages. To begin with, the body is held rigid, the neck extended, and a slight trembling begins to become apparent, particularly affecting the forearms and hands. The eyes stare fixedly but later the eyelids are seen to flutter and droop. The trembling seems to be synchronous with the music, if any, though it is also present if the medium is entering trance without the assistance of drumming. (Gell, 1980, p. 234)

The question is what function possession trance serves in culture. This question has been addressed in several ways. The most influential response to this inquiry is that by Lewis (1989). He argued that as women are the most susceptible to spirit possession, the phenomenon can be traced to the innate conflict between men and women in certain types of societies where men monopolize the social structure. This monopolization of the social structure by men means that women are subordinated to men in the social hierarchy, and this results in women being peripheral. In essence, possession trance is predicated on sexual rivalry, conflict and tension between the sexes. Possession trance is then seen as a means of addressing power inequality in male-dominated societies. This position is not without its critics. For example, Peter Wilson (1967) made the point that patriarchy is alive and well in Western society, yet on Lewis's account, spirit possession has declined in Western society, its therapeutic function having been taken over by various forms of psychotherapy.

Another approach has been to view possession trance as a system of communication between a minimal triad of three 'persons' – host, spirit and intermediary (Lambek, 1980).

In the following example from Malagasy speakers of Mayotte, the therapeutic role of possession trance is overt, and the communicative aspects foregrounded:

> Possession in Mayotte is characterized by temporary and periodic trance states during which the social identity of the individual being possessed (the host) is replaced by that of the possessing spirit. It is said that the spirit rises into the head of the host and takes temporary control of the body. A sharp distinction is maintained between the identities of spirit and host. Indeed, while most (but not all) hosts in Mayotte are women, the spirits who replace them are usually (but, again, not always) male. . . . Possession is defined in Mayotte as an affliction, and it is frequently indicated by symptoms of physical or mental distress which do not respond to other forms of treatment. The 'cure' is a lengthy process which involves not the exorcism but the socialization of the spirit – establishing the spirit's particular identity and entering into an exchange relationship with it. The spirit demands expensive feasts and presents in return from releasing the patient from pain, weakness and other distress. Once the cure is effected, the spirit generally continues to visit periodically – both at the public feasts of other hosts undergoing cures and in the privacy of the host's home – as something of a family intimate. (Lambek, 1980, p. 319)

In this last example, possession is identified as a disturbance in the individual, and this stands in contrast to the preceding discussions, where possession trance is not conceived of as a sign of psychological disturbance or distress requiring amelioration. Rather, possession is part of socially sanctioned ritual of patterned behaviour with comprehensible cultural or religious underpinnings. Oesterreich's (2013) account of possession focuses, almost exclusively, on the form of possession that occurs in a disturbed individual whose possession signals either demonic possession or an errant psychology. The semiotics of possession of this kind are not dissimilar to the ritualized forms described earlier. Oesterreich describes transformation of the physiognomy, for example.

> [T]hat Asmodeus (a demon) was not long in manifesting his supreme rage, shaking the girl backwards and forwards a number of times and making her strike like a hammer with such great rapidity that her teeth rattled and sounds were forced out of her throat. That between these movements her face became completely unrecognizable, her glance furious, her tongue prodigiously large, long, and hanging out of her mouth, livid and dry to such a point that the lack of humour made it appear furred, although it was not at all bitten by the teeth and the breathing was always regular. (p. 18)

Oesterreich also describes changes in the voice, accompanying the changed countenance described earlier, the intonation corresponding to the character of the possessing agent. Oesterreich quotes one of Pierre Janet's cases.

> It was a very extraordinary spectacle for us who were there present to see this wicked spirit speak by the mouth of the poor woman and to hear now the sound of a masculine, now that of a feminine voice, but so distinct the one from the other that it was impossible to believe that only the woman was speaking. (p. 20)

Finally, Oesterreich describes the content of speech as 'betraying a coarse and filthy attitude, fundamentally opposed to all accepted ethical and religious ideas' (p. 22). An example given is as follows:

> In this state the eyes were tightly shut, the face grimacing, often excessively and horribly changed, the voice repugnant, full of shrill cries, deep groans, coarse words; the speech expressing the joy of inflicting hurt or cursing God and the universe, addressing terrible threats now to the doctor, now to the patient herself, saying with deliberate and savage obstinacy that he would not abandon the body of this poor woman and that he would torture both her and her near ones more and more. (Oesterreich, 2013, p. 22)

The role of authority figures in shaping and enabling the character and boundaries, namely the structure, of possession in any individual has been well described by Sluhovsky (1996). His study focused on the possession and exorcism of a 16-year-old girl, Nicole Obry (1565–1566), 'a pretty, pious, and good-natured girl' (p. 1039) who was said not to be very intelligent. She lived in the diocese of Laon in Picardy, France, having moved there three months after her marriage. She complained that the spirit of her recently deceased grandfather appeared to her while she was praying in the local church close to where her grandfather was buried. She claimed that her grandfather told her that he was suffering in purgatory because he had died suddenly before he had time to confess. Her grandfather asked Nicole to mobilize his family to pray for his soul and to give charity on his behalf. At this stage, Nicole was not possessed but merely in receipt of apparitions. The situation changed after her family were unable to make the required pilgrimage to Santiago, and Nicole started to suffer with involuntary seizures. It was in response to questioning by the local teacher that it became apparent that the spirit was not simply outside Nicole's body but was in fact within her body. Examination by a visiting cleric, Friar Pierre de la Motte, concluded that '[a] devil possessed this body' (p. 1040). Exorcism of her possessing demon was conducted in public, during which the demon admitted that his name was Beelzebub. This case is reported as having set the tone for numerous other cases of spirit possession in France.

Sluhovsky argued that there was a distinction between possession and witchcraft. Possession involved involuntary interaction between a human being and a possessing entity, and its termination by exorcism resulted in a healed person who was re-integrated into society. Witchcraft, in contrast, involved a voluntary pact with the devil, usually signed not by the possessed person but through a third participant. Accusations of maleficence were associated with witchcraft (Sluhovsky, 1996). In the sixteenth century, possession was defined by a set of well-established behaviours, including the ability to understand foreign languages, to manifest unnatural strength, to react with horror to sacred objects and to suffer from involuntary convulsions, gestures, seizures, vomiting, fits, faints and paralysis.

Finally, possessed people 'operated within very constrained boundaries, which were defined by the Church. They had to convince clerics, inquisitors, exorcists, doctors, and lay viewers that they were, indeed, possessed and not witches, melancholic, epileptic, or simply mad' (Sluhovsky, 1996, p. 1045).

Possession states as described and defined in psychiatry have to be understood against this background of ritualized possession trance, demonic possession in individuals and the role of authority figures in determining the nature and origins of particular patterned behaviours. As Sluhovsky put it, 'Theologians and doctors in the sixteenth century tried continuously and unsuccessfully to delineate clear distinctions among these different manifestations [witches, melancholic, epileptic or simply mad] of supernatural intervention' (Sluhovsky, 1996, p. 1045). The quest for distinctions continues to date.

The early psychiatric literature on demonic possession was almost exclusively confined to France. Yap (1960) reviewed this literature in 1960 and identified Jacques Jean Llhermitte (1877–1959) as the leading authority of the subject. Llhermitte divided possession into true possession and false possession, a distinction that was not widely held by other French psychiatrists. Llhermitte saw possession as a complex state that was not itself a nosological entity or a legitimate syndrome; rather, it was only a picturesque colouration given to psychoneuroses. Furthermore, he distinguished between two types of possession: one occurred in episodes or attacks and was characterized by clouding of consciousness, and the other was insidious in onset and characterized by lucidity, and the patient was capable of giving an account of the psychological and psychical aspects of the experience of being possessed.

Contemporary conceptualizations group possession and trance states as part of dissociative disorders, emphasizing the temporary loss of personal identity, a narrowing of awareness of immediate surroundings or narrow and selective focusing on environmental stimuli and conviction that the subject has been taken over by a spirit, power, deity or other person. Usually, there is the proviso that these experiences occur outside of religious or culturally accepted situations.

14.2.1 Case Reports

Case 1

A woman of 45, married to a railroad worker and with five children, had come down to Hong Kong by herself. For 4 years she had been treated in a tuberculosis hospital. She had only about 5 years' schooling and had before marriage worked in a kindergarten. Two of her sisters had died of phthisis in their youth. For a number of years she had been troubled by a dream, during which she would find herself in a room with one of her dead sisters, each lying on a bed, and the sister would pull her over, whereupon she would wake up in a fright. . . . Latterly she had been greatly influenced by evangelists of the Assembly of God, both Chinese and western. This revivalist sect believed firmly in the possibility of possession by God and the cure through this means of various illnesses. The patient was suffering from chronic pulmonary tuberculosis with cavitation and had recently been advised to have a thoracoplasty operation done. She was rather troubled by this and was made all the more uneasy by the fact that the evangelists visiting the hospital had told her that she was sinful and that if she believed in God she would be saved; the Holy Ghost would possess her and thereby cure her without need for an operation at all. While normally she appeared to have made up her mind and would press for her transfer to a general hospital for the operation, she at other times became confused and would not consider it at all. She wandered about during these episodes, mostly at night, sometimes appeared to pray, and at odd times said that she was taking on herself the task of driving away devils from the other patients. She said she could see God when she had her eyes closed. This continued for several days and then she became lucid again. However, after a further 10 days she became mute and tearful at different times and started to speak in what purported to be English and Hebrew. She declared that she was possessed by two different Gods. One of these was Jesus Christ and when possessed she declared that the patient was to follow Him, and He would return among men, and that she was to be well and have eternal life. The other God was obscure in nature, but told her and her audience in a mixture apparently of English and Hebrew (which she later 'interpreted') that she should be a prophetess to help to remove pain and sorrow from all the world. She was then admitted into the mental hospital and made an uneventful [sic] recovery after two weeks with sedation and psychotherapy.   (Yap, 1960, p. 131)

Case 2

S.D., [a] 32-year-old married lady, with no formal education, presented with the complaint of abnormal behaviour for 12 days. . . . 12 days before admission while attending a *kirtan* the patient felt uneasy. She had giddiness and a tendency to fall down on getting up. She had limpness of the neck. That night she could not sleep properly. Next day, at noon she again felt uneasy and her neck became limp and the face became pale. One of the neighbours who was called upon to see suggested that she appeared to be possessed by a spirit. That night she started behaving as if possessed by the spirit of one of the earlier tenants of the house who died 4–5 years ago. Her voice changed and she spoke and behaved like a man. She ordered her husband that he should change the residence and threatened him with dire consequences if he did not do so. Next day a 'faith healer' was called to treat her but he failed to drive away the spirit. The abnormal behaviour continued and another 'faith healer' was consulted and he too failed in his mission. . . . On the third day, they moved into a relative's house. After 6 days the family doctor was consulted and persuaded them to remove the loop which the patient had got inserted for family planning purpose 15 days earlier; the husband felt that the blocked blood might have gone into patient's head with resultant abnormal behaviour. . . . Mental examination revealed an untidy, uncooperative lady with a moderate degree of excitement. She talked irrelevantly in a state of possession and was not accessible to reason. In the state of possession she shouted at her husband in a male voice (the possessor's), 'I will eat you up, you should leave my home. I will not stop following you till you leave this city'. . . . During her stay in the ward, sometimes she also behaved as if possessed by goddess *Durga*. . . . During detailed interviews with her and during the narcoanalytic sessions, the following information was collected. She had learnt, a few days prior to getting upset, that a man previously living in the premises that they were presently occupying had died there. (The man had actually died elsewhere but the patient somehow wrongly interpreted it to be so.) Thereafter the patient started fearing the place. Sometimes she thought that the spirit might still be lurking around the house. She feared that the departed spirit might be upset by her children passing urine, etc. in the house. Her fears came into the open when during her illness, she became possessed by that man's spirit. Within three days of possession, they moved into a relative's house.

(Teja & Khanna, 1970, pp. 75–6)

14.2.2 Explanatory Hypotheses

Possession trance and related phenomena are conceptualized as resulting from *dissociation*, a term which is itself not fully understood but which, nonetheless, has a significant role in characterizing conditions such as possession states and dissociative identity disorders, among many others. Pierre Janet (1859–1947) conceptualized dissociation as evidence of division within personality and at the same time discussed notions of dissociation as evidence of alterations in the field of consciousness. It is never clear whether dissociation is a normal psychological process that is part of a continuum operating normally or abnormally in given circumstances.

Henri Ellenberger (1905–1993), in his magisterial text, *The Discovery of the Unconscious* (Ellenberger, 1981), examines Pierre Janet's (1859–1947)

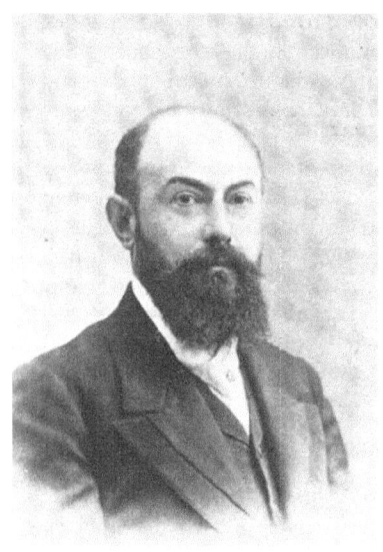

Pierre Janet 1859–1947

considerable contribution to our understanding of the phenomenon termed *psychological automatism* in the nineteenth and twentieth century. Janet developed the notion of the field of consciousness and its narrowing as an important ingredient in the understanding of phenomena that occurred in hysteria and also developed the notion of split parts of personality to explain hysterical symptoms such that the split parts became endowed with autonomous life manifest as the demonstrable symptoms of hysteria. Janet's accounts drew on his studies of anaesthesia, amnesia, abulia, motor disturbance and other abnormalities in hysteria. He was aware of the contributions of Jean-Martin Charcot (1825–1893), Alfred Binet (1852–1911) and Fredric Myers (1843–1901), among others. Janet wrote:

> Psychological life not only consists of a succession of phenomena coming one after the other, and forming a long series in one direction, but each of these successive states is in reality a complex state. . . . We have proposed to call [the] *'field of consciousness*, or maximum extension of consciousness', the largest number of simple, or relatively simple phenomena, which might be gathered at every moment, which might be simultaneously connected with our personality in one and the same personal perception. This field of consciousness, thus understood, is very variable. A chief orchestra, hearing simultaneously all the instruments, and following by reading or his memory the partition of the opera, unites in each his states of consciousness an immense number of facts. The individual who, when asleep, dreams, and the patient during a crisis of ecstasy, have, on the contrary, in their conscious thought only a very limited number of facts. (Janet, 2018)

Jante is here drawing a distinction between the synthetic capacity of the mind, as described earlier, and the effects of dissociation that produces a delimitation of the field of consciousness, resulting in focus on relatively simple sensations or memories. More specifically, Janet used the term *dédoublement* ('undoubling') to refer to the disintegration of psychological processes that results in the failure of unity of personal consciousness. Janet concludes that hysteria is a form of mental depression characterized by the retraction of the field of consciousness and a tendency of personal dissociation and emancipation of the system of ideas and functions that constitute personality (Janet, 2019).

Even more explicitly, Janet goes on to say

> [A] certain number of elementary phenomena, sensations and images, cease to be perceived and appear suppressed by the personal perception; the result is a tendency to a complete and permanent division of the personality, to the formation of several groups independent of each other; these systems of psychological factors alternate some in the wake of others or coexist; in fine, this lack of synthesis favors the formation of certain parasitic ideas which develop completely and in isolation under the shelter of the control of the personal consciousness and which manifest themselves by the most varied disturbances, apparently only physical. (Janet, 2018, pp. 527–8)

The question is whether the altered states of consciousness that manifest in possession trance and related states and are attributed to a specific psychological mechanism, namely dissociation, have underlying neural correlates. Vaitl, Birbaumer & Gruzelier (2005) reviewed the literature on the psychobiology of altered states of consciousness including possession trance. They classified altered states of consciousness as follows:

1. Spontaneously occurring,
2. Physically and physiologically induced,

3. Psychologically induced,
4. Disease induced and
5. Pharmacologically induced.

The psychologically induced altered states include those induced by drumming and dancing and hence include the states described in ritual possession trance, as mentioned earlier. They describe the trance-like states induced by drumming and dancing as characterized by narrowing of awareness of immediate surroundings or unusually narrow and selective focusing on environmental stimuli. Rhythmic bodily movements, namely dancing, become synchronized with the musical beat, resulting in the cessation of self-reflective thinking and the subject becoming increasingly absorbed in the physical activity. Distortions of time sense and unusual bodily sensations supersede, and vivid imagery and strong positive emotions occur in conjunction with feeling one with the rhythm.

Electroencephalogram (EEG) studies show an auditory drive with drumming inducing EEG waves of the same frequency as the drumming and an accompanying increased theta activity while listening to rhythmic, monotonous and patterned drumbeats. Kawai et al. (2017) examined the EEGs of participants during naturally induced possession trance at a dedicatory ritual drama in Bali, Indonesia, and showed that during possession trance state there were increased theta (4–7.5 Hz), alpha-1 (8–9.5 Hz), alpha-2 (10–12.5 Hz) and Beta (13–30 Hz) signals. This suggested that the spontaneous EEG patterns may reflect activation of reward-generating neuronal systems emanating from thalamic and brainstem structures coupled with deactivation of the cerebral cortex. These changes were associated with increases in plasma concentrations of noradrenaline, dopamine and beta-endorphins (Kawai et al., 2001). Independent confirmation of enhanced alpha and theta frequency bands was reported by Oohashi et al. (2002).

In addition to the induction of possession trance by rhythmic drumming, the social setting, the rhythmic bodily movements, shifts in body fluids, synchronicity of respiration with body movement and the induction of heart rate oscillation, the so-called respirator sinus arrhythmia, all play a role in inducing possession trance. Furthermore, respiratory-cardiovascular synchronization with increased blood pressure oscillations cause barorecep-tor stimulation and reduced cortical arousal and excitability.

It is unclear how relevant our understanding of hypnosis is in aiding our understanding of the underlying mechanisms of possession trance. Janet's formulation of dissociation arose out of observation of hypnotic subjects and the study of patients presenting with analgesia and other abnormalities in the context of what used to be termed *hysteria*. This suggests that greater appreciation of the processes underpinning hypnosis may be helpful. Regrettably, hypnosis is not well understood, and there is as yet no neurophysiological measure able to reliably categorize data from hypnotized subjects. One of the most consist-ent models has implicated frontal inhibition, particularly of the left dorsolateral prefrontal cortex (Gruzelier, 1998). Studies investigating hypnosis-induced analgesia show that there is dissociation between somatosensory and affective information during hypnotic analgesia. Hence, drawing attention once again to the role of dissociation in altered states of con-sciousness, of which possession is merely an example. Deeley et al. (2014) model cultural possession phenomena with suggestion and show that experimentally induced models of loss of agency are associated with changes in brain activity and/or connectivity. Increased connectivity was largely confined to the right hemisphere, including the temporal and frontal regions as well as the anterior cingulum and cuneus in the model of possession trance which the authors termed *internal personal agency*. The authors conclude that this suggests that beliefs, expectancies and attributions exercise their effects on cognition and that brain function can be accessed through a variety of means.

A profitable approach to further our understanding of the nature of altered states of consciousness is to examine the structural phenomenology of altered states of consciousness and then to explore which brain systems underpin those structural domains. Vaitl et al. (2005) have done just this. Firstly, they characterized the four dimensions that they believed were the essential features of altered states of consciousness, namely (1) *subjective sense of activation*, such as being alert, awake and responsive (and the dimension vary from high arousal to low arousal); (2) *awareness span*, which refers to the variability of the content of consciousness available to attention and conscious processing; (3) *self-awareness*, which refers to the degree to which an individual is in a reflective attitude and recognizes subjective experience as 'mine' or subjective experience appears to be part of a lager whole such that the subject feels as if they have 'forgotten one's self'; and (4) *sensory dynamics*, which refers to the variety of changes in the sensory and perceptual components of subjective experience, whereby sensations may be reduced or enhanced. In this schema, possession trance is characterized by increased activation/arousal, increased awareness span, reduced self-awareness and increased sensory dynamics. This model allows us to predict that in possession trance there is likely to be reticular and midline thalamic involvement because of their roles in modulating selective attention and consciousness. The goal of this model is to predict which pathways are involved in particular causal mechanisms of various altered states of consciousness. Its value is in setting possession trance alongside other forms of altered states of consciousness. See Vaitl et al. (2005) for a fuller discussion.

14.2.3 Clinical Aspects

Venkataramaiah and Mallikarjunaiah (1981) conducted a house-to-house survey in West Karnataka and reported a one-year prevalence of possession syndrome of 3.7 per cent. When 20 cases from a single school (part of an epidemic) were excluded, the prevalence dropped to 2 per cent. The majority of cases (74 per cent) were female, and the mean age was 19 years. There were no cases of possession in people with higher education, and the majority of cases (77 per cent) had received fewer than eight years of formal education. It is notable that 90 per cent of the population sampled believed in spirit possession.

Yap (1960) reported on 66 cases presenting to Hong Kong Mental Hospital between 1954 and 1956 inclusive. This number constituted 2.4 per cent of all hospital admissions. The majority were female (75.7 per cent) and aged under 35 years. Most of the patients (60 per cent) were married, and a large proportion was illiterate (21.5 per cent). Although the majority of patients endorsed Taoist-Buddhist-Confucian religion (80 per cent), there were still a significant number endorsing Christianity (either Catholicism or Protestant faiths; 9 per cent), a proportion much greater than within the general population. The author speculated whether those Chinese taking to organized Christianity were a self-selected group with strong emotional needs. The clinical diagnosis was hysteria in 32 patients (48.4 per cent), followed by schizophrenia in 16 (24 per cent). Only 7 patients (10.6 per cent) displayed the full degree of possession state as manifest by clouding of consciousness, skin anaesthesia, changed demeanour and tone of voice and subsequent amnesia for the event. Twenty-eight patients (42 per cent) are described as presenting as histrionic – demonstrating an absence of clouding of consciousness, absence of skin anaesthesia, absence of change of demeanour or tone of voice, the possibility of immediate recall to reality and the gaining of attention demonstrable by giggling, belching and other attention-seeking behavioural devices.

The full range of behaviours of the incomplete cases included gagging, torticollis-like movement, chanting, shutting of the eyes, lying stuporose on the ground, rolling about on the ground, climbing up windows, panting, somersaulting, attacking people, scratching the tongue, walking on knees and the imaginary throwing of rice grains. In the most severe cases, the behaviour was determined by the nature of the possessing spirit. For example, a person possessed by a fox spirit barked and pawed, and another possessed by a snake spirit hissed.

Gaw et al. (1998) reported on 20 Chinese patients from Hebei Province. Most patients were female (85 per cent), and the mean age was 37 years. The patients were mostly married (85 per cent), and 45 per cent had no formal education. These patients reported loss of control over their actions, behaviour change, loss of awareness of their surround- ings, loss of personal identity, problems distinguishing reality from fantasy, change in tone of voice and so on. The possessing spirit included a turtle, the spirit of a deceased person, a deity, a snake and the devil. The precipitating causes included interpersonal difficulties with spouse, family illness, death of a relative, financial difficulty and stepping on a snake or urinating into a snake pit next to a tomb.

Spirit possession can also present as a mass phenomenon sometimes involving several members of the same family. Sethi and Bhargava (2009) described one such case in which a chain of events was set in motion by an aunt of the primary presenting patient becoming possessed by a deity and threatening the primary patient's family with harm. Thereafter, the primary patient, her two elder daughters, her husband and another daughter and a son all had become possessed by varying agencies, including deities and deceased relatives. In another report, four individuals became possessed by *Mohini* (female spirits) in the context of suicides of two females by jumping into a well in a remote village of 200 dwellings, of which 60 belonged to Harijan families (Chandrashekar, 1981). These cases evolved within the sociocultural dynamics of beliefs about the malfeasance of spirits of people who die by unnatural means and prophesy by an itinerant fortune teller that young men in the village would become possessed by the *Mohini* of the deceased females who had died by suicide.

An investigation of mass spirit possession among schoolgirls in southern Thailand showed the importance of individual vulnerability, notably of prior psychiatric disorder, problematical character traits and a past history of recurrent trance states in determining the development of spirit possession (Trangkasombat & Su-Umpan, 1998).

A study of a cluster of spirit possession events in Nepal showed that possessed women had more traumatic experiences than non-possessed women and also higher levels of symptoms of psychiatric disorder, namely of anxiety, depression and post-traumatic stress disorder (Sapkota et al., 2014). Despite the high rates of observed psychiatric disorder, the possessed individuals, their families and traditional healers did not attribute possession to psychiatric illness but rather viewed it as an affliction that was a mode of communication between humans and spirits. This study once again demonstrates how possession trance and possession states within psychiatry are multidimensional in nature, involving the intersection of cultural idiom, distress and psychopathology. This intersec- tion is amplified by the study of spirit possession in the aftermath of mass political violence in Mozambique (Igreja, Dias-Lambranca & Hershey, 2010). In a survey of 941 individuals, 18.6 per cent had experienced possession by at least one spirit, and

5.6 per cent had experienced multiple simultaneous spirit possessions. In females who experienced spirit possession, there were significantly reproductive difficulties such as menstrual problems, fertility issues and miscarriages. There were also more physical symptoms such as headaches, stomach pains, pain in the ribs, poor appetite, breathing difficulties and war-related nightmares about sexual assaults perpetrated by males. The role of childhood trauma (i.e., child abuse and/or neglect and trauma) in females who experience spirit possession is confirmed in a study reported from Turkey (Sar, Alioğlu & Akyüz, 2014). An epidemiological survey of trauma-related disorders in war-affected regions of northern Uganda showed that in children abducted and forcibly recruited as child soldiers, there was significant association with spirit possession (Neuner, Pfeiffer & Schauer-Kaiser, 2012). High levels of spirit possession were significantly associated with extreme poverty, sexual trauma, forced commission of murder, abduction and exposure to trauma such perpetration of violence after witnessing family violence. Suicide risk was markedly elevated in those who were aged over 18 years, were female and had post-traumatic stress disorder, depression or spirit possession.

The role of trauma in spirit possession is quite significant, but the identified trauma does not solely flow from wartime events but also includes death of family member in childhood, severe physical injury, threat to life through illness or accident, emotional neglect by family of origin and emotional abuse by family of origin (Duijl, Nijenhuis & Komproe, 2010).

Spirit possession is but one example of how different explanatory models can be, for psychological distress and psychopathology between cultural groups. Idioms of distress, culturally sanctioned beliefs (including religious beliefs) can vary, yet the underlying subjective experiences can be identical. *Jinn* possession is an important phenomenon in clinical practice, and Dein and Illaiee (2013) have situated the religious and cultural beliefs around this phenomenon and argue that clinicians need to collaborate with religious authorities where necessary in caring for patients. Their perspective is that of clinicians where belief in *Jinn* is in ethnic minorities, and their conclusions are echoed by Khalifa and Hardie (2005), who describe two illustrative cases.

Kianpoor & Rhoades (2006) report from Baluchstan, Iran, drawing attention to *Djinnati*, the belief in possession by a *Djinn*. In their study, the prevalence of *Djinnati* was 4 per cent during a six-month period in hospital-admitted patients. *Djinnati* occurred in 0.5 per cent of the general population and in 1 per cent of females. In this sample, *Djinnati* was characterized by impaired consciousness and unresponsiveness to external stimuli; complete amnesia following the episode; psychomotor agitation; screaming; appearing frightened; speaking in a changed voice, accent or language; and a change in identity.

Zar is the term used to describe a form of spirit possession that is common in North Africa, East Africa and Middle Eastern countries including Sudan, Ethiopia, Egypt and Iran. Although it is likely that roots of *zar* are similar, if not identical, in these countries, the manifestations have local colourings. Mianji and Semnani (2015) have given a detailed account of *zar* and its variants and argue that prevalence, clinical characteristics and social context differ between different communities. See Young (1975) for a full description of and discussion about Ethiopian *zar* beliefs and practices. The possibility of misdiagnosis exists, as Witztum and Grisaru (1996) argue regarding presentations of *zar* in Ethiopian migrants in Israel who present with involuntary movements, mutism and incomprehensible language and are liable to be misdiagnosed as having psychiatric disorders or neurological disease.

14.3 Dissociative Identity Disorder (Multiple Personality Disorder)

Mitchill (1816) is usually credited with the first description of dissociative identity disorder or multiple personality disorder. The patient was a young English woman, Mary Reynolds, who had emigrated with her family to Pennsylvania. In her early twenties, she

> [u]nexpectedly and without any kind of forewarning ... fell into a profound sleep, which continued several hours beyond the ordinary term. On waking she was discovered to have lost every trait of acquired knowledge. Her memory was *tabula rasa*; all vestiges of words and things were obliterated and gone. It was found necessary for her to learn everything again. ... [A]fter a few months another fit of somnolence invaded her. On rousing from it, she found herself restored to the state she was before the paroxysm; but was wholly ignorant of every event and occurrence that had befallen her afterwards. ... [S]he is as unconscious of her double character as two distinct persons are of their respective natures. ... During four years upwards, she has undergone periodical transitions from one of these states to the other. (quoted in Fahy, 1988, p. 597)

In fact, variants of what is now thought of as dissociative personality had been recognized as part of the phenomenon of possession before the nineteenth century, particularly what were termed *lucid possession* (in which the subject feels within himself or herself the two souls striving against each other) and *somnambulistic possession* (in which the subject loses consciousness of his or her own self while a mysterious intruder seems to take possession of his or her body and acts and speaks with an individuality of which the subject knows nothing when he or she returns to awareness). Ellenberger (1981) makes the point that there are parallelisms between these two forms of possession and dissociative personality – both can be latent, occurring under influence of hypnosis, or develop spontaneously.

Ellenberger (1981) quotes Eberhardt Gmelin's case, published in 1791.

> In 1789, at the beginning of the French Revolution, aristocratic refugees arrived in Stuttgart. Impressed by their sight, a twenty-year-old German young woman suddenly 'exchanged' her own personality for the manners and ways of a French-born lady, imitating her and speaking French perfectly and German as would a French woman. These 'French' states repeated themselves. In her French personality, the subject had complete memory of all that she had said and done during her previous French states. As a German, she knew nothing of her French personality. With a motion of his hand, Gmelin was easily able to make her shift from one personality to the other. (Ellenberger, 1981, p. 127)

The most celebrated account, if I can use that phrase, is that by Morton Prince (1906, p. 1) in *The Dissociation of a Personality: A Biographical Study in Abnormal Psychology*, which was published in 1906. He wrote:

> Miss Christine L. Beauchamp, the subject of this study, is a person in whom several personalities have become developed; that is to say, she may change personality from time to time, often from hour to hour, and with each change her character becomes transformed and her memories altered. In addition to the real, original or normal self, the self that was born and which she intended by nature to be, she may be any of the three persons. I say three different, because, although making use of the same body, each nevertheless, has distinctly different character: a difference manifested by different trains of thought, by different views and temperament, and by different acquisitive tastes, habits, experiences, and memories.

Prince regarded this case as an example of disintegration of personality. He argued that 'no one secondary personality preserves the whole psychical life of the individual. The synthesis of the original consciousness known as the personal ego is broken up, so to speak, and shorn of some of its memories, perceptions, acquisitions, or modes of reaction to the environment' (p. 3). He was careful to distinguish his use of the term *disintegration* from use of the term *degeneration*, which implies destruction through organic means of the mind.

Morton Prince's account has become the classic text on multiple personality disorder. He appeared to be describing a situation in which there were multiple personalities embodied in the one person. His discussion of the case at several points suggests that he was convinced that he was dealing with separate identities with individual characteristics, memories and so on. And he assumed that the body of Miss Beauchamp was incidental to the activities of these personalities; that is, he argued as if the body had no bearing on identity. For Prince, identity was defined by psychology, and psychology was distinct from the physiology of the body. I will return to the role of the body in identity in Chapter 15.

This case attracted a great deal of attention at the time of its publication. There were a handful of other reports in the first half of the nineteenth century. There were no reports between 1846 and 1873. The upsurge of reports was marked by Prince's publication in 1906. Between 1944 and 1969, only 14 cases were reported (Greaves, 1980, 1993), but by 1986, Coons (1988) estimated that 6,000 cases of multiple personality disorder had been diagnosed in North America alone. The reasons for this marked increase in reported cases is unclear, but among the possibilities is that there has been greater disseminated information about the condition, sharper definition and diagnostic criteria and greater awareness of child sexual abuse with which dissociative personality disorder co-varies. But the most important factor is likely to be the enthusiasm of a few clinicians and their penchant for diagnosing this condition.

Harold Merskey (1995a, 1995b) has been one of the most vocal critics of the concept of multiple personality disorder. His arguments are detailed and logical:

1. The sheer size of the assumed case numbers is implausible – 4.4 per cent of inpatient populations in some studies and 5 per cent of college students in another estimate.
2. The condition is rarely diagnosed outside of North America.
3. A leading authority on multiple personality disorder is reported as having said that the Central Intelligence Agency in the United States had implanted multiple personality disorder into children so that some of the altered personalities could carry more information, and the same agency has inspired current criticisms of the concept so that reports of the discovery of these implanted alters will not be believed.
4. In Canada, 68 per cent of psychiatrists had never made the diagnosis, and 41 per cent had never seen a case.

It is plain from the foregoing that this condition is indeed controversial. Merskey further examined 14 cases before 1905, at least two or three of which had significant evidence of organic brain damage, whereas another three had epilepsy. Other cases had fugue or somnambulistic states, and two had been hypnotized. This meant that the leading nineteenth-century cases were examples of bipolar disorder, organic cerebral disease or hypnotic induction. These latter cases were sometimes overt and frequently persistent. Merskey's analysis of the most recent cases led him to the conclusion that he had not found any case that had emerged through unconscious processes without any prior shaping or preparation by external factors such as physicians or the media. His primary concern was that the symptoms of most cases reported after Prince's case study of Miss Beauchamp were either shaped by the clinician's method of interviewing or influenced by contemporary accounts in films and the media. In summary, Merskey's view is that it is unlikely that dissociative personality disorder ever occurs as a spontaneous persistent natural phenomenon in adults, and when it occurs, if at all, suggestion, social encouragement, preparation by expectation and the reward of attention help to produce and sustain the secondary personality (Merskey, 1992).

These earlier findings and conclusions were amplified in further studies by Piper and Merskey (2004a, 2004b), and the authors also respond to critiques of their work. They conclude that

> [w]herever we look – whether at the posttraumatic model; at theories of repression; at the epidemiologic uncertainties and aggrandizements of the disorder; at the persistent prolifer-ation of personalities; at the elusive data that attempt to sustain the claims of exceptional abuse; at the bland presentation assumptions such as cross-sex, cross-species, or cross-ethnic alters; or at the impossibility of proving almost any of the basic claims of the disorder – we encounter propositions that appear to be founded on beliefs and not on facts or logic. That such beliefs could prosper in a society or a discipline represents an embarrassing weakness of the academic and professional establishment of psychiatry.   (p. 681)

Notwithstanding the many concerns about the legitimacy of the notion of multiple person-ality or dissociative identity disorder, there is an indubitable social reality to the phenom-enon, and this means that it merits investigation and consideration.

14.3.1 Case Reports

Case 1

> A twenty-nine-year-old woman whose personality had become split into A and B three years before, followed the shock she had experienced at her father's suicide. For some time thereafter, she had been afflicted with motor disturbances, hallucinations, and a peculiar instability and changes of mood. One evening, while sitting at the piano, she felt as though someone inside her tried to take a deep breath and tried to sing with her voice. Several weeks went by before personality B learned to 'emerge completely and take possession of the body.' Ever since the two personalities have alternated but always remain conscious of one another.
>
> A remains the normal habitual personality and keeps her previous character. She is a bright and cultured woman of good background, but rather shy and inhibited. She sings poorly. She had a rigid upbringing at home as well as at the convent school and, in her education, a strict taboo had been maintained as to sexual questions. B is a seemingly older, bolder but dignified and serious-looking woman who claims to be the reincarna-tion of the soul of a Spanish singer. She sings well and with assurance and speaks English with a strong Spanish accent. At times she speaks a language that she pretends is Spanish but is actually a composite of bits of broken Spanish and of Spanish-sounding word formations. She is extremely egocentric, shows strong passions, and her main interest lies in the sexual instinct. She pretends to be a voluptuous, fascinating beauty and to have been a dancer, a courtesan, and the mistress of a nobleman.
>
> A and B consider themselves on good terms with each other but being completely separate persons, much as two friends would be. Each knows the other only insofar as the

other will wish to be known and is willing to reveal about herself. . . . They may look at the same thing or read the same book simultaneously. However, it would seem that B never sleeps, and she claims to know A's early life better than A herself. She also maintains that she is A's guardian angel and once hypnotized her. She is obviously the dominating personality.

(summarized by Ellenberger, 1981; see also Cory, 1919)

Case 2

Ansel Bourne was born in 1826. The son of divorced parents, he had spent an unhappy childhood and had later become a carpenter working in small Rhode Island towns. An atheist, he publicly declared, on October 28, 1857, that he would rather be deaf and mute than go to church. Moments later he lost his hearing, speech and sight. On November 11, he went to the church, showing a written message announcing his conversion. On the following Sunday, November 15, he rose up in church in the midst of several hundred worshippers and proclaimed that God had cured him of his infirmities. This alleged miracle brought him immense prestige, and henceforth Bourne combined his carpenter trade with the activity of itinerant preacher. Years later, he lost his wife and remarried, but his second marriage was an unhappy one.

Thirty years after his conversion, Ansel Bourne one day disappeared from his home in Coventry, Rhode Island. He had gone to Providence, cashed $551.00 at the bank, paid a visit to his beloved nephew, and from there his track had been lost.

Two weeks later, a certain Albert Brown arrived at Norristown, Pennsylvania; he rented a little store, bought some merchandise and started a small business of stationery, confection, and small articles. The man led a rather inconspicuous and secluded life. On March 14, he woke up early in the morning and was completely disoriented. He had come back to his former personality of Ansel Bourne and was at a loss to understand what he was doing in this strange place. He called his neighbors, who thought he had become mentally deranged. Finally, his nephew arrived, liquidated the stock of merchandise, and took his uncle back to Coventry. Ansel Bourne had no recollection whatever of what he had done during the two months he had spent living under the name Albert Brown.

In 1890, Ansel Bourne was hypnotized by William James and brought back, under trance, to his secondary personality of Albert Brown. Brown knew nothing of Bourne, but gave a coherent account of what he had done during the two months of his existence. Wherever his statements could be checked by an objective enquiry, they were found to be true. Regarding his fugue, he was obviously dissatisfied with life and suffered from his second wife's nagging nature. He disappeared just after having cashed a large sum of money. His new identity (Albert Brown from Newton, N.H.) was a faint disguise of his true one (Ansel Bourne from New York, N.Y.). It is strange that in his secondary state, Albert Brown did not notice anything unusual about the papers, checkbook, and so on, bearing the name Ansel Bourne, which he had with him all that time.

(Summarized by Ellenberger, 1981; see also Hodgson, 1891)

Case 3

The oldest of six siblings, Rachel, grew up in a very disturbing environment. Her parents were aspiring middle class, with her father being a senior manager in a large international company. However, both her parents were sexually abusive and violent to their children. The atmosphere within the home was always unpredictable. Both parents were openly verbally abusive and negative toward the children, who were periodically threatened with violence, even murder. There were regular small incidents of pinching or punching as the children went past their mother, but on occasions she threw knives and other objects at them. The eldest boys were regularly strangled until they lost consciousness. Understandably, there was much fear, crying and screaming from the younger siblings. The children were not allowed to go the lavatory in the night or get out of bed, subsequently the eldest two boys would urinate in a corner of the bedroom and one of them would hide faeces in a drawer. The children were often locked in a small cupboard under the stairs. The parents even allowed friends of the family to also sexually abuse their children. The mother was also sexually inviting to strangers. For example, she would sunbathe naked when the dustmen were coming or parade naked in the front window. She was admitted to a psychiatric hospital in 1964. . . .

Rachel found the unpredictable, violent and explosive nature of her mother's actions terrifying. She felt her whole life was being threatened and that she would die in a very unpleasant way. In order to cope with such persistent abuse, Rachel began to 'sit beside herself' so that it didn't seem to be happening to her. She found a way of watching what happened rather than to endure it herself. . . .

When Rachel was being sexually abused, she also 'dreamed'. She developed the ability to be sitting next to herself or even outside the room. In this way, Rachel felt nothing, either emotionally or physically. She no longer felt pain when she was hit, and she was able to stop crying with fear.

Once she started school, Rachel 'dreamed' a lot. Sometimes she couldn't remember how she had got to school. She often became mentally absent during lessons. . . . As a teenager, Rachel thought she could sleep anywhere at any time. . . . Rachel would often wake up in a different classroom or find herself on the wrong road on the way back from doing the shopping for her mother. She sometimes woke up to find herself walking across the fields near her house. . . . As she progressed into adulthood, Rachel would frequently experience becoming a 6-year-old child. During these periods, she did not know where she was and would tell people that she was 6 years old. Rachel experienced other alters too, but the 6-year-old girl was the most frequently experienced. (Stickley & Nickeas, 2006)

14.3.2 Explanatory Hypotheses

It is well accepted that dissociative identity disorder/multiple personality disorder is fundamentally a dissociative phenomenon. Whereas possession trance is regarded as occurring in the context of an altered state of consciousness, thereby drawing the phenomenon within a wider spectrum of conscious states, this approach to our understanding of possession trance has not been overtly applied to dissociative identity disorder. This is despite the fact that there are historical links between both concepts (see Ellenberger, 1981) and that Golub (1995) has drawn attention to the notion that possession trance and multiple personality disorder are cultural variations of the same underlying phenomenon. The psychobiology model developed by Nijenhuis, Hart and Steele (2002) traverses much of the same territory as do the explanatory hypothesis for possession trance. These authors conceive of dissociative identity disorder as a severe, chronic, complex childhood-onset form of post-traumatic stress disorder in which repeated early traumatization disrupts the unification of identity.

Furthermore, they propose that each individual identity is characterized by its own pattern of perception, reaction and thinking – and that each displays different psychobiological characteristics that are generally not reproduced by subjects who are simulating dissociative identity disorder in such parameters as electro-dermal activity, visual evoked potentials, cerebral blood flow, autonomic nervous system variables, optical variables and arousal. In addition, they draw attention to the varying mechanisms underlying dissociation, namely involvement of neurochemical systems such as endorphins and interactions among neuro-peptides and catecholamines. But it is the putative involvement of neurological structures such as the amygdala, hippocampus, medial frontal cortex, thalamus, cingulate gyrus and insula in the causation of dissociation that has been most amenable to investigation.

There is evidence of significantly smaller hippocampal volume in subjects with dissociative identity disorder versus normal control individuals. These changes were also demonstrable in patients with post-traumatic stress disorder. In addition, there was evidence of a misshapen hippocampus and significantly smaller volume in the hippocampal CA2-3 subfields, the CA4–dentate gyrus and (pre)subiculum in subjects with both post-traumatic stress disorder and dissociative identity disorder. The severity of the volumetric changes was positively correlated with the severity of childhood traumatization and dissociation. The authors conclude that these findings support a childhood-related trauma aetiology for the abnormal volume and morphology of the hippocampus in post-traumatic stress disorder and dissocia-tive identity disorder (Chalavi, Vissia & Giesen, 2015). There is also evidence not only of volumetric changes in the hippocampus but also of the amygdala in dissociative identity disorder. Vermetten, Schmahl and Lindner (2006) reported reduction in the volume of hippocampus by 19.2 per cent and of the amygdala by 31.6 per cent compared to normal control individuals. In addition, the ratio of hippocampal volume to amygdala was signifi-cantly different between dissociative identity disorder and normal control individuals.

Involvement of the orbitofrontal region, the median and superior frontal regions and the occipital regions has been reported. Sar, Unal and Ozturk (2007) showed, using single-photon-emission computed tomography, decreased regional blood flow in the orbitofrontal region bilaterally and increased blood flow in the median and superior frontal and occipital regions bilaterally. They argued that any comprehensive model of dissociative identity disorder will have to explain the interaction between anterior and posterior brain areas.

The phenomenology of dissociation described by Nijenhuis et al. (2002) encompasses what has been established since the pioneering work of Pierre Janet in early twentieth century, namely that dissociation involves retraction of the field of consciousness and low levels of conscious awareness. The distinction encompasses the introduction of the notions of negative and positive dissociation as well as psychoform and somatoform variants of dissociation. Finally, the theory of structural dissociation identifies two states, a neutral identity state that concentrates on functioning in daily life and that limits access to painful memories and a traumatic identity state that is fixated on and has access to and responds to the traumatic memories. Patients, apparently, learn to switch between these states (Reinders et al., 2006).

The structural dissociation paradigm was tested in a provocation study. Subjects were investigated using three biological parameters, namely (1) subjective ratings of emotional and sensorimotor responses; (2) cardiovascular responses, including heart rate, blood pressure and heart rate variability; and (3) regional blood flow as determined by positron-emission tomography. The authors reported that both subjective responses and cardiovascular responses revealed significant effects in relation to the neutral identity states and the traumatic identity states. Finally, the regional cerebral blood flow data revealed different neural networks to be associated with different processing of neutral and trauma-related memory script (Reinders et al., 2006). And the two dissociative identity states, namely the neutral identity state and the trauma-related state, exhibit different blood flow patterns as well as autonomic and subjective reactions when exposed to identical trauma-related stimuli.

The other hypothesis is a social narrative model that conceives of personal identity not merely as the attribute of an individual but as a dynamic process constructed within social relationships through the mechanism of shared narratives. These narratives give temporal continuity to personal identity (Lynn & Pintar, 1997). The authors make the case that a narrative view of dissociation – in contrast to mechanistic conceptualizations, which locate the phenomenon within an individual as a symptom of a disorder or as a defence mechanism outliving its usefulness – locates the phenomenon in the social relations of the victim, both at the moment of the trauma and as a continuing or recurring process. The experience of trauma disrupts not only identity itself but also the social process through which identity is constructed. See also Spanos (1994) for a sociocognitive perspective that sees dissociative identity disorder as a socially constructed phenomenon that is context-bound, goal-directed social behaviour geared to the expectations of significant others.

The details of either of these explanatory hypotheses are outside the scope of this book. Nonetheless, it is clear that both hypotheses rely on trauma and trauma response as being central to the nature of dissociative identity disorder. It is certainly true that dissociation itself as a process occurs not only in the context of trauma but that the phenomenon is also probably part of a wider spectrum of altered states that human beings experience, and the use to which these states can be put is varied and manifold.

14.3.3 Clinical Aspects

Ross (1991) reported that in a survey of a sample of the general population in Winnipeg, Manitoba, 1 per cent showed multiple personality disorder associated with childhood abuse, and 10 per cent of the population had a history of dissociative disorder of some kind. Furthermore, Ross, Anderson and Fleisher (1991) reported that 5 per cent of general adult psychiatric inpatients met the criteria for multiple personality disorder. Bliss (1985) reported a similar prevalence in his survey of psychiatric inpatients and outpatients; namely, 10 per cent of subjects had multiple personality disorder and 5 to 20 per cent had amnesia for previous traumatic experiences. The rates in other countries outside of North America vary considerably: in Japan, there were no reported cases (Takahashi, 1990); in the Netherlands, in a consecutive series of inpatient admissions, 1.6 per cent were reported as having a dissociative identity disorder, both in females, and two males were diagnosed as factitious dissociative identity disorder (Friedl & Draijer, 2000); in Switzerland, the point prevalence is estimated at 0.005 to 0.1 per cent (Modestin, 1992); and in Turkey, a survey of the general population reported a 0.4 per cent minimum prevalence of dissociative identity disorder (Akyüz et al., 1999).

The clinical features of dissociative identity disorder were described by Putnam, Guroff and Silberman (1986). The mean age of their sample of 100 cases was 31.3 years. The majority of cases (95 per cent) had previously received one of more psychiatric or neurological diagnoses prior to the diagnosis of dissociative identity disorder. The patients presented with symptoms including depression, anxiety and eating disorders and experienced both auditory and visual hallucinations. Many patients presented with symptoms such as psychogenic amnesia, fugue states and conversion symptoms. The number of personalities or alters ranged from 1 to 60, and excluding the primary personality, the average was 13 personalities. There was a marked association with suicide and self-mutilation behaviours. Amnesia was a symptom in 95 per cent of cases. The protean nature of dissociative identity disorder raised valid questions about whether or not it is a valid condition or merely an intriguing symptom of a wide range of psychological disturbances (Fahy, Abas & Brown, 1989). Piper (1994) concluded that patients diagnosed by current criteria as having multiple personality disorder belong to a heterogeneous group that has poorly demarcated boundaries with many other psychiatric conditions.

There are several reports of an associated history of childhood sexual abuse and of other kinds of abuse in childhood. In Ross's (1989) investigation of 236 cases, 79.2 per cent reported extensive sexual abuse in childhood, and 74.9 per cent reported other kinds of abuse as children. In addition, at the time of the investigation, the subjects had been in the health-care system for 6.7 years before a diagnosis of multiple personality disorder was made. On average, each subject had 15.7 personalities, and the personalities were characterized as a child (86.0 per cent), a personality of a different age (84.5 per cent), a protector (84.0 per cent) and a persecutor (84.0 per cent). Suicide occurred in 2.1 per cent, and 72 per cent had attempted suicide. The commonest previous diagnoses were affective disorder, personality disorder, anxiety disorders and schizophrenia. Structured interview data on 102 cases from four centres confirmed the essential findings described earlier, as well as suggesting that the diagnosis was stable over time (Ross et al., 1990). With respect to childhood sexual and physical abuse, Ross and colleagues indicated that more than 50 per cent of subjects reported abuse originating before the age of five years, and the abuse went on for 10 years, on average. Subjects were equally likely to be physically abused by their fathers as by their mothers. Sexual abusers were more likely to be male, but a significant amount of abuse was perpetrated by mothers, female relatives and other females (Ross et al., 1991). Lewis, Yeager and Swica (1997) showed that in 12 murderers presenting with dissociative identity disorder, objective documentation of severe abuse was found in 11 and that the subjects had amnesia for the abuse and underreported it. The relationship between physical or sexual abuse was confirmed in a study from Turkey reporting that 71 per cent of subjects had been abused in childhood (Şar, Yargic & Tutkun, 1996).

Multiple personality has a severe impact on functioning. In a report by Rivera (1991), 57 per cent had problems with drug abuse, 12 per cent had a criminal record and 55 per cent required social assistance because of their inability to work.

The diagnostic criteria for dissociative identity disorder include disruption of autobiographical memory, usually manifest as inter-personality amnesia, in which a particular personality state or identity is retrievable by that same identity but not by a different one. Schacter, Kihlstrom and Kihlstrom (1989) showed in a single case report that the subject was able to retrieve episodes from the recent past from her autobiographical memory but could not recollect a single episode prior to age 10 years. In another investigation of a subject with 22 distinct personalities, Nissen et al. (1988) demonstrated that the degree to which there was compartmentalization of knowledge appeared to depend on the extent to which that knowledge is unique to a personality as well as the extent to which processes operating at the time of retrieval are strongly personality dependent. In essence, there was evidence that knowledge was not as compartmentalized as one might have expected if there was true interidentity amnesia, and this fact is confirmed by Huntjens, Postma and Peters (2003) and Huntjens et al. (2003). A slight variation on this conclusion is that dissociative identity disorder is homogeneous in the degree to which there is blocking of episodic memory between the different personalities, with there being a breakthrough of knowledge in some pairings of personalities and no blocking in others (Morton, 2017).

It has been reported that in post-traumatic stress disorder, memories of the traumatic events are fragmented and occur as waves of intense feelings, visual images, olfactory and auditory perceptions and bodily sensations. This differs from memories of non-traumatic but emotionally significant events, where there is a coherent narrative account. Hart and Bolt (2005) showed that in dissociative identity disorder, subjects show somatosensory re-experiencing for both traumatic and non-traumatic emotionally charged events. This pattern was different from that in normal control individuals.

The possibility of malingering or factitious presentations is obviously present in dissociative identity disorder. It is clear that making distinctions between a true case and these other 'false' cases is difficult. Coons and Milstein (1994) were unable to find any difference in demographic characteristics, presenting symptoms or the characteristics of altered personalities. These difficulties are most pronounced in forensic settings. In the context of the 'Hillside Strangler' case in the United States (*Stute v. Birrnchi*), a set of criteria was developed to assist in distinguishing dissociative identity disorder from malingering. The criteria were (1) the structure and content of the various personalities should have been consistent over time; (2) the boundaries between the different person-alities should have been stable and not readily altered by social cues; (3) the response to hypnosis should have been similar to that of other deeply hypnotized subjects; and (4) those who have known the subject over time should have been able to provide examples of sudden, inexplicable changes in behaviour and identity and evidence to corroborate the claims of intermittent amnesia (Orne, Dinges & Orne, 1984). These criteria them-selves are open to criticism, and Kluft (1987) concluded that the general use of these criteria was not supported by the evidence. He also contended that every characteristic thought to distinguish between dissociative identity disorder and malingerers was shared by both, for example, discrepancies between two channels of communication, slow speech, generalizations with few facts, hesitancy, grammatical errors, long answers and refusal to answer questions.

The case of *Stute v. Birrnchi* illustrates the difficulties that can arise within the forensic setting. Kenneth Birrnchi was a defendant who was charged with first-degree murder and suspected of having dissociative identity disorder. The murders occurred over a four-month period in 1977–1978 and involved the killing of young and attractive women, who were raped and strangled, and some victims were conspicuously displayed nude on hillsides in the Los Angeles area. Hence the killer was called the 'Hillside Strangler'. Under hypnosis, Birrnchi 'Steve' emerged, and he took credit for the two Bellingham murders (the offences that had led directly to the arrest). During hypnosis, 'Steve' explained the specifics of the murders and was able to provide details which only the guilty party knew. However, after hypnosis, Birrnchi continued to assert his innocence and lack of knowledge of the events that took place and disclaimed knowledge of 'Steve'. Birrnchi was therefore diagnosed with dissociative identity disorder. After extensive analysis of the materials, the authors con-cluded that Kenneth Birrnchi had personality disorder and that he was almost successful in simulating multiple personality. The details of this complex and important case are reported by Orne et al. (1984).

The practical problems posed in the forensic setting, that is, the task of distinguishing between 'true' dissociative identity disorder and 'false' dissociative disorder, takes us right back to the extraordinary period of the Spanish Inquisition (1231–1826), also known as the 'Tribunal of the Holy Office of the Inquisition'. In that period, there were attempts to distinguish between witches, those merely possessed and the melancholics who were ill.

There are other far-reaching ethical and philosophical issues that arise out of the presentation of dissociative identity disorder within the legal and justice system. Piper (1994) made the following point:

> If a patient with multiple personality disorder commits an antisocial act for which he or she claims amnesia, it does not at first glance seem offensive to hold that individual blameworthy because the patient, if conceptualized as a collection of relatively autonomous personalities, does not have the full resources of the integrated personality available. Thus he or she has a lessened ability to evaluate the rightness and wrongness of the act. . . . If society accepts the separateness or autonomy of differing alters, it ceases to recognize a morally or legally accountable person, but rather a collection of partial persons with no collective capacity for responsibility. This collection could also be a potentially dangerous entity because of its limited capacity to control undesirable conduct. This view of the patient with multiple personality disorder would justify society's taking coercive action to control him or her, since it assumes he or she would not be responsive to the sanctions that control the rest of us. . . . Another problem is that the 'fragmented person' approach casts serious doubt on whether the patient has one of the major moral and legal attributes of personhood – the ability to choose. Can such a collection of personalities legally choose to sign (itself? himself? themselves?) into hospital, voluntarily enter into a sexual relationship, make a legally binding will, or enter into a contract to buy a car? If he truly respects the idea of autonomous personalities, these questions must be answered in the negative.   (p. 607)

14.4 Conclusion

Possession trance and dissociative identity disorder both challenge our normal attitude towards awareness of unity of the self over time and awareness of identity over time. Both conditions can only be understood by an appeal to a psychological notion, namely dissociation. And in this, both conditions raise questions about what it means to have an altered state of consciousness and whether this state is part of normal experience or only induced by distress or trauma. Finally, dissociative identity disorder demonstrates the potential problems in the application of medical diagnoses, clinical reasoning and psychiatric expertise in a juridical space with their distinct purposes and methods. In every way possible, dissociative identity disorder challenges not only our notions of what constitutes a person, what it means to be autonomous and how identity is borne from an integrated and unified psychology both in terms of temporal duration and in the instant of completing an action but also the rules determining how to attribute fault and culpability.

Body Integrity Identity Disorder (Xenomelia)

15

15.1 Introduction

The term *body integrity identity disorder* refers to a condition characterized by the persistent desire to acquire a physical disability, for example, amputation, paraplegia or other severe disability such as blindness. Individuals who suffer from this condition typically report a desire to achieve their sense of 'true self' and that to be successful in obtaining the desired amputation or disability would enable them to feel 'whole' or 'complete'.

The concept of desire for amputation of a healthy limb is not as new as it sounds. The first reported case was in 1785, when an English man first offered a French surgeon 100 guineas to amputate his healthy leg and, upon the refusal, forced him at gunpoint to perform the amputation. Some time later, the surgeon received 250 guineas in the mail, along with a letter: 'You have made me the happiest of all men . . . by taking away from me a limb which put an invincible obstacle to my happiness' (Johnston & Elliott, 2002, p. 431).

Money, Jobaris and Furth (1977) reported on two cases of men who both sought an elective above-knee amputation. They described how five years earlier, in a series of letters published in *Penthouse* magazine, they had identified a paraphilia associated with amputees or self-amputeeism. This syndrome was termed *apotemnophilia* ('amputation love') or *acrotomophilia* ('attraction to amputees'). The two cases were men who suffered from apotemnophilia, and their desire for self-amputation was said to be 'an *idée fixe* rather than a delusion'.

Two decades later, Bruno (1997) proposed a different psychological concept for similar cases, that of *factitious disability disorder*. Bruno noted that internet forums and discussion groups were becoming more frequent, and in such places, people looking for sexual partners who were amputees were known as *devotees*. Other categories were also established, known as *pretenders* (i.e., people who would pretend to have a disability through use of an assisted device such as crutches or a wheelchair) and *wannabees* (i.e., people who themselves sought to acquire a disability, usually through limb amputation). Bruno proposed a psychological explanation for this disorder in that it seemed to provide an opportunity for the person to be loved or attended to and that the disability could be their own or others, real or pretended.

More recently, Brugger, Lenggenhager and Giummarra (2013) put forward the term *xenomelia* as a more appropriate term because it points to the core feature of the condition, namely estrangement of one or more of one's limbs. These authors cite examples of subjective descriptions by people with body integrity identity disorder: 'I can feel exactly the line where my leg should end and my stump should begin'; 'I feel myself complete without my left leg'; 'the soul feels as though it belongs to a body with only one leg, and the body does not correspond to this inner reality'.

Body integrity identity disorder has immense relevance for how we understand the nature of embodiment, the relationship between the self and the body and the basis of many distinct but interrelated anomalies of bodily experience. The body, under normal circumstances, is experienced as an object, like any other object, but is also subjectively experienced as alive and vital, and it constitutes our identity as a person. These two aspects of bodily experience have two distinct terms in German, namely *Körper* and *Leib*. The former is the body as material object, as a dead mass that has all the characteristic dimensions of any material object and that resists all material manipulation. The latter is the experiencing self that senses and perceives, that is alive and vital and that lives in time and space.

The body is central to Merleau-Ponty's phenomenology (Merleau-Ponty & Smith, 1966). These authors wrote: 'I observe external objects with my body, I handle them, examine them, walk round them, but my body itself is a thing I do not observe: in order to be able to do so, I should need the use of a second body which itself would be unobservable' (p. 91). This proposition depends on a unified sense of self and body such that the body, while it is experiencing the world, is taken for granted. In other words, it is not apparent to itself. The illusory nature of this sense of unity is only revealed in the context of pathology. Furthermore, a schema of the body exists, composed of all the sensations including tactile, thermal, visual, postural and visceral. This schema is not mere perception but involves mental representations that are fluid and constantly adjusting, given new data. Hence, changes in posture, alterations of movement and motion, influence the plastic dimension of the schema. If this were not true, we would not be able to identify where on our body we have been touched, nor would we be able to describe where in space our limbs are at any point in time (Schilder, 1936).

The concept of a body schema is fundamental to our understanding of abnormalities of bodily experience. Gibbs (2005) describes body schema as

> the way in which the body actively integrates its posture and position in the environment. We do not ordinarily sense our bodies making postural adjustments as we perceive objects and events and move about the world. Body schemas allow us to walk adroitly without bumping into or tripping over things, to follow and locate objects, to perceive shape, distance, and duration, and to catch a ball with accuracy. These mundane events all take place independent of our conscious thoughts of the body. (Gibbs, 2005, p. 19)

Our sense of personal identity depends upon how sensory information is correlated in experience; as Gibbs puts it, 'I know who I am, and that I am, in part because I see my body ... as I move and experience specific sensations as a result of action' (Gibbs, 2005). And there are socially driven aspects to the body schema. In a study by Pollio et al. (1997) on the phenomenology of embodiment, awareness of the body as presented to other people in posture and dress and awareness of the body as an aspect of identity were two of the situations identified by participants. Furthermore, we engage with others from a first-person perspective but importantly from an embodied first-person perspective. The physical characteristics of our bodies – the height, weight, shape, mannerisms, gait – all influence how we are seen by others and how we relate to them. The body in society has profound implications for health, gender, sexual preference, ethnicity, disability, social status and politics. To summarize, abnormalities of body experience illuminate the complexity of the body both as an object in the world and as a subject experiencing the world (Oyebode, 2018).

To return to the socially driven aspects of the body schema, it seems as if in individuals with amelia, the congenital absence of limbs, observing motor actions in others led to robust activations of cortical areas involved in the planning and execution of mouth and foot movements. In addition, observation of hand movements activated major components of the fronto-parieto-temporal mirror system. This suggests that the mirror neuron is amenable to activation in individuals who do not possess physical limbs and therefore indicates that the body schema may have a neural underpinning that is innate and responsive to sensory and motor inputs (Gazzola et al., 2007; Hilti & Brugger, 2010).

Body integrity identity disorder provides the opportunity to better understand the relationship of the body schema to the actual material body. Phantom limb experience has provided some understanding of the influence of the body schema on subjective experience. It is now so well established that an amputee can continue to experience movement, posture and pain in a limb that has been amputated. This fact signals that the body schema continues to exist irrespective of the absence of sensory input from an actual limb. Furthermore, the fact that people with amelia can experience phantom limbs, despite never having had any limbs, points to the existence of neural systems ready to respond to sensory inflows from limbs. Indeed, Hilti and Brugger (2010) argued that dysmelia/amelia is the mirror opposite of body integrity identity disorder, amelia being animation without incarnation and body integrity identity disorder being incarnation without animation. Phantom limbs in amelia point to the likely correctness of Melzack's (1990) notion of a neuromatrix, a widespread network of thalamocortical and limbic loops that is basically innate and responds and adapts to sensory inputs and motor commands during a person's life.

Body integrity identity disorder points to the possibility of a mismatch between the body schema and the actual material body. It also raises the issue of how compelling it is to rectify this mismatch by altering the physical body in order to achieve harmony with the body schema.

This issue of the urge to rectify the mismatch between the body schema and the lived body is at the root of the discomfort that body integrity identity disorder generates in the public mind and why it has drawn comments from ethicists and lawyers, This is exemplified by reports in September 1997 of a Scottish surgeon, Dr Robert Smith, who performed an elective above-knee amputation on an English patient with a healthy limb. Two years later, in April 1999, he carried out a further above-knee amputation on a similar patient from Germany. Both patients were reported by Smith as belonging to a small subgroup of people who desire elective amputation in order to feel that they only have three limbs, not four (Dyer, 2000). Sufferers of the condition that Smith described found their condition extremely distressing and disabling and would often resort to self-harm in order to get rid of the limb (Dyer, 2000; Fisher & Smith, 2000). The profound desire to achieve harmony between the body schema and the lived body challenges a number notions: (1) whether it can ever be reasonable to amputate a perfectly healthy limb, (2) what are the limits of autonomous decision-making in medicine, and (3) whether a patient's valid consent overrides a doctor's conscientious objection to performing surgery on a healthy body part. The answers to these questions are outside the scope of this book, but the issues that the questions raise are in the background of the discussions of body integrity identity disorder.

15.2 Case Reports

1. [A] 63-year-old right-handed man who reported that since the age of 4 years he had desired bilateral lower limb amputations. Specifically, he indicated that he wanted his right leg to be

amputated four inches below his hip joint and his left leg to be amputated two inches below the knee, and he stated that these parts felt as if they were 'just not' his. He attributed his feelings about his legs to a 'possessive mother', 'an abusive boss' and a desire to 'fit in'. He noted that recently the left-side desire had become particularly strong, while conversely his desire for a right-sided amputation had decreased. He contacted us a year later to report that his desire for an amputation on his right side had almost completely disappeared. Several months after this, he had an elective left below-knee amputation and subsequently he no longer had any desire for a right leg amputation. (McGeoch et al., 2011, p. 1315)

2. [A] 70-year-old ambidextrous man who reported that he had had the desire to be an amputee of some sort since the age of 4 years when he saw another boy whose hand had been amputated. He reported that since then he had been fascinated by amputees and recalled that when he was 12 years old he thought about crushing a leg under a bus, although he could not remember which leg. He also used to pretend to have only one arm when he was a teenager and also contemplated cutting off a finger. He denied any sexual attraction towards amputees. He first realized at the age of 65 years (via the internet) that there were other people with similar desires to his own. He reported that since then, his desire for an amputation had been focused on his right leg around the middle of the thigh. He reported that on three occasions he had attempted to gain an amputation; twice by means of a tourniquet that he aborted due to the pain and once he was on the verge of crushing the leg under his car but stopped at the final moment. He became adept at applying local anaesthetic nerve blocks, and in early 2007 he carried out a right sciatic nerve block, which left him with a permanent palsy of his right common peroneal nerve. This was reflected in his neurological examination. ... [He] had an elective right above-knee amputation. (pp. 1315–16)

15.3 Explanatory Hypotheses

The most important explanatory hypothesis of the phenomenon involves the role of the right parietal lobe in body image. Dysfunction or lesions of the right parietal lobe are known to be associated with varied conditions such as left-sided neglect, anosognosia, anosodiaphora in which there is indifference to paralysis and misoplegia in which there is morbid dislike or hatred of paralyzed limbs in patients with hemiplegia. In addition, the right parietal lobe has a role in somatophrenia, a condition in which patients misattribute ownership of a paralyzed left arm or leg to another person, supernumerary phantom limbs and personification of a limb by giving it a name of its own (McGeoch et al., 2011). It is further argued that left-sided lesions predominate in body integrity identity disorder, that there is an intrinsic feeling that the limb in question is 'foreign' or 'intrusive' and that some patients feel aversive to the limb in question.

Attention has turned in recent times to probing and examining the neurological aspects of body integrity identity disorder. There is reported evidence of a heightened skin conductance response to pinprick below the desired line of amputation in two individuals who had a long-standing desire for amputation of a limb (Brang, McGeoch & Ramachandran, 2008). This finding was interpreted as arising from a congenital dysfunction of the right superior parietal lobule and its connections to the insula. Earlier, Ramachandran and McGeoch (2007) had proposed that body integrity identity disorder was probably due to dysfunction of the right superior parietal lobule. This view, as discussed earlier, was principally based upon the reported preponderance of left-sided bias for the limb in question and the similarity between body integrity identity disorder and somatophrenia (a condition that follows right parietal stroke and leads to rejection of the left arm as 'alien'). Furthermore, tactile stimulation of regions above and below the desired amputation line produced statistically reduced activation in the right superior parietal lobule using magneto-encephalographic scans (McGeoch et al., 2011). This was interpreted as evidence of inadequate activation of the right superior parietal lobule, a brain area thought to integrate disparate sensory inputs into a coherent body image. The authors proposed that body integrity identity disorder should be renamed 'xenomelia' to reflect the sense of estrangement of the affected limb. In a separate but similar investigation using functional magnetic resonance imaging, it was shown that individuals with body integrity identity disorder showed heightened responsivity of a large somatosensory network, including the parietal cortex and right insula, regardless of whether the stimulated limb felt 'alien' or not (Dijk, Wingen & Lammeren, 2013). Saetta et al. (2020) showed atrophy of the left premotor cortex and impaired functional connection between the right superior parietal lobe and the rest of the brain. This was interpreted as showing the pivotal role of the right parietal lobe in feelings of body ownership. And Blom et al. (2016) showed reduced grey matter volume in the left dorsal and ventral premotor cortices and a larger grey matter volume in the cerebellum in individuals with body integrity identity disorder. This was interpreted as demonstrating the importance of the premotor cortex and the cerebellum in the experience of body ownership and the integration of multisensory information. Dysfunction in these integrative systems is thought to result in a feeling of mismatch between the mental and physical body shape.

Assessments of temporal order judgements of tactile stimulation, proximal and distal to the desire amputation line, revealed defective spatiotemporal integration specifically on the parts of the body that are undesired. It is already known that spatiotemporal integration is mediated by the parietal lobes, and my conclusion is that the undesired body part captures the patient's attention unduly, in a pathologically exaggerated manner; hence the findings are thought to support the notion that body integrity identity disorder is a parietal lobe syndrome (Aoyama, Krummenacher & Palla, 2012).

These findings seem to indicate that abnormal neural processes are likely to be at play in body integrity identity disorder (Sedda, 2011; Sedda & Bottini, 2014), although it is probably premature to foreclose other possibilities (Giummarra, Bradshaw & Nicholl, 2011). Finally, there is evidence of reduced cortical thickness in the superior parietal lobule and reduced cortical surface area in the primary and secondary somatosensory cortices in the inferior parietal lobule, as well as in the anterior insular cortex (Hilti et al., 2013).

It has been suggested that the similarity between somatophrenia secondary to parietal lobe stroke means that body integrity identity disorder might be amenable to caloric vestibular stimulation, just as somatophrenia transiently responds to calorific vestibular stimulation (Ramachandran & McGeoch, 2007). However, this has proven not to be the case (Lenggenhager et al., 2014). Nonetheless, there is evidence from the 'rubber foot' illusion, in which illusory ownership of a fake foot after synchronous and asynchronous stroking of a visible rubber foot and the subject's hidden foot, that individuals with body integrity identity disorder experience an increase in the vividness of the illusion for the undesired foot compared to healthy control individuals (Lenggenhager, Hilti & Brugger, 2015). This finding is interpreted as demonstrating a weakened representation of the affected body part, and it strengthens the possibility that multisensory stimulation may provide therapeutic benefit.

Body integrity identity disorder was originally conceived as a paraphilia, but there is growing evidence that this is not the whole story. Lawrence (2006) described a similarity with transsexualism because both conditions shared a number of features, including profound dissatisfaction with embodiment, sexual arousal from simulation of the sought-after status (pretending to be an amputee or transvestism) and attraction to persons with the same body type as the desired/target body type. This latter feature is said to be prominent in non-homosexual male-to-female transsexuals (transsexual individuals who are not exclusively attracted to males) and is explained by a process termed *erotic target location error*. This process is thought to be present in some cases of body integrity identity disorder. This hypothesis predicts that individuals who desire limb amputation will be noted to also be sexually attracted to amputees, and in part, this is determined by the fact that sexual 'aesthetic preference' for a certain body morphology is dictated by the cortical representation of one's own body image (Ramachandran, Brang & McGeoch, 2009).

In a related but distinct thesis, de Preester (2013) argued for a closer overlap between body integrity identity disorder and paraphilias, making the point that the sexual component is essential to the phenomenology of the condition. De Preester applied Merleau-Ponty's notion of sexual schema interacting with body image to produce the disorder that is manifest as body integrity identity disorder. These ideas are of interest whether or not they apply to body integrity identity disorder. First, Schilder (1936) expressed the view that our body image is part of a community of body images and that there is continuing and reflexive interaction between how people respond to our body and what we incorporate in our body image. These socially determined aspects of the plasticity of the body schema influence how we empathize with others becaue we map onto our own schema another person's body in order to derive meaning from their actions and expressions. Merleau-Ponty's exposition of the sexual is complex, and de Presster's use of this aspect of Merleau-Ponty's work is conjectural indeed, even if interesting. In essence, sexual schema in these terms refers to the manner in which a person relates to particular stimuli because of how they are perceived or experienced. And de Presster derives from this that in body integrity identity disorder, sexual attraction to amputees and sexual arousal associated with imagining being an amputee are understandable given how intimately sexual preference is for identity in a person with body integrity identity disorder (Merleau-Ponty & Smith, 1966; de Preester, 2013).

15.4 Clinical Aspects

First (2005) reported a telephone interview study of 52 individuals who self-identified as having a desire for amputation. It was noted that none of the people included in the study were delusional or psychotic. Their desire for amputation extended back to childhood or adolescence and was associated with distress, attempts at self-amputation or impairment in social or occupational functioning in about three quarters of the sample. In the majority of those interviewed (73 per cent), the primary goal of the amputation was to restore their perceived body identity and not for sexual arousal or gratification, therefore arguing against the idea that the amputation was driven by primary paraphilia (apotemnophilia). Hence apotemnophilia was reconstrued as a disorder of body integrity and identity.

In the initial case reports of Money et al. (1977), both were male, and both identified as bisexual. Though separated, the first had been married and also had homosexual relationships and was able to recall a desire for amputation that began in early childhood and was a fixed desire from age 13 years onwards. He recalled an early childhood injury to the affected leg at the age of two years resulting in him being unable to walk for two years. He was reported as having made a number of attempts to damage his leg either by introducing infection or by using a tourniquet, though the pain was in no way pleasurable for him. The second case recalled onset of desire for amputation from about the age of 11 years. He had attempted to secure an elective amputation a number of times but failed. He had attempted self-amputation.

A better indication of the characteristic age and gender distribution of body integrity identity disorder came from First's telephone survey (First, 2005), which included 52 subjects, 47 of whom were male, four were female and one was male who was intersex at birth. This individual subsequently underwent male-to-female gender reassignment surgery. First noted a degree of potential referrer bias, as approximately two thirds of individuals were recruited into the study via the internet and the others via referral by other subjects. There was a high incidence of homosexual males, possibly explained by the fact that one individual referred a further eight. Excluding those subjects, 72 per cent were heterosexual, 19 per cent were homosexual and 9 per cent were bisexual. All but two of the subjects were Caucasian, and most (90 per cent) had some education beyond high school. At the time of the study, two thirds were in employment, 7 per cent were students and 23 per cent had retired, with an age range of 23–77 years.

A more recent survey of 54 individuals carried out in 2012 (Blom, Hennekam & Denys, 2012) reported findings consistent with First's (2005) report: 80 per cent of subjects interviewed were males, and more than 90 per cent were Caucasian. Two thirds were educated to university degree level, and the age range of participants included in the survey was 18–76 years. Respondents were grouped into amputation versus paralyzation (seeking severance of the spinal cord) groups depending upon the specific desire for disability that they exhibited. Across both groups, the age of onset occurred in childhood or adolescence, with a mean age of 6–7 years.

The actual incidence of individuals who desire self-amputation is unknown, but it is possible that the condition is not as rare as initially thought. Between 2000 and 2003, much media hype followed articles written about Dr Robert Smith and the elective amputations carried out in Scotland. Smith himself knew of other such patients who desired similar operations (Fisher & Smith, 2000; First & Fisher, 2012), and membership of online message board groups reached into numbers of 1,000 to 2,000 (Johnston & Elliott, 2002; First & Fisher, 2012).

Accurate figures are difficult to determine from news articles and reports written about individuals who had sought or had surgical amputation as they have generally remained anonymous, probably due to fears of stigma associated with wishing to acquire a disability. A review of the current internet presence of body integrity identity disorder suggests that some sites continue to exist, such as www.biid.org and www.overground.be; although they are primarily aimed at 'devotees' and 'wannabes', they do contain information relating to body integrity identity disorder and personal stories and accounts of people who have successfully sought amputation. Blog posts by some individuals suggest that the larger groups have 'gone underground' because of the post-millennial explosion of the internet and the increased risk of susceptible individuals being targeted either by people wishing to exploit their interest in finding a surgeon who would perform amputations or to target their desire for such a thing. On Amputee-By-Choice, an internet message board, there are posts offering to put wannabe amputees in touch with willing surgeons all over the world, but for a substantial fee. As can be expected, some responses to these posts are hopeful, whereas others are shams. One magazine article refers to a man known as the 'gatekeeper', who facilitates trips to Asia, where amputations are performed on seemingly ordinary 'tourists' who present with 'symptoms of limb ischemia' and are then give their consent for limb/life-saving surgery. However ordinary this approach to seeking treatment may seem, it is important to remember that unregulated surgical procedures are risky business, and in 1998, US citizen Phillip Bondy paid an unlicensed surgeon in Tijuana, Mexico, $10,000 for a healthy leg amputation and died of gangrene two days later in a San Diego hotel.

The clinical features described here are drawn from the following studies; First (2005), Blom et al. (2012), Bou Khalil and Richa (2012), and First and Fisher (2012). There is a persistent desire to acquire a significant disability, the onset of which occurs during childhood or early adolescence (i.e., between 8 and 12 years of age). The primary motivation is to feel 'whole' or 'complete' and serves to rectify the image of one's own true identity (as an amputee or paraplegic or with a significant disability) without which a sense of intense discomfort or inappropriateness would persist. There is impairment in social or occupational functioning and/or frequent attempts at auto-amputation resulting from significant psychological distress. Presentation at a late age, mostly between the ages 30 and 50 years, and often following a failed self-amputation attempt, despite an early age of onset, is common. This is thought to be due to perceived stigma or adverse judgement from relatives or medical professionals. In addition, there is a predominance of male gender, and it has been suggested recently that females may have a tendency towards a desire for paraplegia rather than amputation.

There appears to be an important sexual component in that the majority of respondents to the survey by First (2005) reported sexual attraction to other amputees, and around half reported that sexual arousal was a secondary reason for desiring amputation. Many patients with body integrity identity disorder also engage in 'pretending' behaviour, such as wrapping up their limbs or using aids and adaptions (Blom et al., 2012). This is often compared with cross-dressing in transsexualism.

There is no evidence that individuals with body integrity identity disorder have a positive family history of psychiatric disorder or co-morbid psychiatric disorder. Bou Khalil and Richa (2012) suggest that there may be an association with *Diagnostic and Statistical Manual of Mental Disorders*, 4th edition (*DSM-IV*), cluster B personality disorders, but this view is based on individual case reports rather than large-scale surveys.

A survey of the Japanese and Chinese literature revealed only two Japanese cases and no Chinese cases at all. The authors are reluctant to conclude that the condition is culture bound; rather, they posit secrecy as the underlying reason for the paucity of case reports (Blom, Vulink & Wal, 2016).

15.5 Conclusion

Body integrity identity disorder refers to a condition characterized by the persistent desire to acquire a physical disability, for example, amputation, paraplegia or other severe disability such as blindness. Individuals who suffer from this condition typically report a desire to achieve their sense of 'true self' and that to be successful in obtaining the desired amputation or disability would enable them to feel 'whole' or 'complete'. The condition probably reflects an underlying distressing mismatch between the body schema and the material body such that extreme measures are sought to rectify the mismatch.

Chapter 16

Côtard Syndrome

16.1 Introduction

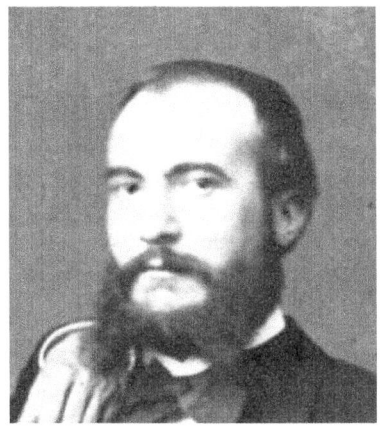

Jules Cotard 1840–1889

Jules Côtard (1840–1889) presented a report entitled, 'Du délire hypochondriaque dans une forme grave de la mélancoli anxieuse', in which he described a 43-year-old female patient on 28 June 1880 at a meeting of the Societé Médico-Psychologique. The woman believed that she had 'no brain, nerves, chest, or entrails, and was just skin and bone ... that neither God or the devil existed ... and that she was eternal and would live forever' (Berrios & Luque, 1995, p. 218). In addition, she said that she did not need food and asked to be burnt alive. She had made various suicide attempts. Côtard initially diagnosed *lypémanie* and formed the view that this was a new type of *lypémanie* consisting of anxious melancholia, ideas of damnation or possession, suicidal behaviour, insensitivity to pain, delusions of non-existence and delusions of immortality. In 1882, he introduced the term *délire des négations* (translated into English as 'nihilistic delusions') to refer to patients in whom there was a tendency to denying everything, including denying the existence of self or world. Côtard wrote:

> I would tentatively suggest the name 'nihilistic delusion' (*délire des negations*) to describe the condition of the patients to whom Griesinger was referring, in whom the tendency towards negation is carried to its extreme. If they are asked their name or age, they have neither – where were they born? They were not born. Who were their father, mother, wife or children. Have they a headache or pain in the stomach, or in any other part of the body? They have no head or stomach and some even have no body. If one shows them an object, a rose or some other flower, they answer, 'that is not a rose, not a flower at all'. In some cases negation is total. Nothing exists any longer, not even themselves.   (Oyebode 2018, pp. 353)

In 1893, Emil Régis coined the term *Côtard's syndrome*, and this term was popularized by Jules Séglas (1856–1939). Berrios et al. (1995) concluded from their conceptual history of the term that Côtard opted for a view that *délire des negations* was a type of depressive disorder, but in the wake of his death, the condition was conceived of as a syndrome that could be associated with agitated depression or anxious melancholia in Côtard's terms or with general paralysis. The central features were anxiety, delusions of negation, damnation and enormity.

Côtard syndrome exemplifies the tight relationship between the self and the body. Self-awareness is composed of (1) awareness of being or existing (ego vitality), which is experienced as a deep sense of being alive and existing and is ultimately fundamental to any other aspect of self-awareness; (2) awareness of activity that derives from the experience of being an agent in the world, acting, executing and operating in the world; (3) awareness of identity of the self that is manifest in an autobiographical narrative, in the persistence of a singular and enduring physiognomy and embodied in a single body; (4) awareness of unity and coherence of the self at any one time and over a duration; and (5) awareness of boundaries of the self that are manifest in being distinct from other material objects and from other persons (Oyebode, 2018).

Côtard syndrome speaks directly to the foundational knowledge that as human beings in the world we are alive and that we exist in the world. This foundational belief is probably partly dependent on sensory inputs from the external world but also from our viscera. It is this profoundly ultimate foundation of our being in the world that Côtard syndrome appears to contradict. One of Minkowski's patients put it this way:

> I do not sense myself anymore. I do not exist anymore. When someone speaks to me, I feel as if he were speaking to a dead person. I have to look at myself to be sure that it is I. I have the feeling of being an absent person. In sum, I am a walking shadow. I have the feeling that I am not the same man when I am lying in bed as I am when I am standing. I am certain of existing only when I am lying down, and even this is not quite true. I don't feel that my body is mine anymore. I do not feel anymore. I have the feeling that I am not here in my room or even under my skin. I do not exist; I am immaterial; I exist less and less; (sees that I am smiling and adds) it would make me smile too, if I heard someone else say something like this. (Minkowski, 1970)

This suggests that the awareness of vitality precedes sensory inputs since even when the patient's attention is drawn to the external world by the use of visual or auditory confirmation, the central false belief remains incorrigible and intractable. Hence the apparent primacy of the body, both in installing and in sustaining, the sense of being indubitably alive, is violated in Côtard syndrome. It is important that we distinguish, very clearly, Côtard syndrome from depersonalization. The first is a delusion, a false belief that is held with conviction and that is resistant to counterargument, whereas the latter is an anomalous experience that is described using the analogical language 'as if'.

Raymond Gibbs's (2005) influential thesis rightly places emphasis on the role of action or enactment on consciousness. In this proposition, conscious experience is grounded in perceptually guided activity in the environment. Gibbs makes the following claim:

> The things that we are most conscious of are those that offer opportunities for action. The affordances that arise from our bodily interactions with objects produce in us a fleeting, and usually inhibited, inner movement that brings them into consciousness. This perceptual grounding, together with our subjective experience of our bodies supports the experience of consciousness. The serial and unitary nature of conscious experience is a fundamental consequence of the embodied and situational character of the mind. (Gibbs, 2005)

Côtard syndrome is important precisely not only because it undermines our commonsense notions of what it is to be alive, but also because it makes it clear that all of the sensory inputs from the body and the continuing presence of action, not merely the intention to act but gross actions, are insufficient to confirm that a subject of experience is alive. It is a profound paradox of the syndrome that subjects of experience can declare with certainty that they are dead and do not evince doubt or surprise at their own declarations in the face of veritable facts.

Berrios and Luque (1995) reported on 100 published cases and, on the basis of factor analysis, found three groups: (1) psychotic depression with loadings for age, anxiety, delusions of guilt, depression and auditory hallucinations; (2) Côtard type 1 with loadings for age, hypochondriacal delusions and nihilistic delusions concerning the body, concepts and existence; and (3) Côtard type 2 with loadings from anxiety, delusions of immortality, auditory hallucinations, nihilistic delusions concerning existence and suicidal behaviour. The authors concluded that Côtard type 1 is likely to represent pure cases of Côtard syndrome and that the nosological origin of these cases was in delusional disorder and not affective disorder. In essence, this investigation supported the notion that pure cases of Côtard syndrome exist, even if they are rare (Berrios & Luque, 1995).

16.2 Case Reports

Case 1

An honourable lady of almost 70 years sat fit and healthy in the kitchen and was preparing the meal as a draught coming through the kitchen-door struck her so forcefully on the neck that she was suddenly completely paralysed on one side as if hit by a stroke. She almost resembled a dead body during the following days. Four days later language returned and she demanded that the women should dress her in a shroud and place her in her coffin since she was in fact already dead. Every effort was made to dissuade her from this ridiculous delusion. Her daughter and servants made it clear to her that she was not dead but still alive. All was in vain, the 'dead' woman became agitated and began to scold her friends vigorously for their negligence in not offering her this last service; and as they hesitated even longer, she became extremely impatient, and began to press her maid with threats to dress her as a dead person. Eventually everybody thought it was necessary to dress her like a corpse and to lay her out in order to calm her down. The lady tried to make herself look as neat as possible, rearranging tucks and pins, inspecting the seam of her shroud, and was expressing the dissatisfaction with the whiteness of her linen. In the end she fell asleep, and was then undressed and put into bed. She was barely awake, when the delusion, that she was really dead and should be buried, recurred. The paroxysm lasted a long time.   (Förstl & Beats, 1992, p. 417)

Case 2

We have before us a patient 68 years old presenting signs of a certain degree of intellectual deterioration: memory failure, judgemental disorders, and partial disorientation in time (her spatial orientation remains relatively well preserved). The behaviour of the patient corresponds to this deficiency; almost constantly she chews bits of string and paper that she picks up all around and finally swallows; she has signs of scratching all over her face and hands. The disorder has persisted for many years. . . . The clinical picture . . . is dominated by a depressive foundation. She whines, laments, complains about everything. We find that she has hypochondriacal delusions to the extent of negative ideas, delusions of ruin, and some delusions of guilt: she doesn't see well anymore, doesn't go to the toilet anymore, doesn't urinate, has nothing in her stomach, doesn't eat anything anymore except paper and scarps, has an empty head, has a cyst or a cancer in her rear, her brain has dried up, she has no more ideas, has water on the brain, has no money except for the forty cents in her pocket, no clothes except for what she has on, no apartment, no name, no address – in a word, she has nothing.   (Minkowski, 1970, pp. 306–7)

16.3 Explanatory Hypotheses

Ramachandran, Blakeslee and Dolan (1998) put forward the notion that Côtard syndrome may arise from a disconnection between the limbic cortex and the whole of the sensory area leading to a lack of emotional contact with the world and resulting in the patient feeling emotionally dead. Another proposal is that of Serino et al. (2013), linking Côtard syndrome with lesions of the temporoparietal junction, a multimodal area associated with bodily self-consciousness integrating inputs from tactile, proprioceptive, visual and vestibular systems. Semantic anomia was put forward by Mendez and Ramírez-Bermúdez (2011) to explain the presentation of Côtard syndrome in semantic dementia. Nonetheless, none of these three attempts sufficiently explains Côtard syndrome.

There is starting to be a degree of coherence in the neurological findings associated with Côtard syndrome, focusing on frontal structures, the temporoparietal junction, the insula and with involvement of subcortical structures, including the thalamus. Charland-Verville, Bruno and Bahri (2013) reported on a single-positron-emission computed tomographic investigation and found hypometabolism in a bilateral frontoparietal network encompassing the precuneus and adjacent posterior cingulate cortices, mesiofrontal and adjacent anterior cingulate cortices, posterior parietal and dorsolateral frontal lobes and right temporoparietal junction. There was hypermetabolic activity in the cerebellum, brainstem and bilateral thalami. The authors concluded that the regions that were observed to be hypometabolic are those relevant to conscious awareness and include key parts of the default-mode network in which integrated self is instantiated. They therefore hypothesized that their finding corresponds to profound disturbance in core consciousness in Côtard syndrome. Ozkan and Caliyurt (2016) investigated a single case and confirmed these findings: hypometabolism in the fronto-parieto-temporal association cortex and hypermetabolism in the basal ganglia.

Another study using cranial computed tomographic imaging revealed dilatation of the lateral and third ventricles, and magnetic resonance imaging showed central atrophy and lateral ventricle dilatation. In the same report, single-positron-emission computed tomography demonstrated left temporal, left frontal and left parietal lobe hypoperfusion (Caliyurt, Vardar and Tuglu, 2004). The relevance of these findings for our understanding of the nature and origin of Côtard syndrome was not discussed by the authors. In another single-positron-emission computed tomographic study in a single case, there was no demonstrable change in regional blood flow, but there was reduced striatal D_2 receptor binding (De Risio, De Rossi & Sarchiapone, 2004). The authors interpreted the reduced dopamine receptor binding as a marker of psychosis.

In an investigation of a single case presenting with neuroleptic malignant syndrome, catatonia and Côtard syndrome in the context of depressive psychosis, structural magnetic resonance imaging revealed leukoencephalopathy that was interpreted as secondary to perinatal injury at birth (Weiss, Santander & Torres, 2013).

Restrepo-Martínez and Espinola-Nadurille (2019) investigated a 19-year-old male patient with positron-emission tomography and demonstrated a marked decrease in the occipital lobe and insular cortices bilaterally and moderate hypometabolism in the anterior cingulate cortex and prominent hypermetabolism in both frontal and medial temporal lobes. Following treatment and clinical improvement, the positron-emission tomographic changes normalized in frontal and medial frontal metabolism, but there was no substantial change in the insular metabolism. The authors integrate their findings into what is already known about brain imaging changes that are demonstrable in Côtard syndrome. Their view is that the insula is central in processing emotional and sensory stimuli, focusing specifically on interoception, our awareness of internal sensations. Their postulate is that disruption in the processing of internal and external stimuli in the insular cortex and other limbic structures results in the subjective experience that lays the groundwork for Côtard syndrome.

In a review of the characteristics of 12 patients seen at the Mayo Clinic, Sahoo and Josephs (2018) reported that on neuroimaging, four patients had frontal lobe changes, four had generalized volume loss and seven had right-sided or bilateral hemisphere lesions. They concluded that Côtard syndrome occurred in the context of a wide spectrum of neurological change, and right-sided lesions appeared to predominate. They put forward the idea of disconnection in the neural circuits involved in the perception of self, similar to the explanatory hypothesis for delusional misidentification syndromes (see Chapter 1), emphasizing the inability to link perceptions of external or internal stimuli with internally generated autobiographical memories.

In a case study of a 56-year-old woman with semantic dementia, Mendez and Ramirez-Bermudez (2011) introduced language/semantic failure as an additional mechanism underpinning Côtard syndrome. The patient had progressive loss of semantic abilities, surface dyslexia and prosopagnosia. Neuroimaging demonstrated bilateral anterior temporal lobe atrophy, most prominent on the left, and single-photon-emission tomography showed hypoperfusion in the anterior temporal lobes, again more prominent on the left. The authors argue that Côtard syndrome had arisen from the patient's inability to know the meaning or source of somatic and internal sensations. The patient had lost the ability to describe her experiences and also lost the identity of the body parts from which these experiences emanated. For example, she did not know the meaning of terms such as chin, knee, nose or hair and could not recognize organs such as heart, stomach, liver or intestines. What this case does is remind us that the origins and mechanism underlying Côtard syndrome may be multifold and dissociation of somatic sensations from semantic knowledge in the setting of a failure of evaluation of beliefs may be important, too.

In summary, there is as yet no definitive mechanism put forward for Côtard syndrome, but there are indications of where the likely structural and functional abnormalities lie.

16.4   Clinical Aspects

There are no good epidemiological studies; hence the incidence and prevalence of Côtard syndrome are not established. In a thorough survey of a service for old age psychiatric patients in Hong Kong, Chiu (1995) reported a prevalence of 0.57 per cent for Côtard syndrome. The catchment area size was 750,000 people, with 8.7 per cent aged over 65 years. There were only two patients with Côtard syndrome, and both cases occurred in the context of depression. This survey, at least, confirms that Côtard syndrome is relatively rare. Other surveys have more or less confirmed this relative rarity. Ramirez-Bermudez (2010) reported a prevalence of 0.11 per cent in all inpatients in neurology and 0.63 per cent in psychiatric inpatients in Mexico.

Berrios and Luque (1995a) established the clinical features of Côtard syndrome in their analysis of 100 published cases. The mean age of the published cases was 52 years. The most common symptoms were depression (89 per cent), nihilistic delusion concerning the body (85 per cent), delusion of guilt (63 per cent), nihilistic delusion concerning existence (69 per cent), hypochondriacal delusion (58 per cent), anxiety (65 per cent) and delusion of immortality (55 per cent). In a related report on the conceptual history of Côtard syndrome, the same authors made the important point that the term *délire des negations* was not merely nihilistic delusions but a symptom cluster, explaining and emphasizing that the French concept of *délire* was not fully captured by the English term *delusion* (Berrios and Luque, 1995b).

Côtard syndrome has been described in the context of mood disorders, including recurrent depression and bipolar disorder, and schizophrenia. In schizophrenia, it is estimated to occur in 0.87 per cent of cases (Cipriani et al., 2019). It has been associated with dementia and learning disability (Kearns, 1987; Lerner, Bergman & Greenberg, 1995); acquired brain injury (Young, Robertson & Hellawell, 1992); ischaemic stroke (Sottile et al., 2015); following right subdural haematoma (Perez, Fuchs & Epstein, 2014); in delirium (Oberndorfer, Schönauer & Eichbauer, 2017), Parkinson's disease (Factor & Molho, 2004; Solla et al., 2015), multiple sclerosis (Shaan, Rizvi & Sharma, 2018), Hashimoto's thyroiditis (Hajnal & Lazary, 2019), migraine (Parks et al., 2014), and epilepsy (Drake, 1988); intracerebral tumors (Bhatia, 1993; Gonçalves & Tosoni, 2016), and anti-NMDA encephalitis (Funayama & Takata, 2018). There are reports of Côtard syndrome in the context of treatments for medical conditions including as a side effect of the use of valacyclovir and acyclovir (Lindén & Helldén, 2013) and following treatment with radioactive iodine (Kaya & Bulut, 2019).

Although Côtard syndrome is usually reported in adults, there are increasing reports in children and adolescents (Fillastre et al., 1992; Cohen, Cottias & Basquin, 1997; Allen & Pfefferbaum, 2000; Soultanian, Perisse & Révah-Levy, 2005).

Patients with Côtard syndrome often refuse to eat or drink. This behaviour derives from their delusional belief that they are already dead and hence do not need any sustenance from victuals or derives from the belief in their immortality, which means that they have no need for food or drink (Silva, Leong & Weinstock, 2000; Nejad, 2002; Teixeira & Araújo, 2015 ; Solimine, Chan & Morihara, 2016). The same beliefs may underlie self-mutilation, suicidal behaviours and aggressive acts (Ghaffari, Kerdegari & Reyhani 2007; Huber & Agorastos, 2012).

There are a number of unusual presentations of Côtard syndrome. Reif, Murach and Pfuhlmann (2003) reported on a female patient presenting with the delusional belief of paralysis in whom antipsychotic drugs had devoured her nerve ganglia, and Walloch et al. (2007) reported on a pregnant woman who denied being pregnant despite the clinically obvious signs of advanced pregnancy. These cases illustrate the need to be cognizant of the nature of the wider meaning of 'negation' in psychosis, taking account of psychotic denial of physical function and of pregnancy and the expressed explanations for these beliefs.

There are several reports of coexisting cases of Côtard syndrome and delusional misidentification syndromes, particularly Capgras syndrome, Frégoli syndrome and occasionally reduplicative paramnesia (Joseph & O'Leary, 1986; Young, Leafhead & Szulecka, 1994; Yalin, Varol Taş & Gunevır, 2008; Mashayekhi & Ghayoumi, 2015; Sottile et al., 2015). These reports are important because they suggest that there may well be aetiological links between these conditions. In delusional misidentification syndromes, particularly Capgras syndrome, there is disconnection between face recognition memory and the autonomic arousal system that is confirmatory for true identification. As described earlier, it may be that a similar disconnection is present in Côtard syndrome – sensory inputs from exteroceptors and interoceptors are disconnected from limbic structures underling conscious awareness of the body. This tentative explanation of the co-occurrence of Côtard syndrome and delusional misidentification syndromes allows for further investigation of these conditions. But there are several outstanding questions, for example, why do the conditions not occur jointly more often? What mechanism underpins the episodic nature of these conditions?

There is a need to be aware of cultural inflections on the presentation of Côtard syndrome. Nejad, Anari and Pouya (2013) described a 42-year-old woman who 'felt that something strange had happened to her. She felt she is nothing and is dead, as that she has been murdered by a ghost (Aal)'. Aal is female mythical creature who causes harm to women just after they deliver a baby. This mythical creature is said to dissect the victim's abdomen and eat the victim's liver. In other words, in this particular case, the patient used a local acceptable and comprehensible myth to explain her predicament.

Yarnada, Katsuragi and Fujii (1999) suggested that Côtard syndrome could be described in three stages: germination, blooming and chronic. The condition of their 46-year-old female patient's evolved gradually over a 12-month period or so. There was no doubt that during what the authors termed the 'blooming' stage her condition was well established, and she reported that 'I can't taste what I am eating. I can't identify the pleasant smell of bread and coffee. I can't see the rain outside the window I can't hear the sound of clocks' (p. 397). She also said

> Food wouldn't go down my throat. My bowels don't work, and my body can't excrete urine or faeces. Ability to memorize or think completely disappeared, and the brain was broken. Unless I say now, I will not be able to even speak tomorrow. . . . Why should I commit suicide? Now I have a body that does not die. (p. 397)

The chronic stage was essentially a worsening of the clinical condition to include persecutory delusions and social withdrawal. The condition ultimately responded to treatment. It is important to say that this description does not conform to the evolution of the majority of cases described in the literature. Despite being a novel approach and conceptually elegant, I do not believe that there is an empirical basis for adopting this system of staging.

There may be a role for attribution style in determining whether anomalous experience is ascribed to a change in the world or in oneself. Wright and Young (1993) reported on a patient who developed Côtard and Capgras syndromes sequentially. The patient presented with Côtard syndrome when she was depressed and Capgras syndrome when she had persecutory delusions. This case was explained as demonstrating the importance of attribution style determined by depressed mood, which in this case exaggerated negative effects. This proposal was tested on a 24-year-old female patient who presented with Côtard syndrome in the context of herpes simplex encephalitis. She was reported to have a significantly greater proportion of internalizing attributions than the control group both overall and for negative events specifically. The authors interpret their findings as support for the role of attributions in determining the nature of abnormal beliefs in the context of anomalous subjective experiences (McKay & Cipolotti, 2007).

16.5 Conclusion

Côtard syndrome exemplifies the tight relationship between the self and the body. The awareness of vitality, an aspect of awareness of the self, depends upon sensations from our viscera and probably also from awareness of activity that is reliant on agency and action in the world. What Côtard syndrome does is to undermine our assumptions that our belief in being alive depends upon these mechanisms because even when these matters are drawn to the attention of patients with Côtard syndrome, their stated false belief that they are already dead remains fixed and incorrigible. This suggests that central mechanisms exist that underpin the sense of vitality and disruption of these mechanisms probably underlie Côtard syndrome.

Confabulation

17.1 Introduction

Confabulation is a falsification of memory that occurs in clear consciousness and in association with an organic derived amnesia (Berlyne, 1972). It is probably best to consider it as a loose term that covers a range of qualitatively different memory disturbances (Oyebode, 2018). It covers such disparate phenomena as mild distortions of an actual memory, including intrusions, embellishments, elaborations, paraphrasing and high false-alarm rates on tests of anterograde amnesia. It can also refer to highly implausible, bizarre descriptions of false realities such as claiming to be a space traveller temporarily resident on planet Earth (Gilboa & Moscovitch, 2002). The term also has been used to include (1) memory confabulations; (2) confabulations about intentions and actions in subjects who had undergone commissurotomy resulting in split-brain phenomenon or in hemianosognosia or somatophrenia, where individuals deny obvious disability; (3) perceptual confabulations that occur in Anton syndrome, which is characterized by unawareness of blindness (Martín Juan et al., 2018); and (4) confabulations deriving from emotions (see Hirstein [2009] for a fuller review). In addition, the term has been extended by some authors to include explanations for aspects of delusions and autism (McKay & Kinsbourne, 2010; Spitzer et al., 2017). In many respects, the recent widening of the scope of the term has been unhelpful.

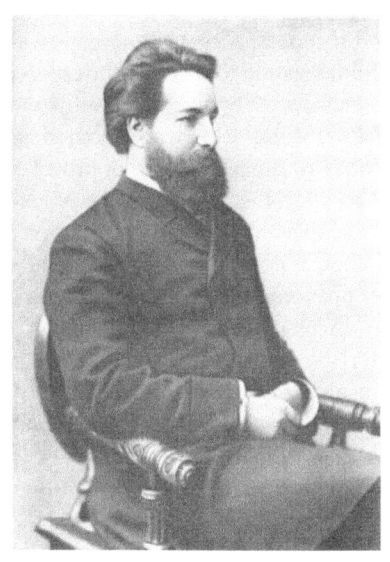

Sergei Sergeievich Korsakoff 1854–1900

Traditionally, the term *confabulation* is associated with the memory disturbance originally identified by Sergei Sergeievich Korsakoff (1854–1900) in the condition that he originally termed *psychosis polyneuritica seu cerebropathia psychica toxaemica* and described in 1890. Korsakoff described the condition as follows:

> The patient begins to tell implausible stories about himself, tells of his unusual voyages, confuses old recollections with recent events, is unaware of where he is and who are the people around him. Sometimes in addition, there occur illusions of sight and hearing which confuse the patient still further. . . . Together with the confusion, nearly always a profound disorder of memory is observed, although the disorder of memory occurs in pure form. In

such instances the disorder of memory manifests itself in an extraordinarily peculiar amnesia, in which the memory of recent events, those which just happened, is chiefly disturbed, whereas the remote past is remembered. ... At first, during conversation with such a patient, it is difficult to note the presence of a psychic disorder; the patient gives the impression of a person in complete possession of his faculties; he reasons about everything perfectly well, draws correct deductions from given premises, makes witty remarks, plays chess or a game of card, in a word, comports himself as a mentally sound person. ... This confusion does not involve that which the patient perceives at the present moment but affects only the recollection of the past events. Thus, when asked to tell how he has been spending his time, the patient would very frequently relate a story altogether different from that which actually occurred, for example, he would tell that yesterday he took a ride in town, whereas in fact he has been in bed for two months, or he would tell of conversations which have never occurred, and so forth. On occasion, such patients invent some fiction and constantly repeat it, so that a peculiar delirium develops, rooted in false recollection (pseudo-reminiscences). (Victor & Yakovlev, 1955, pp. 397–99)

The phenomenon that Korsakoff termed *pseudo-reminiscences* was later called *confabulation* by Bonhoeffer (1901) and by Wernicke, Pick and Kraepelin (Lorente-Rovira et al., 2011). Berlyne (1972) cites Bonhoeffer (1901) as describing two types of confabulation, namely a momentary form and a spontaneous form. The momentary form is often provoked by questions that probe the patient's memory for events, and if this exposes memory gaps with the attendant embarrassment, it can then result in ad hoc confabulation to cover up the exposed memory lapse. This phenomenon reveals that the patient remains socially aware of the situation. The spontaneous form is characterized by descriptions of adventurous experiences, sometimes of a fantastic nature. These two terms overlap somewhat with Kopelman's notions of provoked or spontaneous confabulation (Kopelman, 1987). In this account, the provoked type of confabulation is said to be common in amnesic patients and resembles errors produced in normal subjects after a prolonged period of retention and may reflect a normal response to a faulty memory. Spontaneous confabulation, in contrast, is a rarer phenomenon and probably reflects specific underlying neurological abnormalities (see further discussion later in this chapter).

Gilboa and Moscovitch (2002) describe the characteristic features of confabulation as follows: (1) it is a falsely retrieved memory, often containing false details within its context; (2) the patient is unaware that he or she is confabulating and often unaware of the existence of memory deficits (in other words, confabulation is not intentional); (3) patients may act on their confabulation, confirming their belief in the false memory; and (4) confabulation is most apparent in autobiographical memory.

The terms *Korsakoff syndrome* and *Korsakoff symptom complex* were proposed by Friedrich Jolly in 1897 and *Korsakoff psychosis* by Bonhoeffer in 1901 to describe the combination of a severe defect of learning, a loss of memory for recent events, loss of orientation and a tendency to confabulation in the context of habitual use of alcohol (Schnider, 2008). The relationship between Wernicke's encephalopathy and Korsakoff psychosis is another aspect of our understanding of the underlying mechanism of confabulation. Korsakoff had already reported on prodromal agitation and confusion, including features of ophthalmoplegia, nystagmus and ataxia, before the development of what we now recognize as Korsakoff psychosis. In the early twentieth century, animal experiments had suggested an important role for thiamine deficiency in Korsakoff psychosis. The reports of patients investigated at Changi Prison, Singapore, during World War II demonstrated that there was an onset of confusion, ataxia, nystagmus and ophthalmoplegia six weeks after thiamine deficiency and severe amnesia after a further two to three weeks. Confabulation was reported in 25 per cent. The mortality rate was influenced by the availability of thiamine (Wardener & Lennox, 1947; Kopelman, 2015). But it was the work of Victor, Adams and Collins (1971) that finally distinguished between Wernicke encephalopathy and Korsakoff psychosis, drawing attention to the overlap between them and identifying the underlying neuropathology, particularly the role of the thalamus and the mammillary bodies (Victor et al., 1971).

17.2 Case Reports

Case 1

I saw the patient June 1, 1889. At that time the psychic symptoms were alright slight; the patient knew clearly where she was, who were about her, remembered fairly well what was going on, and related correctly details of her illness. However, in a long conversation one could note anomalies in the psychic sphere. These anomalies chiefly concerned the memory. Thus, in telling of something about the past, the patient would suddenly confuse events and would introduce the events related to one period into the story about another period. For example, telling about a trip she had made to Finland before her illness and describing her voyage in fair detail, the patient mixed into the story her recollections of Crimea, and so it turned out that in Finland people always eat lamb and the inhabitants are Tartars. When, I objected, however, she promptly agreed that she had confused the facts. Such muddling of facts not infrequently occurs in this patient, but in most instances she herself notices them. Furthermore, she frequently gives false information in regard to her past illness. Thus, she assures me that she well remembers a physician who came to see her in consultation and describes him as having black hair, whereas he is completely gray. In general the patient does not remember that which occurred during the time of the illness, although gradually the events of her illness become restored in her memory.   (Victor & Yakovlev, 1955, p. 404)

Case 2

BS was a 61-yerar old man, who had been found collapsed on a pavement by a neighbour. He was confused and disorientated, and he showed pronounced nystagmus. He was also very ataxic, and he could stand only with support. At admission, he admitted to consuming a bottle of whiskey a day. He was 'stuck' in the 1970s or early 1980s, thinking that Margaret Thatcher was Prime Minister and Richard Nixon was President of the United States. He confabulated in episodic memory, thinking that he had recently taken a girlfriend home to his parents at Christmas, and that he was still serving in the airforce (as he had done in the 1970s). He also confabulated in personal semantic memory, thinking that his brother had emigrated to Canada, when the brother was in fact visiting on a weekly basis, and also in semantic memory, thinking the Pope had recently been assassinated.   (Kopelman, 2010, p. 16)

Case 3

AB was a 43-year old hospital employee, who was admitted to the Accident and Emergency department, with Wernicke's encephalopathy (confusion, ophthalmoplegia, ataxia, and nystagmus), and she was found to have a half empty bottle of vodka in her handbag. Despite high doses of multivitamins, the patient continued to confabulate floridly, and subsequently cancer of the cervix was diagnosed. She confabulated in episodic memory, saying that she had been admitted for measles, and that her parents were visiting her regularly, despite the fact that they had been dead for 4 and 20 years respectively. She talked about being employed in the hospital, but identified the wrong hospital. She said that her brother was a doctor living on the 22nd floor, when her ward was on the top floor (the 12th). She also confabulated in semantic memory, saying that Stanley Baldwin was still the Prime Minister, and that Robert Maxwell (the newspaper proprietor) had been shot. (Kopelman, Ng & Brouke, 1997, p. 16)

17.3 Explanatory Hypotheses

There are four contending overarching theories that attempt to explain confabulation: (1) those which emphasize context-dependent memory confusions; (2) the proposal of a novel concept of temporal consciousness and the dysfunction thereof; (3) the proposition of errors in strategic search, problems in retrieval and accompanying impairments in monitoring of responses; and (4) the influence of motivational factors in the content of confabulations.

In Korsakoff's original description (see earlier), there was already a suggestion that confabulation arose from the intrusion of 'old recollections with present impressions' (Korsakoff, 1955, p. 397). In other words, it was suggested that the memory errors that were apparent depended on context to become apparent. An example is given in the report by Schnider et al. (2013) on a 57-year-old locksmith with chronic alcohol abuse who had presented with Wernicke-Korsakoff syndrome. The patient was convinced that he had to forge a metal piece for the boat of the Fehlmann sailing team (a famous team in the 1980s).

During the medical rounds, he asked with deep concern for the permission to leave the hospital to respond to this important obligation. On occasions, he spontaneously showed up at the nurses' office to ask, with much insistence, for permission to leave the unit to work on the metal piece. ... As it turned out, the patient, who had worked as a locksmith at a perfume factory, had indeed prepared a particular piece of metal for the Fehlmann sailing boat in 1985. He had worked on it for one month in the evening hours but never spent the whole night or the weekend on it. (Schnider et al., 2013, pp. 93–4)

The authors conclude that the main failure was that a correct memory of 20 years previously was transposed in time and became the inappropriate basis for current behaviour.

Temporal consciousness is defined as a specific form of consciousness that allows individuals to have the phenomenological experience of remembering their personal past, of being oriented in their present world and of predicting their personal future (Dalla Barba & Boisse, 2010; Serra et al., 2014; Barba et al., 2020). The proposition here is that temporal consciousness facilitates the distinction in our apprehension of an object either as a unique object or as a member of a multiplicity of objects. To use the proponents' example, 'this pen on the desk is both *a pen* and *the pen*'. The constructs underpinning this proposition are complex and highly philosophical. In essence, all objects that come into consciousness have to be transposed from being a member of a class to being a unique object at the level of what the proponents term 'temporalization' of the object. In confabulation, it is thought that errors of memory occur because the patients are relying on personal habits and routines to answer questions that have unique answers. Finally, there is an additional proposal which links confabulation specifically to the preservation of the hippocampus irrespective of any other demonstrable neuropathology that is aetiologically associated with confabulation (Dalla Barba & La Corte, 2015). In other words, the suggestion is that the integrity of the hippocampus is required for the normal functioning of temporal consciousness. Amnesic patients with an impaired hippocampus, in this model, do not confabulate, whereas, amnesic patients with a spared hippocampus do confabulate (Dalla Barba & La Corte, 2013).

Gilboa regards confabulation as a deficit in strategic retrieval processes (Gilboa & Moscovitch, 2002; Gilboa, 2010). This explanatory model is built on a particular approach to memory processes, including, on the one hand, the nature of encoding/storage and, on the other hand, retrieval. The model assumes that memory traces, comprising hippocampal-neocortical ensembles, are formed to represent conscious experience. These ensembles do not encode temporal order or thematic/semantic meaning. The frontal lobe structures are critical for endowing information with the semantic organization and temporal order. Faulty encoding due to dysfunction at the level of limbic structures may then contribute to the evolution of confabulation in that they act to impair retrieval processes by providing information poorly or erroneously encoded. For confabulation to occur, these erroneous details will need to be produced by the retrieval process. The retrieval process itself may be dysfunctional either by way of erroneous activations or by failure in monitoring of retrieved information because of impaired functioning of the prefrontal regions. In sum, three basic faulty processes may underlie confabulation: (1) faulty search processes that signal an inability to initiate and maintain an orderly process of exploring long-term memory, (2) faulty associations between memory cues and memory representations, and (3) faulty monitoring, which is itself a necessary and sufficient condition for confabulation.

The role of emotion and motivational factors is beginning to re-emerge as important. This was already nascent in the discussions about confabulation as a means of covering up memory gaps or of responding to embarrassment. The notion is that patients who confabulate are distorting previous experiences in ways that are significantly more pleasant and self-enhancing than control subjects and that the content of confabulation is mostly positive. Furthermore, confabulating subjects are as impaired on recall of information as other amnesic patients, but they showed a selective bias in recalling information that portrayed a more positive image of themselves. The authors conclude that the self-enhancing content of confabulation is probably an exaggeration of normal self-serving memory distortion (Fotopoulou et al., 2008a, 2008b; Fotopoulou, 2010).

The psychological models just described are only useful to the degree that they are comprehensible in light of the neuroanatomical substrate of confabulation and our understanding of the function of the structures implicated in confabulation. There is considerable consensus on the role of the mammillary bodies, anterior and dorsomedial nuclei of the thalamus and structures that include the basal prosencephaly and orbitofrontal cortex in Wernicke-Korsakoff syndrome. The severe amnesia in Wernicke-Korsakoff syndrome is thought to result from involvement of the mammillary bodies and the anterior nuclei of the thalamus, which receives afferents from the hippocampus. The confabulation that characterizes the condition is thought to result from the involvement of the dorsomedial nucleus of the thalamus, which receives inputs from the frontal cortex and from cortical and subcortical structures such as the amygdala (Lorente-Rovira et al., 2011). The actual pathological findings in Wernicke-Korsakoff syndrome are well characterized: there is neuronal loss, gliosis and micro-haemorrhages in the paraventricular and periaqueductal grey matter (Victor et al.,

1971). Victor thought that involvement of the mediodorsal nucleus of the thalamus might be critical in the anterograde amnesia that characterizes Korsakoff psychosis.

Structural neuroimaging studies have confirmed what was already established: alterations in structures such as the thalamus, mammillary bodies, periventricular grey matter and frontal cortex and functional imaging studies demonstrate reduced glucose uptake in the thalamus bilaterally, the hypothalamus, the mammillary bodies and the basal forebrain/ orbitofrontal cortex (Kopelman, 2015).

17.4 Clinical Aspects

It was clear from Korsakoff's original description that alcohol was only one possible cause of the condition that we now know as Korsakoff psychosis. Other causes that he mentioned include intestinal obstruction, persistent vomiting, typhoid, syphilis, pelvic infection, intra-abdominal tumour with associated vomiting, tuberculosis, typhus, lymphadenoma and poisoning with arsenic, lead, hydrogen disulphide, carbon monoxide, ergot and 'spoilt corn' (Korsakoff, 1889, 1955).

There are reports of confabulation in the context of anorexia nervosa (Saad et al., 2010), hunger strike in a prisoner (Durmaz, Aktaş & Akkişi Kumsar, 2020), hypothalamic relapse of a cardiac large B-cell lymphoma (Ospina-García et al., 2018), right frontal lobe epilepsy (Fujikawa et al., 2016), normotensive hydrocephalus (Dalla Barba et al., 2016), limbic encephalitis (Nahum et al., 2010), infarction of the artery of Percheron (Zhou et al., 2015), left thalamopolar infarct (Ghika, 2012), mesial bifrontal stroke (Nersesjan, Bogwardt & Kondziella, 2020), ruptured aneurysm of the anterior communicating artery (Borsutzky et al., 2010), left mediofrontal subcortical haematoma (Iizuka et al., 2005) and following traumatic head injury (Oyama et al., 1998).

There are reports of unusual forms of confabulation. Cocchini et al. (2014) reported on *phantabulation*, which they described as frequent and purposeful interactions with contextually appropriate imagined objects. The case was a 52-year-old man who had presented following rupture of an anterior communicating artery.

> Phantabulations occurred quite regularly and did not appear to be specific to any situation, time, or location. They could occur spontaneously during a conversation with the examiners, relatives, or friends and sometimes during formal testing sessions. . . . On one occasion, for instance, MT held an imaginary bottle, commenting 'it's quite light'. Phantabulations could be triggered by a variety of stimuli, which could be either endogenous (e.g., talking about or imagining an object) or exogenous (e.g., seeing a basin could trigger MT to begin brushing his teeth with an imaginary toothbrush). . . . On one occasion, for example, a nurse guided him to the toilet door, as he had some difficulty in finding his way there. Once alone in front of the toilet door, he started to undress himself to sit on an imaginary toilet. The nurse quickly came back to guide him inside of the room, at which MT looked perplexed, as if he could not understand why he was being asked to move. (p. 585)

The authors conclude that phantabulation results from confusion between real and imagined objects caused by a failure to inhibit florid visual imagery and facilitated by cortical release mechanisms. In this case, the novel phenomena occurred in the context of confabulation and are akin to but distinct from the context-dependent form of confabulation because they are founded on either a visual object such as a door or a visual image of an imaginary object, and the behaviour is context specific.

Another unusual presentation is that termed *graphabulation*, which is discussed as a graphic form of confabulation by Roh et al. (2012). The patient was a 53-year-old woman with Wernicke-Korsakoff syndrome following hyperemesis gravidarum at the age of 35 years. She had severe anterograde amnesia and confabulation. The novel phenomenon was observed in the setting of test of the patient's ability to copy and recall familiar and unfamiliar figures. The authors reported that

> firstly, the patient was able to perfectly copy figures but could recall few of the figures in immediate and delayed recall. . . . [T]he patient filled the memory gaps with irrelevant figures or similar figures using extra strokes. Second, the number of strokes required to draw the figures increased as a function of time delay. . . . Third, there was no difference in the number of strokes between the familiar and unfamiliar tasks.

17.5 Conclusion

Confabulation is a falsification of memory that occurs in clear consciousness and in association with an organic-derived amnesia. The meaning of the term has widened beyond Korsakoff psychosis to include several phenomena. Nonetheless, it is a term that has allowed for an increase in our understanding of the nature of memory disturbance and the neurological underpinning of such disparate phenomena as mild distortions of an actual memory, including intrusions, embellishments, elaborations, paraphrasing or high false-alarm rates on tests of anterograde amnesia.

Ganser State

18.1 Introduction

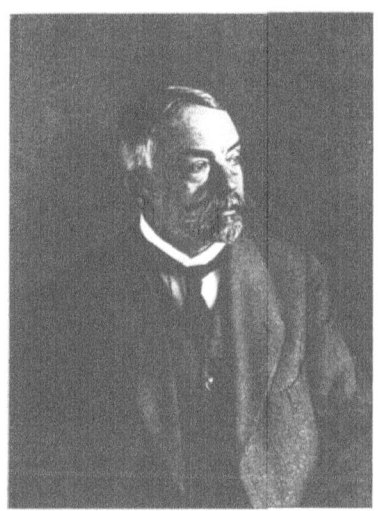

Sigbert Josef Maria Ganser 1853–1931

On 23 October 1897, Sigbert Josef Maria Ganser (1853–1931) presented a paper, entitled, 'A Peculiar Hysterical State', at the Central Psychiatric and Neurological Convention at Halle on a condition that was to later bear his name. He reported

> These patients have a number of common features which justify grouping them together as a distinct entity. . . . The most obvious sign which they present consists of their inability to answer correctly the simplest questions which are asked of them, even though by many of their answers they indicate that they have grasped, in a large part, the sense of the question, and in their answers they betray at once a baffling ignorance and a surprising lack of knowledge which they most assuredly once possessed, or still possess.
>
> As a demonstration I would like to report a conversation which was held with one of these patients: Are you able to count to ten? Yes. (But he does not, and is silent.) Well, then, count. (But he does not, and only counts on being prompted.) 1, 2, 3, 4. (Then he is quiet again.) What follows one? Two, Then? Twelve, 93 and . . . and after 93? (He continues in that fashion.) On another occasion: 1, 2, 3, 4, 5, 7, 8, 9, 10, 11, 14, 18, 19, 20, 21, 24, 27. How much are two and one? Three. Three and two? Seven. Five and two? Four. What is four minus one? Five (Then he corrected the answer to three.) In what city are we? Berlin, in Russia. What are you doing here? We wanted to go hunting, and we unhitched our horses. How many noses do you have? I don't know. Have you any nose at all? I do not know if I have a nose. Have you eyes? I have no eyes. How many fingers do you have? Eleven. How many ears? (He first touches his ears, and then says: Two.) How many legs does a horse have? Three. An elephant? Five. After being shown a coin and asked, What is that? the answer is: A map which a person hangs on his watch chain. Glancing at the eagle stamped upon a coin: I don't know that person. Is this Kaiser Wilhelm? He was shown a dollar and was asked: Do you know a dollar? He said, I don't know a dollar. That is a toy which one gives to children. What is your name? My name is Fürst (incorrect). (Schorer, 1965, pp. 120–1)

The clinical features were based on examination of four patients, all of whom were prisoners at the time of the examination. The other features included (1) auditory and/or visual hallucinations, (2) clouding of consciousness described as a 'twilight state', (3) hysterical stigmata, including analgesia over the whole body, whereby a pinprick evoked no pain sensation or hyperalgesia, (4) sudden resolution of the symptoms, and (5) amnesia for the episode. Ganser added that in all cases there was a strongly operating precipitating trauma, namely an attack of typhus, financial worries and distress and traumatic head injury associated with loss of consciousness. Ganser was aware right from the outset that the clinical picture raised the strong suspicion of malingering, but he was adamant that there was no evidence of malingering in his cases.

> I must say that I never had the impression that these patients sought to deceive me. They never made any spontaneous absurd remarks; only when questioned did any such answers appear, and often they showed how troublesome to them these repeated examinations were. They appeared unwilling to have anyone think of their answers as false and simple-minded, and of themselves as ignorant and foolish, whereas they appeared convinced that whatever they said was correct. (p. 125)

Nonetheless, the possibility of malingering cannot be overlooked, and even though Wertham's statement that 'Ganser reaction is a hysterical pseudostupidity which occurs almost exclusively in jails and in old-fashioned German psychiatric textbooks [and] is now known to be almost always due more to conscious malingering that to unconscious stupefaction' (Wertham, 1949; quoted in Goldin & MacDonald, 1955, p. 275) is an exaggeration, this dimension of the problem needs to be kept in mind.

The central feature of Ganser state is identifiable in discourse. The point here is that the abnormal phenomena arise in the context of conversational speech, that is, in discourse as opposed to phenomena that reveal themselves by the patient on his or her own. The patient's responses to verbal inquiries are off the mark. Goldin and MacDonald (1955) have argued that the current term used to denote these unusual responses, *vorbeireden*, is usually translated into English as 'talking past the point' or 'talking beside the point' or 'talking at cross-purposes' but that none of these translations correctly expresses the meaning that Ganser was attempting to convey. Furthermore, they make the point that Ganser's original term was *vorbeigehen*, meaning 'to pass by'. Other terms used to describe the typical Ganser response are *paralogia* and *approximate answers*. Jaspers (1997) refers to paralogia as having intelligible content that is manifestly related to the question, and even though the intellectual competence is there, nonetheless the answer is incorrect. Whatever term is used, the essence of the verbal responses is that the patient understands the question being asked and makes a response that is in the correct domain but that only approximates the correct answer.

Jaspers thought that *vorbeireden* had diverse origins, and he referred to the possibility of pseudo-dementia or as an aspect of the buffoonery sometimes seen in schizophrenia. On the question of the nature of twilight states in hysteria in general and in Ganser state more specifically, Bleuler (1950) wrote that they are like waking dreams which portray desires, wishes or fears in a direct or symbolic way as already fulfilled, and the overlap between twilight state in schizophrenia and Ganser state is that there may be complete negative rapport with the environment. In schizophrenia, as in Ganser state, the twilight state may be released in prisoners subject to judicial or medical examination. Bleuler goes on to give examples that are indistinguishable from the descriptions previously given by Ganser: 'ordered to open a lock, the patient attempts to push the wrong end of the key into the lock' (p. 219).

The possibility that the Ganser state is merely an example of hysteria pseudo-dementia is put forward by Mayer-Gross et al. They assert that both conditions are coterminous and identical (Slater & Roth, 1970b), but Anderson and Mallinson (1941) argue that a distinction can be made, and this based on the absence of a disorder of consciousness in pseudo-dementia and the proposition that in Ganser state the examiner is never left with the subjective impression that the patient is malingering.

Ganser himself reported his cases as examples of hysterical disorder, but two of his three original cases had suffered serious head injury, and the third was recovering from typhus. Whitlock (1967) demonstrated that Ganser state occurs in the context of both functional and organic psychoses but concedes that it is possible that when Ganser symptoms appear in the functional psychosis, it is possible that hysterical symptoms have been grafted onto the underlying psychotic process, even though he does not favour this conclusion.

18.2 Case Reports

Case1

The patient, male, aged 26 years, a skilled plumber by trade, was admitted to a psychiatric ward three weeks after sustaining a closed head injury with concussion. Physically, he showed inequality of the pupils and an extensor left plantar response. The EEG showed diffuse slow activity, with an abnormality which improved slowly throughout the period of in-patient treatment. Mentally he was pleasant, somewhat facile, and had difficulty concentrating on a given task. On questioning he responded as follows:

Q. 'What is your name?'

A. 'It may be the same as yours.'

Q. 'How old are you?'

A. 'How should I know that?'

Later, he gave his correct age, but gave the year of his birth as 1922 instead of 1933. When this inaccuracy was commented on, he replied in an offhand manner, 'Well, it's nearabouts'. When asked to give his address, he said 'Newcastle upon Tyne, Newcastle'. Asked in what street he lived, he replied, 'It may be the street we have been trying to find tonight'. He was then asked to state the colour of his (blue) pyjamas and he replied that it might be red. The colour of a red chair he gave as brown, but later correctly as red. He appeared to have some difficulty in naming objects correctly and was disoriented in time and place. When asked to say how long he had been in the ward, he replied 'Well, I could have come in this minute, couldn't I?'; he had some difficulty in distinguishing between the words 'world' and 'ward'. Throughout the interview, he was cheerful, off-hand and a little perplexed. The great majority of his answers had the approximate and paralogic quality of the Ganser symptoms. . . . On discharge he was correctly oriented, was able to give the correct answers to most questions, but was still decidedly euphoric. He had a posttraumatic amnesia of five weeks' duration.   (Whitlock, 1967, pp. 23–4)

Case 2

The patient, a female, aged 59, was admitted to a psychiatric ward three days after falling off a ladder. She was completely unconscious for a few minutes following the accident, but managed to walk into the admission ward. At that time she was wholly disoriented, was unable to give her name, and appeared to be confused. Shortly after her admission, she walked out of the hospital and returned home. She was then re-admitted and transferred to the psychiatric unit. At interview, she appeared somewhat distraught and untidy. Physical examination and EEG studies revealed nothing of significance. Mentally she appeared to be somewhat confused; when addressed by her name, she looked over her shoulder as if expecting to see someone of this name in another part of the room. In reply to direct questions, she said that she had four legs and two heads. When a single finger was pointed at her, she said there were two. She appeared wholly disoriented in time and place, believing that she was staying in a hotel, and asked to see the manager. Her capacity to sustain a conversation fluctuated considerably, but over the subsequent ten days, there was an all-round improvement in her condition. She became correctly oriented and was finally discharged. The duration of post-traumatic amnesia was not recorded in this case.

(Whitlock, 1967, p. 24)

Case 3

Admitted on 15/3/67 was a 19-year-old single Indian storekeeper. His father was a telephone operator who had died two years before of heart attack. His mother operated a food stall. He was the eldest in a family of 7 boys and 3 girls, all living in a flat. He was educated in English up to the eighth year, and was a member of the Singapore Volunteer Armed Forces. On 3/1/67 he was knocked down in a traffic accident on his way to work and sustained a mild head injury. Following this he had headache and pain in the right shoulder. He was treated . . . for 'Depression'. On 15/3/67 he attempted suicide by jumping into the sea from a busy pier, for which he was admitted to this hospital. Two days later, when he was examined by the author, he complained he heard voices of people saying all sorts of things about him, and felt people wanting to harm him. He gave incorrect or approximate answers to simple questions. The following was a sample of his responses. Question: 'I give you some numbers and you repeat after me, 74658.' Answer: '7465.' Question: 'Can you count 1, 2, 3, up to 20?' Answer: '1, 2, 3, 20.' He identified objects wrongly: tuning fork = iron; blood pressure set = balloon (pointing to the pump). He was given an identical examination on 21/3/67, when he answered all questions correctly, but he was unable to remember the previous examination. He said he had been very well previously but a little uncomfortable after the accident. On 17/4/67 he returned to work and was certified to be fit for full duties. He wanted a medical certificate to show that he had stayed in Woodbridge Hospital so that he could claim compensation from the insurance.   (Tsoi, 1973, p. 570)

18.3 Explanatory Hypothesis

The most accepted explanation for Ganser state is that it is an example of hysterical dissociation or, in modern terms, a dissociative disorder in which there is a partial or complete loss of the usual integration between memories, awareness of identity and immediate sensations of control of motor activity. It is assumed that it is distinct from malingering as the motivation is unconscious. It is thought that (1) the symptoms are an imperfect representation of the condition that they resemble, (2) they correspond to the mental image that the patient might be expected to have of the illness or emotional state that it resembles, (3) the immediate state can be seen to serve a gainful purposeful for the patient, and (4) there will be previous evidence of episodes of dissociation (Enoch, Trethowan & Barker, 1967). Anderson, Trethowan and Kenna (1959) reported, based on an investigation of simulation of mental illness, that some of the subjects gave approximate answers that were similar to those reported in the Ganser state. Furthermore, in comparison to patients with pseudo-dementia, patients with dementia, and a normal non-simulating group, the group that was simulating mental illness gave more and more normal responses as time passed. It seemed as if fatigue acted to normalize the responses of the simulating subjects, whereas perseveration increased in the dementia group and in the pseudo-dementia group, and the patients became uncooperative.

The apparent association of Ganser state with a history of traumatic head injury or other cerebral insults is not easy to explain away simply by redoubt to psychogenic mechanisms. Cutting (2011) makes the point that Ganser state is often associated with left hemisphere damage and that this suggests that the core feature of Ganser state, namely approximate answers, is an example of impairment of left hemisphere–dependent lexical or semantic knowledge. Cutting developed this notion further by asserting that there is nothing 'hysterical' about someone who cannot count from one to ten or cannot give the correct number of legs that a horse has since the cunning animal itself cannot do so and that does not make it hysterical.

What is clear is that no fully acceptable overarching explanatory hypothesis exists to explain how Ganser state comes to develop, at least in those cases where a pure psychological explanation is insufficient.

18.4 Clinical Aspects

Dalfen and Feinstein (2000) reported on four patients from a sample of 513 (0.7 per cent) in a mild traumatic brain injury outpatient clinic in a one-year period. This underlines the relative rarity of this condition. In this sample, the patients had brief post-traumatic amnesia and no retrograde amnesia. There was no ongoing litigation in three of the four cases, but there was evidence of acute stress disorder or post-traumatic stress disorder. The presence of acute stress disorder or post-traumatic stress disorder did not explain how or why Ganser state occurred in these patients.

Tsoi (1973) reported on 10 cases drawn from Woodbridge Hospital, Singapore, serving at the time a population of 2 million people and seeing more than 1,500 patients annually for the 10-year period of the investigation. This report once again attests to the rarity of Ganser state. The patients were all males and were aged between 19 and 56 years. Two of the 10 patients were seeking compensation for head injuries and three were awaiting trial for murder. There were disproportionately people of Indian ethnicity in the sample compared to the background census data. The author concluded that Ganser state was likely to lie on the continuum from hysteria to malingering.

Milo Tyndel (1956) reported on his observations in the years 1950–1954 as an examiner for the General Disability Insurance Institute in Vienna, Austria. He found 25 people from investigation of several thousand referred for neurological and psychiatric examination. All these people were males. They were aged between 50 and 65 years. All were married or divorced and except for the three examined in their homes, the others were either accompanied by their spouses, daughters or elderly unmarried male friends. The attending relatives were described as overly solicitous and helped them not only with all formalities but with dressing and undressing; they behaved much more in a parental manner than as attendants of sick persons, trying to answer questions for the examinees, interfering with the examination and showing an adverse, in some cases hostile, attitude towards the examiner. Physical examination did not reveal any gross pathology. Psychological investigation showed findings of psychological disturbance in the sense of anxiety and hysteria, without serious difficulties in thinking processes. Various degrees of memory impairment did not exceed to a considerable degree the average impairment of elderly persons. In all but two cases there were more or less obvious signs indicating deliberately incorrect responses (malingering). Nonetheless, Tyndel concludes that there is no sharp delimitation between unconscious and conscious mental processes, and he cautions against determining that these cases are examples of malingering or hysteria.

There is little doubt that Ganser state occurs in the setting of neurological disorder and in psychiatric illness. Snyder and Buchsbaum (1998) reported a case presenting with bizarre visual experiences and absurd verbal responses in which positron-emission tomography revealed bilateral lesions involving occipital association cortex, posterior temporal and parietal lobes most likely to be due to hypoxia secondary to asthmatic attack. There are other reports implicating temporoparietal lesions resulting from intracerebral haemorrhage (Anupama, Rao and Dhananjaya, 2006) and lacunar infarcts of both frontal lobes (Ouyang, Duggal & Jacob, 2003), posterior cerebral infract, frontotemporal dementia (Ladowsky-Brooks & Fischer, 2003) and space-occupying lesion of the dominant hemisphere (Doongaji, Apte & Bhat, 1975).

In addition to the association with neurological disorder, Ganser state also occurs in the context of psychiatric disorder. Mendis and Hodgson (2012) reported from their review of 59 papers, comprising 94 cases, that the majority of cases were males (77.65 per cent), and the mean age was 31.6 years. Approximately 15 per cent of cases were aged under 16 years. Most patients presented with approximate answers (88.3 per cent) and clouding of consciousness (85 per cent). Only 43.6 per cent presented with somatic conversion symptoms and 28.7 per cent with hallucinations. Importantly, only 11.7 per cent had all the four cardinal features of Ganser state. In their sample, 22.3 per cent had a prior history of cerebral insult, and as for past psychiatric history, this was present in 41.5 per cent. Recognizable psychiatric illnesses occurred alongside Ganser state in 47.8 per cent of cases, and the reported conditions were psychosis, organic mental illness, depression, psychotic depression, stress/grief reaction and Tourette syndrome. The context of the Ganser state was a criminal event in 28.6 per cent of cases, and in a further 8.5 per cent of cases there was an ongoing compensation claim. It is notable that almost 20 per cent occurred in the context of domestic or occupational stress.

Andersen, Sestoft and Lillebæk (2001) reported on the possible causal role of solitary confinement in prison in Ganser state. The individual patient was identified in a survey of 268 remand prisoners in Denmark. This case also underlined how rare Ganser state was even in prison and perhaps even more surprising in a sample including 173 prisoners who were in solitary confinement, 53 of whom had been confined in this manner for more than two months.

Ganser state has been reported in children. In 28.6 per cent of cases, there was a history of previous head injury, and in 21.4 per cent, there was a forensic history. In children, Ganser state appears to be associated with Tourette syndrome, psychosis and enuresis (Mendis & Hodgson, 2012). Miller, Bramble and Buxton (1997) reviewed six case reports in children and confirmed the association with head injury, schizophrenia, depression and severe learning disability. They make the additional point that while the full syndrome may resolve quickly, many of the symptoms persist and may be maintained by other mechanisms, such as abnormal illness behaviour and dissociation. They also pointed to the possibility of variation in the semiotics of Ganser state in children and gave the example of brushing the tongue instead of the teeth as a behavioural motor alternative to approximate answers that they termed 'approximate movement'.

The possibility of malingering is never far away during a discussion about the origins and nature of the verbal behaviour of patients presenting with Ganser state. Merckelbach, Peters and Jelicic (2006) reported on a case of Ganser state in which malingering was established. This report raised the value of using a test of simulated or malingered symptoms, especially where there is disability or a compensation claim in the background.

18.5 Conclusion

The classical hallmark feature of Ganser state is 'approximate answers', a symptom of such absurdity that it automatically raises questions about the possibility or even probability of malingering. The ancillary features, including auditory and/or visual hallucinations, clouding of consciousness, hysterical stigmata including analgesia over the whole body, sudden resolution of the symptoms and amnesia for the episode point to the possibility of gross underlying abnormalities. Despite the obvious association with traumatic head injury and severe psychiatric disorders, Ganser state remains very much an enigmatic condition.

Chapter

19

Diogenes Syndrome

19.1 Introduction

Macmillan and Shaw (1966, p. 1032) introduced the term *senile breakdown* to describe

> a small group of individuals who cease to maintain the standards of cleanliness and hygiene which are accepted by their local community. . . . The usual picture is that of an old woman living alone, though men and married couples suffering from the condition are also found. She, her garments, her possessions, and her house are filthy. She may be verminous and there may be faeces and pools of urine on the floor.

The authors found 72 individuals (60 females and 12 males) in the Nottingham area of the United Kingdom. The vast majority (93 per cent) were aged over 70 years, and most were widowed women (51.3 per cent). In addition, 69.4 per cent lived alone and were often also socially isolated. Premorbidly, the pattern that emerged was of a domineering, quarrelsome and independent individual, and adjectives that were applied to them included *independent, unfriendly, stubborn, obstinate, aloof, aggressive, suspicious, secretive* and *quarrelsome*.

Our knowledge of this condition was further extended by the report by Clark, Mankikar and Gray (1975), who described 30 elderly patients (14 males and 16 females), all of whom were admitted into hospital with acute illness and extreme self-neglect. All the patients lived in a state of domestic squalor, and their homes were filthy on the outside, with peeling paint work and dirty, broken windows that had dingy net curtains.

> Inside there was a characteristic strong, stale, and slightly suffocating smell. The patients were usually dressed in layers of dirty clothing sometimes covered by an old raincoat or overcoat, and, when confined to bed, they lay beneath a pile of ragged blankets, clothing or newspapers. They never appeared to undress or wash, the hair being long and unkempt, with exposed surfaces of skin deeply ingrained with dirt. Only two patients apologized about their personal or domestic state. Several hoarded useless rubbish (syllogomania) – newspapers, tins, bottles, and rags, often in bundles and stacks – and in six instances the size of the collection seriously reduced living space.   (p. 366)

Clark and colleagues termed the condition *Diogenes syndrome* after the fourth-century Greek philosopher who is described as the first of the cynics. Diogenes (?412–323 BC), also known as Diogenes the Cynic, was born in Sinopes and died in Corinth. He believed that virtue was better revealed in action than in theory and used his lifestyle and behaviour to criticize the social values and institutions of his day. He made a virtue of poverty. He begged for a living and often slept in a ceramic jar in the marketplace.

Cybulska (1998)has argued that the term *Diogenes syndrome* is a misnomer as Diogenes was a happy, self-sufficient individual in contrast to Diogenes syndrome patients, who were often described as 'angry, suspicious, reclusive and buried under an abundance of inanimate objects, dirt and dust'. Cybulska suggested that Plyushkin in Nikolai Gogol's *Dead Souls* or Mrs Havisham in Charles Dickens' *Great Expectations* were better fits for the condition. Gogol's Plyushkin is an extraordinary literary example of Diogenes syndrome.

Chichikov stepped into a dark, wide entryway, from which the cold blew as if from a cellar. From the entryway he moved into a room that was also dark, although barely illuminated by light issuing from a wide crack beneath a door. On opening this door, he finally found himself in the light and was struck by the disorder that presented itself. It looked as if the floors were being washed, with all the furniture piled up in here temporarily. On one table stood a broken chair, and next to it, a clock whose pendulum had stopped and to which a spider had already attached its web. Here too, leaning sideways against a wall, stood a cupboard containing antique silver, small decanters and Chinese porcelain. On a writing desk, inlaid with mother-of-pearl mosaic which had fallen out in places, leaving shallow, yellowish grooves filled with glue, lay a host of odds and ends: a pile of small papers covered in a small hand, and pressed under a marble paperweight green with age and topped by an egg-shaped handle; an ancient book bound in leather binding and with red edging; a lemon, completely shrivelled and no bigger than a wild hazelnut; the broken-off arm of a chair; a glass containing some liquid and three flies, which was covered with a letter; a scrap of sealing wax; a scrap of rag that had been picked up somewhere; two quills smudged with ink and dried up as if from consumption; a toothpick, completely yellowed, which the owner might perhaps have used to pick his teeth before the French invasion of Moscow. . . .

Far more noteworthy was his attire. By no means or efforts could one ascertain what his dressing gown had been concocted from: the sleeves and the upper parts had become so dirty and shiny that they resembled the black-tarred leather used for boots; dangling from the back were four flaps instead of two, with cotton stuffing leaking out of them. Wound round his neck was something, whether a stocking, or a garter, or a stomacher could not be made out; but certainly it was not a cravat. . . .

Not content with such a state of affairs, he also walked through the streets of his village every day, peering under footbridges, under duckboards, and everything he came upon – an old sole, a peasant woman's rag, an iron nail, a shard of earthenware – he would haul off to his house and place on the heap which Chichikov had noticed in a corner of the room. 'Look, there goes the fisherman, off to catch something!' the muzhiks would say, when they saw him going in pursuit of his booty. And in point of fact, after he had passed there was no need to sweep the street. If an officer riding by happened to lose a spur, said spur was on its way on to the well-known heap in a flash; if a peasant woman was standing by the well gawking at something and forgot her bucket, he would carry the bucket off too. If, however, a sharp-eyed muzhik caught him in the act, he didn't argue and handed the plundered object back; but once it had joined the heap, that was the end of it: he would swear that the object was his and had been bought by him at such-and-such a time, from so-and-so, or had come down to him from his grandfather. In his room he would pick everything up off the floor that he saw: sealing wax, a scrap of paper, a quill, and all this he would put on the writing desk or the window sill. (Gogol, 1961, pp. 126–30)

Alternative terms have been proposed, including *senile squalor syndrome, messy house syndrome, senile recluse, disposophobia* and *Havisham syndrome* (Byard, 2014), but *Diogenes syndrome* has endured despite its imperfection.

19.2 Case Reports

Case1

Mr A is a 68-year-old man living on the ground floor of a block of flats in the east end of a major city. He was first referred to the psychiatric services in December 1994 when his general practitioner expressed concern that he may have become depressed following the death of his flatmate some months previously. It was suggested that he may have some form of dementia. When seen on a domiciliary visit by the psychiatrist he was somewhat agitated and this made his rather bizarre way of speaking difficult to interpret – he spoke rapidly in a sing-song voice with various odd oaths interrupting his speech. To compound these difficulties he gave many wrong answers to questions deliberately, as we discovered after getting to know him better – for example, at a later date he not only told us that he had been asked the name of the Prime Minister, but told us the wrong answer, he had replied then, as well as the correct one. After further contacts it was evident that there were no obvious signs of dementia or of depressive illness; and his agitation settled once he became familiar with us. His accommodation was in a very neglected and filthy state, with dirty walls and floors, dilapidated furniture and with assorted crockery, cutlery and bottles strewn around. Mr A himself had long, uncombed hair and a long straggly beard; his clothes looked as if they had not been washed for decades. The general feeling of neglect was emphasized by the presence of his cat ('more intelligence than humans, they care about you', as he said); at the first visit he had two adult cats, which were soon followed by three kittens. The cat food was laid out on newspapers on a table in the living room for the cats to help themselves. The cats, somewhat incongruously, well were groomed. . . . Mr A's way of living has, however, caused great concern to the local social work department and to various other agencies over many years; this compounded by his habit of making visits to neighbours' doors on a number of occasions – he states he goes out looking for company. He goes out in his bare feet. When he goes to doors of those who know him there is no great problem but he has been known to knock at the wrong door where he presents a frightening spectre with his dirty appearance, long hair and beard and his odd speech, worse when he becomes flustered at their reaction.   (Jackson, 1997, pp. 115–15)

Case 2

A 61-year-old obese Caucasian female with a previous history of bipolar 1 disorder and hypothyroidism presented for an out-patient psychiatric follow-up review accompanied by her Community Psychiatric Nurse. She was found to have pressured speech, elated mood, increased energy, and very poor personal hygiene. She was dishevelled, unkempt, wearing dirty clothes, and was foul smelling. She was very agitated, and was verbally and physically abusive to staff. She had no insight and refused any form of treatment. She was diagnosed with having a manic relapse secondary to non-adherence to medication, and was involuntarily admitted to the in-patient psychiatric ward. . . . The following day she was adamant about having to go feed her cats and dogs, and eventually gave permission for a Community Psychiatric Nurse enter her house to attend to her pets. Upon entering the house, it was found to be in complete disarray. The house was crammed with filthy clothes, garbage, dirty dishes, and rotting food. There was no kitchen sink in sight, and it looked as if some dishes were being cleaned in the toilet. Any clear space of floor was strewn with cat and dog faeces. An unbearable stench emanated from the entire two-storey home. Upon questioning the patient regarding her home and her personal hygiene, the patient had no insight into any problems.

(Irvine & Nwachukwu, 2014, pp. 1–2)

19.3 Explanatory Hypotheses

Diogenes syndrome is not a homogeneous condition. This means that there is as yet no overarching explanatory hypothesis that makes comprehensible the collection of symptoms that characterize this behavioural syndrome. Lee et al. (2014) investigated a case series of people living in squalor and showed that living in squalor is associated with impaired executive function. Furthermore, there is a suggestion that behavioural variant frontotemporal dementia may provide a window into the neurobiology of Diogenes syndrome. Finney and Mendez (2017) reported on five patients with behavioural variant frontotemporal dementia who presented with Diogenes syndrome. The authors make the case for understanding (1) decline in self-awareness, (2) decline in self-care, and (3) collecting behaviour that leads to a tendency for a cluttered and disordered environment as symptoms that may hint at underlying mechanisms. The proposal is that the decline in self-care and self-awareness is mediated by frontal lobe deficits, and the collecting behaviour may be mediated by a combination of impairment of frontal activity, specific impairment of frontolimbic–striatal limbic connectivity and abnormal activity in the anterior cingulate and its supervisory attentional systems. The end result is decreased concern for personal care, compulsive behaviour and disinhibition of responsiveness to environmental items of interest. It is invariably true that Diogenes syndrome has been reported in individuals with frontotemporal dementia and in others with frontal lobe lesions, but nonetheless, there are many other patients who do not seem to have any demonstrable underlying neurological or psychiatric disorders.

In a novel investigation into the underlying mechanisms of Diogenes syndrome, Ashworth, Rose and Wilson (2018) reported on TD, a 53-year-old male patient who was a 'blue baby' at birth and had never left home but continued to live in the family home with his brother after his mother died. His situation was drawn to the attention of the services after a fall and acute illness with pneumonia. The home environment on inspection was found 'in appalling condition with access almost impossible given that the whole environment was one of squalor. There were faeces everywhere, cockroaches and rodents throughout the house, food mouldy and out of date, some dating back to the time of their mother's death. Newspapers and rubbish were stacked high in every room.' The authors questioned the possibility of a role for a deficit in recognizing and processing disgust in the aetiology of Diogenes syndrome – the argument being if one has a deficit in recognizing or processing disgust, this may lead to an individual not being able to recognize a situation as disgusting as found in the squalor that patients live in and hence may experience a lack of shame. The authors demonstrated that TD had significant global executive functioning difficulties, showed evidence of poor self-awareness, had problems with smell detection that may compromise the ability to sense disgusting smells, was unable to detect perceptual expressions of disgust in others and had abnormally low shame responses to shameful scenarios. There was no impairment of the ability to imagine or describe the consequences of living in squalor, there was no impairment in his ability to use his emotions to make decisions and there was no impairment of his sensitivity to perception of disgusting scenarios. There was no evidence of dementia. The authors did not come to a conclusive judgement about the relationship between disgust, shame and Diogenes syndrome. Nonetheless, their findings hint at the possibility that there is a role for recognition and processing of disgust in achieving a comprehensive understanding of Diogenes syndrome.

19.4 Clinical Aspects

In their original paper, Macmillan and Shaw (1966) estimated the incidence rate as 0.5 per 1,000 per year and concluded that Diogenes syndrome is a rare condition. In Hong Kong, Chan, Leung and Chiu (2007) reported 18 cases collected over the six-year period 1996–2001 from a sample of 4,000 patients seen in that period. Macmillan and Shaw (1966) reported that only 16 per cent of cases were male, whereas Clark et al. (1975:h9) reported that in their series, 46.6 per cent were male. The Hong Kong case series had 38.8 per cent males. In summary, the Diogenes syndrome probably occurs equally in males and females. The mean age at first presentation is over the age of 70 years (Clark et al., 1975; Macmillan & Shaw, 1966). It is strikingly associated with social isolation and being widowed or single (Macmillan & Shaw, 1966) (Clark et al., 1975) (Chan et al.,).

Diogenes syndrome has been associated with frontal lobe lesions (Beauchet, Imler, Cadet, Blanc – La Revue de, & 2002,), learning disability, dementia including frontotemporal dementia, schizophrenia, mood disorder (Fond, Jollant, & Abbar, 2011), obsessive compulsive disorder and, personality disorder (Amanullah, Oomman, & Datta, 2009).

The Eastern Baltimore Mental Health survey of a representative sample of households did not find any severe cases of social breakdown syndrome but showed that social breakdown syndrome was associated with increasing age, being present in 41% of those aged over 85 years and when combined with dementia was present in the oldest age group. Moderate social breakdown syndrome was most common in those aged 65–74 years and was rarely associated with dementia. The authors make the point that only a small fraction of social breakdown syndrome in the community is associated with dementia except in the very old, that is those aged over 85 years (Radebaugh, Hooper, & Gruenberg, 1987). The role of frontotemporal dementia in the development of Diogenes syndrome has been discussed above. It is worth emphasizing the fact that the consensus statement on the clinical diagnostic criteria for frontotemporal lobar degeneration includes a) early loss of insight, b) decline in personal hygiene and grooming, c) perseverative and stereotyped behaviour which includes hoarding and d) utilization behaviour (Neary et al., 1998).

In a sample of patients with obsessive compulsive disorder, Drummond et al. report that 8% presented with self-neglect, domestic squalor and hoarding behaviour (Drummond, Turner, Reid, 1997). Fontenelle reported on a patient presenting with Diogenes syndrome in association with both obsessive-compulsive disorder and Tourette syndrome. He makes the point that since hoarding was not part of the clinical picture, perhaps hoarding behaviour is not a fundamental feature of Diogenes syndrome (Fontenelle, 2008).

Even though Diogenes syndrome occurs most often in socially isolated individuals, it can also present in couples or in siblings who live together. Macmillan and Shaw reported on a couple aged 81 and 76 years, who lived in a basement room of their large house in indescribable squalor. The wife was admitted into hospital and subsequently died but, surprisingly the husband was successfully re-housed and kept his new accommodation clean and tidy (Macmillan & Shaw (1966). Sometimes Diogenes syndrome becomes evident after the death of the individuals involved. Byard (2014) argued that it is important to be aware of the possibility of Diogenes syndrome when attending a death scene of people who die in isolation and lie undiscovered for a period. He makes the point that Diogenes syndrome can be involved in a large number of deaths, including hypothermic deaths in socially isolated individuals, and bleeding from an undiagnosed rectal carcinoma in a reclusive man may suggest foul play when natural causes are more likely. Furthermore, decomposition may introduce artefacts at autopsy, and postmortem animal depredation may simulate inflicted injury and complicate the autopsy.

Zivković and Nikolić (2014) reported on two brothers who died during the winter and were found in a flat that was in poor condition – dirty and filled with rubbish and also lacking in heat. The cause of death was difficult to establish but was assumed to be hypothermia, and this was confirmed by Wischnewski spots, dark brown erosions on the gastric mucosa linked to hypothermia. This case was an example of *Philemon and Baucis death*, a term derived from the Greek myth of the couple Philemon and Baucis who after showing hospitality to Zeus and Hermes were granted their wish to die together at the same time, turning into trees whose leaves intertwined, proving their eternal love, even in death. The term can also be used in relation to natural deaths which occur at the same place and at the same time to two individuals who had been living together and who had been emotionally connected.

Some patients with Diogenes syndrome collect/hoard a large number of animals while at the same time neglecting the basic care of those animals. This variant of Diogenes syndrome has been termed *Noah syndrome*. Saldarriaga-Cantillo and Rivas Nieto (2015) reported an 83-year-old widow who had lived in solitude for 20 years and who came to attention following a fall. Her home showed poor sanitary conditions. She lived with 15 dogs and 16 cats, and animal faeces were present in the house, and the house was infested with cockroaches and flies. The dogs and cats were malnourished and in poor health.

Hurley et al. (2000) provided an observational study in the greater Dublin area of people who refused statutory and voluntary service support. The majority were women (54.5 per cent) and were over the age of 65 years (69.5 per cent). Forty-seven per cent of the subjects met criteria for Diogenes syndrome, and 54.1 per cent exhibited hoarding behaviour. This study highlighted the importance of recognizing the possibility of Diogenes syndrome in individuals who refuse offer of services. And in a different vein, a survey of health departments in the State of Massachusetts in the United States, covering a population of 1.79 million people, found that 64 per cent of the health department officers had received at least one report of hoarding behaviour. These cases involved multiple community agencies with considerable cost to the community. Only about a half the reported cases recognized the lack of sanitation in their homes, and only a third cooperated with the health departments. Thirty-two per cent of cases where data were available involved the hoarding of animals (Noah syndrome), and these cases were thought to pose even greater risk to the health of the community (Frost, Steketee & Williams, 2000).

19.5 Conclusion

Diogenes syndrome is a behavioural disorder with diverse causation that occurs notably in elderly individuals who both live alone and are socially isolated. It is characterized by extreme squalor and is associated with hoarding behaviour. The association with frontotemporal dementia is perhaps its most established feature.

References

Abbate, C., Trimarchi, P. D., Salvi, G. P., et al. (2012). Delusion of inanimate doubles: Description of a case of focal retrograde amnesia. *Neurocase* 18(6), 457–77. doi:10.1080/13554794.2011.627344

Abelson, R. P. (1979). Differences between belief and knowledge systems. *Cognitive Science* 3(4), 355–66. doi:10.1207/s15516709cog0304_4

Abrams, K. M., & Robinson, G. E. (1998). Stalking: I. An overview of the problem. *Can J Psychiatry* 43(5), 473–6. doi:10.1177/070674379804300504

Ackner, B. (1954a). Depersonalization: I. Aetiology and phenomenology. *J Ment Sci* 100, 838–53.

Ackner, B. (1954b). Depersonalization: II. Clinical syndromes. *J Ment Sci* 100, 853–72.

Adachi, N. (1996). Charles Bonnet syndrome in leprosy: Prevalence and clinical characteristics. *Acta Psychiatr Scand* 93(4), 279–81. doi:10.1111/j.1600-0447.1996.tb10648.x

Adachi, N., Watanabe, T., Matsuda, H., & Onuma, T. (2000). Hyperperfusion in the lateral temporal cortex, the striatum and the thalamus during complex visual hallucinations: Single photon emission computed tomography findings in patients with Charles Bonnet syndrome. *Psychiatr Clin Neurosci* 54(2), 157–62. doi:10.1046/j.1440-1819.2000.00652.x

Adachi, N., Nagayama, M., Anami, K., et al. (1994). Asymmetrical blood flow in the temporal lobe in the Charles Bonnet syndrome: Serial neuroimaging study. *Behav Neurol* 7(2), 97–9. doi:10.3233/BEN-1994-7209

Adinkrah, M. (2008). Husbands who kill their wives: An analysis of uxoricides in contemporary Ghana. *Int J Offender Ther Comp Criminol* 52(3), 296–310.

Adityanjee, A. M. (1995). Delusion of pregnancy in males: A case report and literature review. *Psychopathology* 28(6), 307–11. doi:10.1159/000284942

Adler, A., & Magruder, W. W. (1946). Folie à deux in identical twins treated with electroshock therapy. *J Nerv Ment Dis* 103, 181–6.

Adler, J., Schabinger, N., Michal, M., et al. (2016). Is that me in the mirror? Depersonalisation modulates tactile mirroring mechanisms. *Neuropsychologia* 85, 148–58.

Ahmed, H., Blakeway, E. A., Taylor, R. E., & Bewley, A. P. (2015). Children with a mother with delusional infestation: Implications for child protection and management. *Pediatr Dermatol* 32(3), 397–400. doi:10.1111/pde.12441

Ahn, B. H., Kim, J. H., Oh, S., et al. (2012). Clinical features of parricide in patients with schizophrenia. *Aust NZ J Psychiatry* 46(7), 621–9. doi:10.1177/0004867412442499

Aizenberg, D., Schwartz, B., & Zemishlany, Z. (1991). Delusional parasitosis associated with phenelzine. *Br J Psychiatry* 159, 716–17. doi:10.1192/bjp.159.5.716

Ajzen, I. (2005). *Attitudes, Personality, and Behavior.* McGraw-Hill Education, London.

Akyüz, G., Doğan, O., Şar, V., et al. (1999). Frequency of dissociative identity disorder in the general population in Turkey. *Comp Psychiatry* 40(2),151–9.

Alao, A. O., & Hanrahan, B. (2003). Charles Bonnet syndrome: Visual hallucination and multiple sclerosis. *Int J Psychiatry Med* 33(2), 195–9. doi:10.2190/0NUQ-Y5Q9-TA6H-RJHH

Aldridge, M. L., & Browne, K. D. (2003). Perpetrators of spousal homicide: A review. *Trauma, Violence, & Abuse* 4(3), 265–76.

Allen, J. R., Pfefferbaum, B., Hammond, D., & Speed, L., (2000). A disturbed child's use of a public event: Côtard's syndrome in a ten-year-old. *Psychiatry* 63(2), 208–13. doi:10.1080/00332747.2000.11024912

Álvaro, L. C. (2005). Hallucinations and pathological visual perceptions in

Maupassant's fantastical short stories: A neurological approach. *J Hist Neurosci* 14(2), 100–15. doi: 10.1080/096470490523399

Amanullah, S., Oomman, S. K., & Datta, S. S. (2009). Diogenes syndrome revisited. *Ger J Psychiatr* 12(1), 38–44.

Andersen, H. S., Sestoft, D., & Lillebæk, T. (2001). Ganser syndrome after solitary confinement in prison: A short review and a case report. *Nordic J Psychiatry* 55(3), 199–201. doi:10.1080/08039480152036083

Anderson, D. N., & Williams, E. (1994). The delusion of inanimate doubles. *Psychopathology* 27(3–5), 220–5.

Anderson, E. W., & Mallinson, W. P. (1941). Psychogenic episodes in the course of major psychoses. *J Ment Sci* 87(368), 383–95.

Anderson, E. W., Trethowan, W. H., & Kenna, J. C. (1959). An experimental investigation of simulation and pseudo-dementia. *Acta Psychiatric Scand Suppl* 34(132), 14–35.

Anupama, M., Rao, K. N., & Dhananjaya, S. (2006). Ganser syndrome and lesion in the temporoparietal region. *Ind J Psychiatry* 48(2), 123–5.

Anyasodor, M., Goulding, J., & Bewley, A. (2015). Penoscrotodynia is a somatoform disorder and requires psychiatric treatment. *Br J Dermatol* 41(5), 474–9.

Anyasodor, M. C., Taylor, R. E., Bewley, A., & Goulding, J. M. R. (2016). Dysaesthetic penoscrotodynia may be a somatoform disorder: Results from a two centre retrospective case series. *Clin Exp Dermatol* 41(5), 474–9. doi:10.1111/ced.12824

Anzellotti, F., Onofrj, V., Maruotti, V., & Ricciardi, L. (2011). Autoscopic phenomena: Case report and review of literature. *Behav Brain Funct* 7(1), 2. doi:10.1186/1744-9081-7-2

Aoyama, A., Krummenacher, P., Palla, A., et al. (2012). Impaired spatial-temporal integration of touch in xenomelia (body integrity identity disorder). *Spatial Cognit Comput* 12(2–3), 96–110. doi:10.1080/13875868.2011.603773

Arai, T., Hasegawa, Y., Tanaka, T., et al. (2014). [Transient Charles Bonnet syndrome after excision of a right occipital meningioma: A case report]. *No Shinkei Geka* 42(5), 445–51.

Arias, M., Constela, I. R., Iglesias, S., et al. (2007). The autoscopic phenomena in neurological clinic: A study of two cases. *J Neurol Sci* 263(1–2), 223–5.

Arnold, L. D., Bachmann, G. A., Kelly, S., et al. (2006). Vulvodynia: Characteristics and associations with co-morbidities and quality of life. *Obstet Gynecol* 107(3), 617–24.

Arnone, D., Patel, A., & Tan, G. M. (2006a). The nosological significance of folie à deux: A review of the literature. *Ann Gen Psychiatry* 5, 11. doi:10.1186/1744-859X-5-11

Arnone, D., Patel, A., & Tan, G. M.-Y. (2006b). The nosological significance of folie à deux: A review of the literature. *Ann Gen Psychiatry* 5(1), 11. doi:10.1186/1744-859X-5-11

Aronson, G. (1952). Delusion of pregnancy in a male homosexual with an abdominal cancer. *Bull Menninger Clin* 16(5), 159–66.

Ashraf, N., Antonius, D., Sinkman, A., et al. (2011). Fregoli syndrome: An underrecognized risk factor for aggression in treatment settings. *Case Rep Psychiatry* 2011, 351824. doi:10.1155/2011/351824

Ashwin, P. T., & Tsaloumas, M. D. (2007). Complex visual hallucinations (Charles Bonnet syndrome) in the hemianopic visual field following occipital infarction. *J Neurol Sci* 263(1–2), 184–6. doi:10.1016/j.jns.2007.05.027

Ashworth, F., Rose, A., & Wilson, B. A. (2018). TD: The case of Diogenes syndrome – Deficit or denial? *Neuropsychol Rehabil* 28(2), 244–58. doi:10.1080/09602011.2017.1391104

Aspell, J., Lenggenhager, B., & Blanke, O. (2009). Keeping in touch with one's self: Multisensory mechanisms of self-consciousness. *PLoS One.* https://journals.plos.org/plosone/doi:org/10.1371/journal.pone.0006488

Aspell, J., Lenggenhager, B., & Blanke, O. (2011). Multisensory perception and bodily self-consciousness: From out-of-body to inside-body experience. In M. M. Murray &

M. T. Wallace (eds.), *The Neural Basis of Multisensory Processes*. CRC Press/Taylor & Francis, Boca Raton, FL.

Augustin, J., Guegan-Massardier, E., Levillain, D., et al. (2001). [Musical hallucinosis following infarction of the right middle cerebral artery]. *Rev Neurol (Paris)* 157(3), 289–92.

Ayling, K., & Ussher, J. M. (2008). 'If sex hurts, am I still a woman?' The subjective experience of vulvodynia in heterosexual women. *Arch Sex Behav* 37(2), 294–304. doi:10.1007/s10508-007-9204-1

Azizi, M., & Elyasi, F. (2017). Biopsychosocial view to pseudocyesis: A narrative review. *Int J Reprod Biomed (Yazd)* 15(9), 535–42.

Bachmann, G. A., Rosen, R., Pinn, V. W., et al. (2006). Vulvodynia: A state-of-the-art consensus on definitions, diagnosis and management. *J Reprod Med* 51(6), 447–56.

Bailey, C. H., Andersen, L. K., Lowe, G. C., et al. (2014). A population-based study of the incidence of delusional infestation in Olmsted County, Minnesota, 1976–2010. *Br J Dermatol* 170(5), 1130–5. doi:10.1111/bjd.12848

Baillarger, M. (1891). M Baillarger. *J Ment Sci* 37(157), 333.

Baker, D., Hunter, E., Lawrence, E., et al. (2003). Depersonalisation disorder: Clinical features of 204 cases. *Br J Psychiatry* 182, 428–33.

Banissy, M. J., Walsh, V., & Ward, J. (2009). Enhanced sensory perception in synaesthesia. *Exp Brain Res* 196(4), 565–71. doi: 10.1007/s00221-009-1888-0

Banissy, M. J., Kadosh, R. C., Maus, G. W., & Walsh, V. (2009). Prevalence, characteristics and a neurocognitive model of mirror-touch synaesthesia. *Exp Brain Res* 198(2–3), 261–72. doi:10.1007/s00221-009-1810-9

Barba, G. D., Brazzarola, M., Marangoni, S., & Alderighi, M. (2020). Confabulation affecting temporal consciousness significantly more than knowing consciousness. *Neuropsychologia* 140, 107367. doi:10.1016/j.neuropsychologia.2020.107367

Barnett, K. J., Finucane, C., Asher, J. E., et al. (2008). Familial patterns and the origins of individual differences in synaesthesia.

Cognition 106(2), 871–93. doi:10.1016/j.cognition.2007.05.003.

Baron-Cohen, S., Burt, L., Smith-Laittan, F., et al. (1996). Synaesthesia: Prevalence and familiality. *Perception* 25(9), 1073–9. doi:10.1068/p251073

Barrett, D. (1988). Trance-related pseudocyesis in a male. *Int J Clin Exp Hypn* 36(4), 256–61. doi:10.1080/00207148808410516

Barton, J. L., & Barton, E. S. (1986). Misidentification syndromes and sexuality. *Bibl Psychiatr* 164, 105–20.

Batinic, B., Duisin, D., & Barisic, J. (2013). Obsessive versus delusional jealousy. *Psychiatr Danub* 25(3), 334–9.

Bauer, R. M. (1984). Autonomic recognition of names and faces in prosopagnosia: A neuropsychological application of the guilty knowledge test. *Neuropsychologia* 22(4), 457–69.

Beall, A. E., & Sternberg, R. J. (1995). The social construction of love. *J Soc Pers Relat* 12(3), 417–38.

Beauchet, O., Imler, D., Cadet, L., et al. (2002). Diogenes syndrome in the elderly: Clinical form of frontal dysfunction? Report of 4 cases. *Rev Med Interne* 23(2), 122–31. doi:10.1016/s0248-8663(01)00527-6

Beaulicu, R. A., Tamboli, D. A., Armstrong, B. K., et al. (2018). Reversible Charles Bonnet syndrome after oculoplastic procedures. *J Neuroophthalmol* 38(3), 334–6. doi:10.1097/WNO.0000000000000477

Begum, M., & McKenna, P. J. (2011). Olfactory reference syndrome: A systematic review of the world literature. *Psychol Med* 41(3), 453–61.

Benson, D. F., Gardner, H., & Meadows, J. C. (1976). Reduplicative paramnesia. *Neurology* 26(2), 147–51.

Berlyne, N. (1972). Confabulation. *Br J Psychiatry* 120(554), 31–9.

Bernard, J. W. (1986). Messiaen's synaesthesia: The correspondence between color and sound structure in his music. *Music*

Perception: An Interdisciplinary Journal 4(1), 41–68.

Berrios, G. E. (1982). Tactile hallucinations: Conceptual and historical aspects. *J Neurol Neurosurg Psychiatry* 45(4), 285–93.

Berrios, G. E. (1990). Musical hallucinations: A historical and clinical study. *Br J Psychiatry* 156(2), 188–94.

Berrios, G. E. (1996). *The History of Mental Symptoms: Descriptive Psychopathology Since the Nineteenth Century.* Cambridge University Press, Cambridge, UK.

Berrios, G. E., & Brook, P. (1984). Visual hallucinations and sensory delusions in the elderly. *Br J Psychiatry* 144, 662–4. doi:10.1192/bjp.144.6.662

Berrios, G. E., & Kennedy, N. (2002). Erotomania: A conceptual history. *Hist Psychiatry* 13(52 Pt 4), 381–400. doi:10.1177/0957154X0201305202

Berrios, G. E., & Luque, R. (1995a). Côtard's syndrome: Analysis of 100 cases. *Acta Psychiatr Scand* 91(3), 185–8. doi: 10.1111/j.1600-0447.1995.tb09764.x

Berrios, G. E., & Luque, R. (1995b). Côtard's delusion or syndrome?: A conceptual history. *Compr Psychiatry* 36(3), 218–23.

Berson, R. J. (1982). Capgras' syndrome. CUNY Academic Works, New York.

Bhaskaran, R., Kumar, A., & Nayar, P. C. (1990). Autoscopy in hemianopic field. *J Neurol Neurosurg Psychitry* 53(11), 1016–17.

Bhate, S. M., Spear, J. C. M., & Robertson, P. E. (1989). Coexistence of delusions of pregnancy and infestation in a male. *Br J Psychiatry* 155, 423–4.

Bhatia, M. S. (1993). Côtard's syndrome in parietal lobe tumor. *Indian Pediatr* 30(8), 1019–21.

Bidault, E., Luauté, J. P., & Tzavaras, A. (1986). Prosopagnosia and the delusional misidentification syndromes. *Bibl Psychiatr* 164, 80–91.

Bitton, G., Thibaut, F., & Lefevre-Lesage, I. (1991). Delusions of pregnancy in a man. *Am J Psychiatry* 148(6), 811–12. doi:10.1176/ajp.148.6.811

Bivin, G. D., & Klinger, M. P. (1937). *Pseudocyesis.* Principia Press, San Francisco.

Blackmore, S. (1986). Out-of-body experiences in schizophrenia. *J Nerv Ment Dis* 174(10), 615–19.

Blakemore, S. J., Bristow, D., Bird, G., et al. (2005). Somatosensory activations during the observation of touch and a case of vision-touch synaesthesia. *Brain* 128(7), 1571–83.

Blanke, O. (2012). Multisensory brain mechanisms of bodily self-consciousness. *Nature Rev Neurosci* 13, 556–71.

Blanke, O., & Arzy, S. (2005). The out-of-body experience: Disturbed self-processing at the temporo-parietal junction. *Neuroscientist* 11(1), 16–24.

Blanke, O., & Mohr, C. (2005). Out-of-body experience, heautoscopy, and autoscopic hallucination of neurological origin: Implications for neurocognitive mechanisms of corporeal awareness and self-consciousness. *Brain Res Rev* 50(1), 184–99.

Blanke, O., Landis, T., Spinelli, L., & Seeck, M. (2004). Out-of-body experience and autoscopy of neurological origin. *Brain* 127(2), 243–58.

Bleuler, E. (1950). *Dementia Praecox or the Group of Schizophrenias.* International University Press, Madison, CT.

Bleuler, E., & Lehmann, K. (1881). Zwangsmässige lichtempfindungen durch Schall und Verwante erscheinungen auf dem Gebiete der andern sinnesempfindungen. *J Nature* 24, 51.

Blom, J. D., Coebergh, J. A., Lauw, R., & Sommer, I. E. (2015). Musical hallucinations treated with acetylcholinesterase inhibitors. *Front Psychiatry* 6, 46. doi:10.3389/fpsyt.2015.00046

Blom, R. M., Hennekam, R. C., & Denys, D. (2012). Body integrity identity disorder. *PLoS One.* doi: 10.1371/journal.pone.0034702

Blom, R. M., Vulink, N. C., Wal, S. J. V. D., et al. (2016). Body integrity identity disorder crosses culture: Case reports in the Japanese and Chinese literature. *Neuropsychiatric Dis Treat* 12, 1419–23.

Blom, R. M., Wingen, G. A. V., Wal, S. J. V. D., & Luigjes, J. (2016). The desire for amputation or paralyzation: Evidence for structural brain anomalies in body integrity identity disorder (BIID). *PLoS One*. doi: 10.1371/journal. pone.0165789

Boettcher, B. (2001) Ganser syndrome: A case study. www.iap.org.au.

Bogren, L. Y. (1983). Couvade. *Acta Psychiatr Scand* 68(1), 55–65.

Bogren, L. Y. (1984). The Couvade syndrome: Background variables. *Acta Psychiatr Scand* 70(4), 316–20.

Bolakale, A. S., Ibrahim, A., & Amusa, A. (2015). Pseudocyesis vera in a health institution, north western Nigeria. *J Public Health Afr* 6(2), 532. doi:10.4081/jphia.2015.532

Bonhoeffer, K. (1901). *Die akuten Geisteskrakheiten der Gewohnheistrinker*. Gustav Fischer, Jena.

Bornstein, J., Cohen, Y., Zarfati, D., et al. (2008). Involvement of heparanase in the pathogenesis of localized vulvodynia. *Int J Gynecol Pathol* 27(1), 136–41.

Borsutzky, S., Fujiwara, E., Brand, M., & Markowitsch, H. J. (2010). Susceptibility to false memories in patients with ACoA aneurysm. *Neuropsychologia* 48(10), 2811–23. doi:10.1016/j. neuropsychologia.2010.05.023

Bos, E. M., Spoor, J. K. H., Smits, M., & Schouten, J. W. (2016). Out-of-body experience during awake craniotomy. *World Neurosurg* 92, 586.e9–e13.

Bou Khalil, R., & Richa, S. (2012). Apotemnophilia or body integrity identity disorder: A case report review. *Int J Low Extrem Wounds* 11(4), 313–19. doi:10.1177/ 1534734612464714

Bouckoms, A., Martuza, R., & Henderson, M. (1986). Capgras syndrome with subarachnoid hemorrhage. *J Nerv Ment Dis* 174(8), 484–8.

Bourgeois, M. L., Duhamel, P., & Verdoux, H. (1992). Delusional parasitosis: Folie a deux and attempted murder of a family doctor. *Br J Psychiatry* 161(5), 709–11.

Bourguignon, E. (1973). *Religion, Altered States of Consciousness, and Social Change*. Ohio State University Press, Columbus, OH.

Boyer, P. N., Devlin, M., & Boggild, M. (2018). Rare and rarer: Co-occurrence of stroke-like migraine attacks after radiation therapy and Charles Bonnet syndromes. *Oxf Med Case Rep* 2018(10), 349–52. doi:10.1093/omcr/ omy077

Brang, D., McGeoch, P. D., & Ramachandran, V. S. (2008). Apotemnophilia: A neurological disorder. *NeuroReport* 19(13), 1305–6.

Breckler, S. J. (1984). Empirical validation of affect, behavior, and cognition as distinct components of attitude. *J Pers Soc Psychol* 47(6), 1191–205.

Breen, N., Caine, D., & Coltheart, M. (2000). Models of face recognition and delusional misidentification: A critical review. *Cogn Neuropsychol* 17(1), 55–71. doi:10.1080/ 026432900380481

Brewer, G., & Riley, C. (2009). Height, relationship satisfaction, jealousy, and mate retention. *Evol Psychol* 7(3), 530–44. doi: 10.1177/147470490900700310

Brewer, J. D., Meves, A., Bostwick, J. M., et al. (2008). Cocaine abuse: Dermatologic manifestations and therapeutic approaches. *J Am Acad Dermatol* 59(3), 483–7. doi:10.1016/j.jaad.2008.03.040

Brewer, V. E., & Paulsen, D. J. (1999). A comparison of US and Canadian findings on uxoricide risk for women with children sired by previous partners. *Homicide Studies* 3(4), 317–32.

Broca, P. (1861). Remarks on the seat of the faculty of articulated language, following an observation of aphemia (loss of speech). *Bull Soc Anatomique* 6, 330–57.

Brockington, I. F. (1996). *Motherhood and Mental Health*. Oxford University Press, New York.

Brown-Vargas, D., & Cienki, J. J. (2012). Occipital lobe epilepsy presenting as Charles Bonnet syndrome. *Am J Emerg Med* 30(9), e5–e6. doi:10.1016/j. ajem.2012.03.008

Brown, E., & Barglow, P. (1971). Pseudocyesis: A paradigm for psychophysiological interactions. *Arch Gen Psychiatry* 24(3), 221–9.

Brown, M., King, E., & Barraclough, B. (1995). Nine suicide pacts: A clinical study of a consecutive series 1974–93. *Br J Psychiatry* 167(4), 448–51.

Brüggemann, B. R., & Garlipp, P. (2007). A special coincidence of erotomania and Fregoli syndrome. *Psychopathology* 40(6), 468. doi:10.1159/000108127

Brugger, P. (1994). Are 'presences' preferentially felt along the left side of one's body. *Percept Mot Skills* 79(3 Pt 1), 1200–2.

Brugger, P., Lenggenhager, B., & Giummarra, M. J. (2013). Xenomelia: A social neuroscience view of altered bodily self-consciousness. *Front Psychol* 4(204). doi:10.3389/fpsyp.2013.00204

Brugger, P., Regard, M., & Landis, T. (1997). Illusory reduplication of one's own body: Phenomenology and classification of autoscopic phenomena. *Cogn Neuropsychiatry* 2(1), 19–38. doi/pdf/10.1080/135468097396397

Brugger, P., Agosti, R., Regard, M., & Wieser, H. G. (1994). Heautoscopy, epilepsy, and suicide. *J Neurol Neurosurg Psychiatry* 57(7), 838–9.

Brugger, P., Blanke, O., Regard, M., et al. (2006). Polyopic heautoscopy: Case report and review of the literature. *Cortex* 42(5), 666–74.

Brüne, M. (2001). De Clerambault's syndrome (erotomania) in an evolutionary perspective. *Evol Hum Behav* 22(6), 409–15.

Bruno, R. L. (1997). Devotees, pretenders and wannabes: Two cases of factitious disability disorder. *Sex Disabil* 15, 243–60. doi:10.1023/A:1024769330761

Budur, K., Mathews, M., & Mathews, M. (2005). Couvade syndrome equivalent. *Psychosomatics* 46(1), 71–2. doi:10.1176/appi.psy.46.1.71

Bullen, F. S. J. (1899). Olfactory hallucinations in the insane. *J Ment Sci* 45(190), 513–33.

Burke, W. (2002). The neural basis of Charles Bonnet hallucinations: A hypothesis. *J Neurol Neurosurg Psychiatry* 73(5), 535–41.

Buss, D. M., & Schmitt, D. P. (1993). Sexual strategies theory: An evolutionary perspective on human mating. *Psychol Rev* 100(2), 204–32.

Buunk, A. P., & Castro Solano A. (2011). Gender differences in the jealousy-evoking effect of rival characteristics: A study in Spain and Argentina. *J Cross Cult Psychol* 42(3), 323–39. doi: 10.1177/0022022111403664

Byard, R. W. (2014). Diogenes or Havisham syndrome and the mortuary. *Forensic Sci Med Pathol* 10, 1–2. doi:10.1007/s12024-013-9458-y.

Byrd, R. P., & Roy, T. M. (1993). False pregnancy: An unusual paraneoplastic syndrome associated with bronchogenic neoplasm. *J Ky Med Assoc* 91(11), 501–3.

Cacioppo, S. (2016). What happens in your brain during mental dissociation? A quest towards neural markers of a unified sense of self. *Curr Behav Neurosci Rep* 3, 1–9. doi: 10.1007/s40473-016-0063-8.

Caliyurt, O., Vardar, E., & Tuglu, C. (2004). Côtard's syndrome with schizophreniform disorder can be successfully treated with electroconvulsive therapy: Case report. *J Psychiatr Neurosci* 29(2), 138–41.

Capgras, J. (1923). L'illusion des sosies dans un delire systematique chronique. *Bull Soc Clin Med Ment*, 2, 6–16.

Carabellese, F., Rocca, G., Candelli, C., & Catanesi, R. (2014). Mental illness, violence and delusional misidentifications: The role of Capgras' syndrome in matricide. *J Forensic Leg Med* 21, 9–13. doi:10.1016/j.jflm.2013.10.012

Caribé, A. C., Daltro-Oliveira, R., Araújo, R. H., et al. (2013). Systemic lupus, folie a trois and homicide. *Compr Psychiatry* 54(7), 1032–3. doi:10.1016/j.comppsych.2013.04.011

Carpiniello, B., Pinna, F., & Tuveri, R. (2011). Delusional infestation in a patient with renal failure, metabolic syndrome, and chronic cerebrovascular disease treated with aripiprazole: A case report. *Case Rep Med* 2011, 103652. doi:10.1155/2011/103652

Chagnon, N. A., & Irons, W. (1979). *Evolutionary Biology and Human Social Behavior*. Duxbury Press, North Scituate, MA.

Chalavi, S., Vissia, E. M., & Giesen, M. E. (2015). Abnormal hippocampal morphology in dissociative identity disorder and post-traumatic stress disorder correlates with childhood trauma and dissociative symptoms. *Hum Brain Map* 36(5), 1692–1704. doi: 10.1002/hbm.22730.

Chan, S. M. S., Leung, P. Y. V., & Chiu, F. K. H. (2007). Late-onset Diogenes syndrome in Chinese: An elderly case series in Hong Kong. *Neuropsychiatr Dis Treat* 3(5), 589–96.

Chandrashekar, C. R. (1981). A victim of an epidemic of possession syndrome. *Indian J Psychiatry* 23(4), 370–2.

Charland-Verville, V., Bruno, M. A., & Bahri, M. A (2013). Brain dead yet mind alive: A positron emission tomography case study of brain metabolism in Côtard's syndrome. *Cortex* 49(7), 1997–9.

Chatterjee, S. S., Khonglah, D., Mitra, S., & Garg, K. (2018). Gulliver's world: Persistent lilliputian hallucinations as manifestation of Charles Bonnet syndrome in a case of cataract and normal pressure hydrocephalus. *Indian J Psychiatry* 60(3), 358–60. doi:10.4103/psychiatry.IndianJPsychiatry_236_18

Chaturvedi, S. K. (1989). Delusions of pregnancy in men: Case report and review of the literature. *Br J Psychiatry* 154, 716–18. doi:10.1192/bjp.154.5.716

Chimbos, P. D. (1978). *Marital Violence: A Study of Interspouse Homicide*. R & E Research Associates, San Francisco.

Chiu, H. F. K. (1995). Côtard's syndrome in psychogeriatric patients in Hong Kong. *Gen Hosp Psychiatry* 17(1), 54–5.

Choi, E. J., Lee, J. K., Kang, J. K., & Lee, S. A. (2005). Complex visual hallucinations after occipital cortical resection in a patient with epilepsy due to cortical dysplasia. *Arch Neurol* 62(3), 481–4. doi:10.1001/archneur.62.3.481

Chowdhury, A. N., Mukherjee, H., Ghosh, K. K., & Chowdhury, S. (2003). Puppy pregnancy in humans: A culture-bound disorder in rural West Bengal, India. *Int J Soc Psychiatry* 49(1), 35–42. doi:10.1177/0020764003049001536

Christodoulou, G. N. (1978a). Syndrome of subjective doubles. *Am J Psychiatry* 135(2), 249–51.

Christodoulou, G. N. (1978b). Course and prognosis of the syndrome of doubles. *J Nerv Ment Dis* 166(1), 68–72.

Christodoulou, G. N., & Malliara-Loulakaki, S. (1981). Delusional misidentification syndromes and cerebral 'dysrhythmia'. *Psychiatr Clin (Basel)* 14(4), 245–51.

Christodoulou, G. N., Margariti, M., Kontaxakis, V. P., & Christodoulou, N. G. (2009). The delusional misidentification syndromes: Strange, fascinating, and instructive. *Curr Psychiatr Rep* 11(3), 185–9.

Cipriani, G., Logi, C., & Di Fiorino, A. (2012). A romantic delusion: De Clerambault's syndrome in dementia. *Geriatr Gerontol Int* 12(3), 383–7.

Cipriani, G., Nuti, A., Danti, S., & Picchi, L. (2019). 'I am dead': Côtard syndrome and dementia. *Int J Psychiatry Clin Pract* 23(2), 149–56. doi:10.1080/13651501.2018.1529248

Clark, A. N. G., Mankikar, G. D., & Gray, I. (1975). Diogenes syndrome: A clinical study of gross neglect in old age. *Lancet* 305(7903), 366–8.

Clinton, J. F. (1986). Expectant fathers at risk for couvade. *Nurs Res* 35(5), 290–5.

Cocchini, G., Lello, O., McIntosh, R. D., & Della Sala, S. (2014). Phantabulation: A case of visual imagery interference on visual perception. *Neurocase* 20(5), 581–90. doi:10.1080/13554794.2013.826689

Coebergh, J. A. F., Lauw, R. F., Sommer, I. E. C., & Blom, J. D. (2019). Musical hallucinations and their relation with epilepsy. *J Neurol* 266(6), 1501–15. doi:10.1007/s00415-019-09289-x

Coebergh, J. A. F., Lauw, R. F., Bots, R., et al. (2015). Musical hallucinations: Review of treatment effects. *Front Psychol* 6, 1501–15. doi:10.3389/fpsyg.2015.00814.

Cohen, D., Cottias, C., & Basquin, M. (1997). Côtard's syndrome in a 15-year-old girl. *Acta Psychiatr Scand* 95(2), 164–5. doi:10.1111/j.1600-0447.1997.tb00391.x

Cohen, L. M. (1982). A current perspective of pseudocyesis. *Am J Psychiatry* 139(9), 1140–4. doi:10.1176/ajp.139.9.1140

Cohen, S. Y., & Le Gargasson, J. F. (2006). [Adaptation to central scotoma: III. Visual hallucinations and Charles Bonnet syndrome]. *J Fr Ophtalmol* 29(3), 329–35. doi:10.1016/s0181-5512(06)73794-9

Coleman, S. M. (1933). Misidentification and non-recognition. *J Ment Sci* 79, 42–51.

Collacott, R. A., & Napier, E. M. (1991). Erotomania and Fregoli-like state in Down's syndrome: Dynamic and developmental aspects. *J Ment Defic Res* 35(Pt 5), 481–6.

Contardi, S., Rubboli, G., Giulioni, M., et al. (2007). Charles Bonnet syndrome in hemianopia, following antero-mesial temporal lobectomy for drug-resistant epilepsy. *Epileptic Disord* 9(3), 271–5. doi:10.1684/epd.2007.0110

Cook, F., Dougherty, S., Moreton, R., & Khorsandi, M. (2017). Keep an eye out: A rare case of acute-onset Charles Bonnet syndrome after Stanford type A aortic dissection repair surgery. *Scott Med J* 62(2), 66–9. doi:10.1177/0036933017696661

Coons, P. M. (1988). Misuse of forensic hypnosis: A hypnotically elicited false confession with the apparent creation of a multiple personality. *Int J Clin Exp Hypnosis* 36(1), 1–11. doi:10.1080/00207148808409323

Coons, P. M., & Milstein, V. (1994). Factitious or malingered multiple personality disorder: Eleven cases. *Dissociation* 7(2), 81–5.

Cope, T. E., & Baguley, D. M. (2009). Is musical hallucination an otological phenomenon? A review of the literature. *Clin Otolaryngol* 34(5), 423–30. doi:10.1111/j.1749-4486.2009.02013.x

Cordeiro, Q., Corbett, C. E., & Cordeiro, Q. (2003). [Delusional parasitic infestation and folie à deux: Case report]. *Arq Neuropsiquiatr* 61(3B), 872–5.

Cory, C. E. (1919). A divided self. *J Abnorm Psychol* 14(4), 281–91.

Côtard, J. (1974). Nihilistic delusions. In S. R. Hirsch & M. Shepherd (eds.), *Themes and Variations in European Psychiatry*. John Wright & Sons, Bristol, UK.

Courbon, P. (1927). Syndrome d'illusion de Fregoli et schizophrenie. *Bull Soc Clin Med Ment* 15, 121–5.

Courbon, P., & Fail, G. (1927). Syndrome 'd'illusion de Frégoli' et schizophrénie. *Bull Soc Clin Med*, pp. 121–5.

Courbon, P., & Tusques, J. (1932) Illusion d'intermetamorphose et de charme. *Ann Med Psychol* 90, 401–5.

Cox, T. M., & ffytche, D. H. (2014). Negative outcome Charles Bonnet syndrome. *Br J Ophthalmol* 98(9), 1236–9. doi:10.1136/bjophthalmol-2014-304920

Craike, W. H., & Slater, E. (1945). Folie à deux in uniovular twins reared apart. *Brain: A Journal of Neurology* 68(3), 213–21.

Crane, D. L. (1976). More violent Capgras. *Am J Psychiatry* 133(11), 1350.

Craske, S., & Sacks, B. I. (1969). A case of 'double autoscopy'. *Br J Psychiatry* 115, 343–5.

Cutting, J. (1991). Delusional misidentification and the role of the right hemisphere in the appreciation of identity. *Br J Psychiatry Suppl* 14, 70–5.

Cutting, J. (2011). *A Critique of Psychopathology*. Forest Publishing, East Sussex, UK.

Cybulska, E. (1998). Senile squalor: Plyushkin's not Diogenes' syndrome. *Psychiatric Bull* 22(5), 319–20.

Cytowic, R. E. (1997). Synaesthesia: Phenomenology and neuropsychology – A review of current knowledge. *Psyche* 2(10), 17–39.

Cytowic, R. E., Eagleman, D., Eagleman, D. M., & Nabokov, D. (2009). *Wednesday Is Indigo Blue*. MIT Press, Cambridge, MA.

Dalfen, A. K., & Feinstein, A. (2000). Head injury, dissociation and the Ganser syndrome. *Brain Injury* 14(12), 1101–5. doi:10.1080/02699050050203595

Dalla Barba, G., & Boisse, M. F. (2010). Temporal consciousness and confabulation: Is the medial temporal lobe 'temporal'? *Cogn Neuropsychiatry* 15(1), 95–117. doi:10.1080/13546800902758017

Dalla Barba, G., & La Corte, V. (2013). The hippocampus, a time machine that makes errors. *Trends Cogn Sci (Regul Ed)* 17(3), 102–4. doi:10.1016/j.tics.2013.01.005

Dalla Barba, G., & La Corte, V. (2015). A neurophenomenological model for the role of the hippocampus in temporal consciousness: Evidence from confabulation.

Front Behav Neurosci 9(218), 82–6. doi:10.3389/fnbeh.2015.00218

Dalla Barba, G., Barbera, C., Brazzarola, M., & Marangoni, S. (2016). Recovery from confabulation after normotensive hydrocephalus shunting. *Cortex* 75, 82–6. doi:10.1016/j.cortex.2015.11.016

Dally, P., & Gomez, J. (1979). Capgras: Case study and reappraisal of psychopathology. *Br J Med Psychol* 52(3), 291–5.

Daly, M., & Wilson, M. (1997). Crime and conflict: Homicide in evolutionary psychological perspective. *Crime and Justice* 22, 51–100.

Daly, M., Wilson, M., & Weghorst, S. J. (1982). Male sexual jealousy. *Ethol & Sociobiol* 3(1), 11–27.

Damas-Mora, J., Skelton-Robinson, M., & Jenner, F. A. (1982). The Charles Bonnet syndrome in perspective. *Psychol Med* 12(2), 251–61.

Dantendorfer, K., Maierhofer, D., & Musalek, M. (1997). Induced hallucinatory psychosis (folie à deux hallucinatoire): Pathogenesis and nosological position. *Psychopathology* 30(6), 309–15. doi:10.1159/000285071

Darby, R. R., Laganiere, S., Pascual-Leone, A., et al. (2017). Finding the imposter: Brain connectivity of lesions causing delusional misidentifications. *Brain* 140(2), 497–507. doi:10.1093/brain/aww288

Daulatabad, D., Sonthalia, S., Srivastava, A., et al. (2017). Folie a deux and delusional disorder by proxy: An atypical presentation. *Australas J Dermatol* 58(3), e113–e116. doi:10.1111/ajd.12490

David, R. R., & Fernandez, H. H. (2000). Quetiapine for hypnogogic musical release hallucinations. *J Geriatr Psychiatry Neurol* 13(4), 210–11. doi:10.1177/089198870001300406

Davis, J. L., Kurek, J. A., Sethi, K. D., & Morgan, J. C. (2017). Delusional infestation in Parkinson's disease. *Mov Disord Clin Pract* 4(1), 111–15. doi:10.1002/mdc3.12352

Davison, K. (1964). Episodic depersonalization: Observations on 7 patients. *Br J Psychiatry* 110, 505–13.

de Clerambault, C. G. (1921/1942). Les psychosis passionelles. In *Oeuvre psychiatrique [Psychiatric works]* (pp. 315–22). Presses Universitaires de France, Paris.

de Koning, E., & Piette, M. H. (2014). A retrospective study of murder-suicide at the Forensic Institute of Ghent University, Belgium: 1935–2010. *Med Sci Law* 54(2), 88–98. doi:10.1177/0025802413518018

de Morsier, G. (1967). [The Charles Bonnet syndrome: visual hallucinations in the aged without mental deficiency]. *Ann Med Psychol (Paris)* 2(5), 678–702.

de Morsier, G. (1969). Diencephalic visual hallucinations, part II. *Psychiatr Clin* 2(4), 232–51.

de Pauw, K. W. (1994). Delusional misidentification: A plea for an agreed terminology and classification. *Psychopathology* 27(3–5), 123–9.

de Pauw, K. W., & Szulecka, T. K. (1988). Dangerous delusions: Violence and the misidentification syndromes. *Br J Psychiatry* 152, 91–96.

de Pauw, K. W., Szulecka, T. K., & Poltock, T. L. (1987). Frégoli syndrome after cerebral infarction. *J Nerv Ment Dis* 175(7), 433–8.

de Preester, H. (2013). Merleau-Ponty's sexual schema and the sexual component of body integrity identity disorder. *Medicine Health Care & Philosophy* 16(2), 171–84. doi:10.1007/s11019-011-9367-3.

de Risio, S., de Rossi, G., & Sarchiapone M. (2004). A case of Côtard syndrome: 123I-IBZM SPECT imaging of striatal D_2 receptor binding. *Psychiatr Res* 130(1), 109–12.

Deeley, Q., Oakley, D. A., Walsh, E., et al. (2014). Modelling psychiatric and cultural possession phenomena with suggestion and fMRI. *Cortex* 53, 107–19.

Dein, S., & Illaiee, A. S. (2013). Jinn and mental health: Looking at Jinn possession in modern psychiatric practice. *Psychiatrist* 37(9), 290–3.

Dening, T. R., & Berrios, G. E. (1994). Autoscopic phenomena. *Br J Psychiatry* 165(6), 808–17. doi:10.1192/bjp.165.6.808

Devinsky, O., Feldmann, E., & Burrowes, K. (1989). Autoscopic phenomena with seizures. *Arch Neurol* 46(10), 1080–8.

Devinsky, O., Khan, S., & Alper, K. (1998). Olfactory reference syndrome in a patient with partial epilepsy. *Neuropsychiatr Neuropsychol Behav Neurol* 11(2), 103–5.

Dewhurst, K., & Todd, J. (1956). The psychosis of a association: Folie à deux. *J Nerv Ment Dis* 124(5), 451–9.

Dewhurst, W. G., & Eilenberg, M. D. (1961). Folie a trios: Case report. *J Ment Sci* 107, 486–90.

Dick, P. K. (2011). *A Scanner Darkly*. Houghton Mifflin Harcourt, Boston.

Dijk, M. T. V., Wingen, G. A. V., & Lammeren, A. V. (2013). Neural basis of limb ownership in individuals with body integrity identity disorder. *PLoS One*. 10.1371/journal.pone.0072212

Dijkstra, P., Barelds, D. P. H. (2010). An inventory and update of jealousy-evoking partner behaviours in modern society. *Clin Psychol Psychother* 17(4), 329–45. doi:10.1002/cpp.668

Dippel, B., Kemper, J., & Berger, M. (1991). Folie à six: A case report on induced psychotic disorder. *Acta Psychiatr Scand* 83(2), 137–41.

Dixon, J. C. (1963). Depersonalization phenomena in a sample population of college students. *Br J Psychiatry* 109, 371–5.

Dixon, M. J., Smilek, D., & Merikle, P. M. (2004). Not all synaesthetes are created equal: Projector versus associator synaesthetes. *CABN* 4(3), 335–43.

Dobash, R. E., Dobash, R. P., Cavanagh, K., & Medina-Ariza, J. (2007). Lethal and nonlethal violence against an intimate female partner: Comparing male murderers to nonlethal abusers. *Violence Against Women* 13(4), 329–53.

Docherty, J. P., & Ellis, J. (1976). A new concept and finding in morbid jealousy. *Am J Psychiatry* 133(6), 679–83. doi:10.1176/ajp.133.6.679

Doja, A. (2005). Social thought and commentary: Rethinking the Couvade. *Anthropol Q* 78(4), 917–50.

Doongaji, D. R., Apte, J. S., & Bhat, R. (1975). Ganser state (syndrome): An unusual presentation of a space occupying lesion of the dominant hemisphere. *Neurol India* 23(3), 143–8.

Dostoevsky, F. (1846). *The Double: A Petersburg Poem.*

Dostoyevsky, F. (2009). *Notes from Underground and The Double* (trans. R. Wilks). Penguin Books Ltd., London.

Douen, A. G., & Bourque, P. R. (1997). Musical auditory hallucinosis from *Listeria* thrombencephalitis. *Can J Neurol Sci* 24(1), 70–2.

Drake, M. E., Jr, & Revue, M. E. (1988). Côtard's syndrome. *Psychiatr J Univ Ottawa* 13, 36–9.

Draper, B., & Cole, A. (1990). Folie à deux and dementia. *Aust NZ J Psychiatry* 24(2), 280–2. doi:10.3109/00048679009077694

Drummond, L. M., Turner, J., & Reid, S. (1997). Diogenes' syndrome: A load of old rubbish? *Irish J Psychol Med* 14(3), 99–102.

Duarte, C., Choi, K. M., & Li, C. L. (2011). [Delusional parasitosis associated with dialysis treated with aripiprazole]. *Acta Med Port* 24(3), 457–62.

Duijl, M. V., Nijenhuis, E., & Komproe, I. H. (2010). Dissociative symptoms and reported trauma among patients with spirit possession and matched healthy controls in Uganda. *Culture Med & Psychiatry* 34(2), 380–400. doi:10.1007/s11013-010-9171-1

Durmaz, O., Aktaş, S., & Akkişi Kumsar, N. (2020). From psychosis to Wernicke encephalopathy: A case of hunger strike in prison. *Neurocase* 26(4), 248–51. doi:10.1080/13554794.2020.1786587

Dyer, C. (2000). Surgeon amputated healthy legs. *BMJ* 320(7231), 332.

Dyer, S. J., Abrahams, N., Hoffman, M., & van der Spuy, Z. M. (2002). 'Men leave me as I cannot have children': Women's experiences with involuntary childlessness. *Hum Reprod* 17(6), 1663–8. doi:10.1093/humrep/17.6.1663

Eccles, J. A., Garfinkel, S. N., Harrison, N. A., et al. (2015). Sensations of skin infestation linked to abnormal frontolimbic brain reactivity and differences in self-representation. *Neuropsychologia* 77, 90–6. doi:10.1016/j. neuropsychologia.2015.08.006

Edelstyn, N. M., Oyebode, F., & Barrett, K. (1998). Delusional misidentification: A neuropsychological case study in dementia associated with Parkinson's disease. *Neurocase* 4(3), 181–8.

Edelstyn, N. M., Riddoch, M. J., Oyebode, F., et al. (1996). Visual processing in patients with Frégoli syndrome. *Cogn Neuropsychiatry* 1(2), 103–24. doi:10.1080/135468096396587

Edwards, L. (2004). Subsets of vulvodynia: Overlapping characteristics. *J Reprod Med* 49(11), 883–7.

Edwards, L., Mason, M., Phillips, M., et al. (1997). Childhood sexual and physical abuse: Incidence in patients with vulvodynia. *J Reprod Med* 42(3), 135–9.

Ehlers, I., Hipler, U. C., Zuberbier, T., & Worm, M. (2002). Ethanol as a cause of hypersensitivity reactions to alcoholic beverages. *Clin Exp Allergy* 32(8), 1231–5. Retrieved from https://onlinelibrary.wiley.com /doi/abs/10.1046/j.1365-2745.2002.01457.x

Ehrström, S., Kornfeld, D., & Rylander, E. (2009). Chronic stress in women with localised provoked vulvodynia *J Psychosom Med* 30(1), 73–9. doi:10.1080/ 01674820802604359

Ekbom, K. A. (1938). Der prasenile dermatozoenwahn. *Acta Psychiatr Neurol Scand* 13, 227–59.

El Gaddal, Y. Y. (1989). De Clerambault's syndrome (erotomania) in organic delusional syndrome. *Br J Psychiatry* 154(5), 714–16.

El Ouazzani, B., El Hamaoui, Y., Idrissi-Khamlichi, N., & Moussaoui, D. (2008). [Recurrent pseudocyesis with polydipsia: A case report]. *Encephale* 34(4), 416–18. doi:10.1016/j.encep.2007.09.006

Ellenberger, H. F. (1981). *The Discovery of the Unconscious*. Basic Books, New York.

Ellis, H. D. (1994). The role of the right hemisphere in the Capgras delusion. *Psychopathology* 27(3–5), 177–85.

Ellis, H. D., & Young, A. W. (1990). Accounting for delusional misidentifications. *Br J Psychiatry* 157(2), 239–48.

Ellis, H. D., de Pauw, K., Christodoulou, G. N., et al. (1992). Recognition memory in psychotic patients. *Behav Neurol* 5(1), 23–6. doi:10.3233/BEN-1992-5104

Ellis, H. D., Luauté, J. P., & Retterstøl, N. (1994). Delusional misidentification syndromes. *Psychopathology* 27(3–5), 117–20.

Ellis, H. D., Whitley, J., & Luauté, J. P. (1994). Delusional misidentification: The three original papers on the Capgras, Frégoli and intermetamorphosis delusions. (Classic Text No. 17). *Hist Psychiatry* 5(17 Pt 1), 117–46. doi: 10.1177/0957154X9400501708; PMID: 11639277.

Ellis, H. D., Young, A. W., Quayle, A. H., & De Pauw, K. W. (1997). Reduced autonomic responses to faces in Capgras delusion. *Proc Biol Sci* 264(1384), 1085–92. doi:10.1098/ rspb.1997.0150

Ellis, P., & Mellsop, G. (1985). De Clérambault's syndrome: A nosological entity. *Br J Psychiatry* 146(1), 90–3.

Enoch, M. D., Trethowan, W. H., & Barker, J. C. (1967). *Some Uncommon Psychiatric Syndromes*. John Wright, Bristol, UK.

Euripides. (1963). *Medea and Other Plays; Medea; Hecabe; Electra; Heracles* (trans with introduction by P. Vellacott). Penguin Books Ltd., London.

Evans, D. L., & Seely, T. J. (1984). Pseudocyesis in the male. *J Nerv Ment Dis* 172(1), 37–40. doi:10.1097/00005053-198401000 00008

Evans, P., & Merskey, H. (1972). Shared beliefs of dermal parasitosis: Folie partagée. *Br J Med Psychol* 45(1), 19–26.

Evans, W. N. (1951). Simulated pregnancy in a male. *Psychoanal Q* 20(2), 165–78.

Factor, S. A., & Molho, E. S. (2004). Threatening auditory hallucinations and Côtard syndrome in Parkinson disease. *Clin Neuropharmacol* 27(5), 205–7.

Fahy, T. A., Abas, M., & Brown, J. C. (1989). Multiple personality. *Br J Psychiatry* 154, 99–101.

Fair, B. (2010). Morgellons: Contested illness, diagnostic compromise and medicalisation. *Sociol Health Illn* 32(4), 597–612. doi:10.1111/j.1467-9566.2009.01227.x

Feinberg, T. E., & Roane, D. M. (2005). Delusional misidentification. *Psychiatr Clin North Am* 28(3), 665–83, 678. doi:10.1016/j. psc.2005.05.002

Fénelon, G., Soulas, T., & Langavant L. C. D. (2011). Feeling of presence in Parkinson's disease. *J Neurol Neurosurg Psychiatry* 82(11), 1219–24.

Fennig, S., Chelban, J., Naisberg-Fennig, S., & Neumann, M. (1993). Pseudopregnancy and postpartum psychosis: A case study. *Psychopathology* 26(2), 113–16. doi:10.1159/ 000284809

Fernando, F. P., & Frieze, M. (1985). A relapsing folie à trois. *Br J Psychiatry* 146, 315–16.

Ffytche, D. H. (2007). Visual hallucinatory syndromes: Past, present, and future. *Dialogues Clin Neurosci* 9(2), 173–89.

Ffytche, D. H. (2008). The hodology of hallucinations. *Cortex* 44(8), 1067–83. doi:10.1016/j.cortex.2008.04.005

Ffytche, D. H., & Howard, R. J. (1999). The perceptual consequences of visual loss: Positive pathologies of vision. *Brain* 122(7), 1247–60.

Fillastre, M., Fontaine, A., Depecker, L., & Degiovanni, A. (1992). Five cases of Côtard's syndrome in adolescents and young adults: Symptoms of bipolar manic-depressive psychosis. *L'encephale* 18(1), 65–6.

Filley, C. M., & Jarvis, P. E. (1987). Delayed reduplicative paramnesia. *Neurology* 37(4), 701–3.

Finney, C. M., & Mendez, M. F. (2017). Diogenes syndrome in frontotemporal dementia. *Am J Alzheimers Dis Other Demen* 32(7), 438–43. doi:10.1177/1533317517717012

First, M. B. (2005). Desire for amputation of a limb: Paraphilia, psychosis, or a new type of identity disorder. *Psychol Med* 35(6), 919–28.

First, M. B., & Fisher, C. E. (2012). Body integrity identity disorder: The persistent desire to acquire a physical disability. *Psychopathology* 45(1), 3–14.

Fischer, I. C. (1962). Hypothalamic amenorrhea: Pseudocyesis. In *Psychosomatic Obstetrics, Gynecology and Endocrinology* (pp. 291–7). Charles C Thomas, Springfield, IL.

Fisher, B. K. (1997). The red scrotum syndrome. *Cutis* 60(3), 139–41.

Fisher, J. D. (2019). Emergency department presentation of 'delusional parasitosis by proxy': Delusional parent, injured child. *Am J Emerg Med* 37(9), 1806.e1–e2. doi:10.1016/j. ajem.2019.05.058

Fisher, K., & Smith, R. (2000). More work is needed to explain why patients ask for amputation of healthy limbs. *BMJ* 320(7242), 1147.

Fitzgibbon, B. M., & Giummarra, M. J. (2010). Shared pain: From empathy to synaesthesia. *Neurosci Biobehav Rev* 34(4), 500–12.

Fitzgibbon, B. M., Enticott, P. G., & Rich, A. N. (2012). Mirror-sensory synaesthesia: Exploring 'shared' sensory experiences as synaesthesia. *Neurosci Biobehav Rev* 36(1), 645–57.

Flanagan, P. J., & Harel, Z. (1999). Pseudocyesis in an adolescent using the long-acting contraceptive Depo-Provera. *J Adolesc Health* 25(3), 238–40.

Fleminger, S. (1992). Seeing is believing: The role of 'preconscious' perceptual processing in delusional misidentification. *Br J Psychiatry* 160, 293–303.

Fleminger, S. (1994). Delusional misidentification: An exemplary symptom illustrating an interaction between organic brain disease and psychological processes. *Psychopathology* 27(3–5), 161–7.

Fleury, V., Wayte, J., & Kiley, M. (2008). Topiramate-induced delusional parasitosis. *J Clin Neurosci* 15(5), 597–9. doi:10.1016/j. jocn.2006.12.017

Flournoy, H. (1923). Hallucinations Lilliputiennes atypiques chez un vieillard atteint de cataracte. *L'encephale* 18, 566–79.

Fond, G., Jollant, F., & Abbar, M. (2011). The need to consider mood disorders, and especially chronic mania, in cases of Diogenes syndrome (squalor syndrome). *Int Psychogeriatr* 23(3), 505.

Fontenelle, L. F. (2008). Diogenes syndrome in a patient with obsessive-compulsive disorder without hoarding. *Gen Hosp Psychiatry* 30(3), 288–90. doi:10.1016/j. genhosppsych.2007.10.001

Förstl, H., & Beats, B. (1992). Charles Bonnet's description of Côtard's delusion and reduplicative paramnesia in an elderly patient (1788). *Br J Psychiatry* 160(3), 416–18.

Förstl, H., Besthorn, C., Burns, A., et al. (1994). Delusional misidentification in Alzheimer's disease: A summary of clinical and biological aspects. *Psychopathology* 27(3–5), 194–9.

Förstl, H., Almeida, O. P., Owen, A. M., & Burns, A. (1991). Psychiatric, neurological and medical aspects of misidentification syndromes: A review of 260 cases. *Psychol Med* 21 (4), 905–10.

Förstl, H., Burns, A., Jacoby, R., & Levy, R. (1991). Neuroanatomical correlates of clinical misidentification and misperception in senile dementia of the Alzheimer type. *J Clin Psychiatry* 52(6), 268–71.

Foster, A. A., Hylwa, S. A., Bury, J. E., et al. (2012). Delusional infestation: Clinical presentation in 147 patients seen at Mayo Clinic. *J Am Acad Dermatol* 67(4), 673.e1–e10. doi:10.1016/j.jaad.2011.12.012

Fotopoulou, A. (2010). The affective neuropsychology of confabulation and delusion. *Cogn Neuropsychiatry* 15(1), 38–63. doi:10.1080/13546800903250949

Fotopoulou, A., Conway, M. A., Solms, M., et al. (2008a). Self-serving confabulation in prose recall. *Neuropsychologia* 46(5), 1429–41. doi:10.1016/j.neuropsychologia.2007.12.030

Fotopoulou, A., Conway, M. A., Tyrer, S., et al. (2008b). Is the content of confabulation positive? An experimental study. *Cortex* 44(7), 764–72. doi:10.1016/j.cortex.2007.03.001

George, F. S. J. (1910). *Totemism and Exogamy: A Treatise on Certain Early Forms of Superstitution and Society*. Wentworth Press, Sydney, Australia.

Freedman, D. G. (1979). *Human Sociobiology*. Free Press, New York.

Freudenmann, R. W., & Lepping, P. (2009a). Delusional infestation. *Clin Microbiol Rev* 22(4), 690–732.

Freudenmann, R. W., & Lepping, P. (2009b). Delusional infestation. *Clin Microbiol Rev* 22(4), 690–732. doi:10.1128/CMR.00018-09

Freudenmann, R. W., Kölle, M., Schönfeldt-Lecuona, C., et al. (2010). Delusional parasitosis and the matchbox sign revisited: The international perspective. *Acta Derm Venereol* 90(5), 517–19. doi:10.2340/00015555-0909

Friedl, M. C., & Draijer, N. (2000). Dissociative disorders in Dutch psychiatric inpatients. *Am J Psychiatry* 157(6), 1012–13. doi:10.1176/appi.ajp.157.6.1012

Friedmann, A. C., Ekeowa-Anderson, A., Taylor, R., & Bewley, A. (2006). Delusional parasitosis presenting as folie à trois: Successful treatment with risperidone. *Br J Dermatol* 155(4), 841–2. doi:10.1111/j.1365-2133.2006.07424.x

Frost, R. O., Steketee, G., & Williams, L. (2000). Hoarding: A community health problem. *Health Social Care Commun* 8(4), 229–34. doi:10.1046/j.1365-2524.2000.00245.x

Fujikawa, M., Nishio, Y., Kakisaka, Y., et al. (2016). Fantastic confabulation in right frontal lobe epilepsy. *Epilepsy Behav Case Rep* 6, 55–57. doi:10.1016/j.ebcr.2016.08.003

Funayama, M., & Takata, T. (2018). Côtard's syndrome in anti-*N*-methyl-D-aspartate receptor encephalitis. *Psychiatr Clin Neurosci* 72(6), 455–6.

Galton, F. (1881). Visualised numerals. *J Anthropol Inst Great Britain and Ireland* 10, 85–102.

Galton, F. (1883). *Inquiries into Human Faculty and Its Development*. Macmillan, London.

Gama-Marques, J., Jesus, G., & Brissos, S. (2014). [Olfactory reference syndrome and hyperhidrosis: Comorbidity in one patient]. *Rev Neurol* 59(12), 575.

Gander, T., Lübbers, H. T., Zemann, W., & Jacobsen, C. (2014). Charles Bonnet syndrome in cranio-maxillofacial surgery: Case report. *Oral Maxillofac Surg* 18(1), 95–8. doi:10.1007/s10006-013-0406-5

Ganser, S. J. M. (1898). A peculiar hysterical state. *Arch Psychiatr Neuen-Krankheit* 30(2), 633–40.

Garcia-Mingo, A., Dawood, N., Watson, J., & Chiodini, P. L. (2019). Samples from cases of delusional parasitosis as seen in the UK Parasitology Reference Laboratory (2014–2015). *Open Forum Infect Dis* 6(10). doi:10.1093/ofid/ofz440

Gaskin, I. M. (2012). Has pseudocyesis become an outmoded diagnosis. *Birth* 39(1), 77–9. doi:10.1111/j.1523-536X.2011.00521.x

Gaub, H. D. (1767). *De regimine mentis.* University of Lausanne, Lausanne, Switzerland.

Gaw, A. C., Ding, Q., Levine, R. E., & Gaw, H. (1998). The clinical characteristics of possession disorder among 20 Chinese patients in the Hebei province of China. *Psychiatr Serv* 49(3), 360–5. doi:10.1176/ps.49.3.360

Gazzola, V., Worp, H. V. D., Mulder, T., et al. (2007). Aplasics born without hands mirror the goal of hand actions with their feet. *Curr Biol* 17(14), 1235–40.

Gell, A. (1980). The gods at play: Vertigo and possession in Muria religion. *J R Anthropol Instit Man,* 15(2), 219–48.

Ghaffari, N. A. R., Kerdegari, M., & Reyhani, K. H. (2007). Self-mutilation of the nose in a schizophrenic patient with Côtard syndrome. *Arch Iran Med* 10(4), 540–2.

Ghaziuddin, M. (1991). Folie a deux and mental retardation: Review and case report. *Can J Psychiatry* 36(1), 48–9.

Ghika, J. (2012). [Acute amnestic syndrome: Left thalamo-polar infarct]. *Rev Med Suisse* 8 (336), 782, 784–5.

Giannini, A. J., Slaby, A. E., & Robb, T. O. (1991). De Clérambault's syndrome in sexually experienced women. *J Clin Psychiatry* 52(2), 84–6.

Gibbens, T. C. N. (1958). Sane and insane homicide. *J Crim L Criminol & Police Sci.* 49(110),1958–9.

Gibbs, Jr, R. W. (2005). *Embodiment and Cognitive Science.* Cambridge University Press, Cambridge, UK.

Gibson, E., & Klein, S. (1961). *Murder .* HM Stationery Office, London.

Giesecke, J., Reed, B. D., Haefner, H. K., et al. (2004). Quantitative sensory testing in vulvodynia patients and increased peripheral pressure pain sensitivity. *Obstet Gynecol* 104 (1), 126–33.

Gilboa, A. (2010). Strategic retrieval, confabulations, and delusions: Theory and data. *Cogn Neuropsychiatry* 15(1), 145–180. doi:10.1080/13546800903056965

Gilboa, A., & Moscovitch, M. (2002). The cognitive neuroscience of confabulation: A review and a model. In A. D. Baddeley, M. D. Kopelman & B. A. Wilson (eds.), *Handbook of Memory Disorders* (2nd ed., pp. 315–42). John Wiley & Sons, Chichester, UK.

Gillett, T., Eminson, S. R., & Hassanyeh, F. (1990). Primary and secondary erotomania: Clinical characteristics and follow-up. *Acta Psychiatr Scand* 82(1), 65–9.

Gilmour, G., Schreiber, C., & Ewing, C. (2009). An examination of the relationship between low vision and Charles Bonnet syndrome. *Can J Ophthalmol,* 44(1), 49–52. doi:10.3129/i08-169

Ginsberg, L. (1923). A case of synaesthesia. *Am J Psychol* 34, 582–9.

Giummarra, M. J., Bradshaw, J. L., & Nicholl, M. E. R. (2011). Body integrity identity disorder: Deranged body processing, right fronto-parietal dysfunction, and phenomenological experience of body incongruity. *Neuropsychol Rev* 21(4), 320–33.

Glassman, J. N., Magulac, M., & Darko, D. F. (1987). Folie à famille: Shared paranoid disorder in a Vietnam veteran and his family. *Am J Psychiatry* 144(5), 658–60. doi:10.1176/ajp.144.5.658

Glazer, H. I. (2000). Dysesthetic vulvodynia: Long-term follow-up after treatment with surface electromyography-assisted pelvic floor muscle rehabilitation. *J Reprod Med* 45(10), 798–802.

Glazer, H. I., Jantos, M., Hartmann, E. H., & Swencionis, C. (1998). Electromyographic comparisons of the pelvic floor in women with dysesthetic vulvodynia and asymptomatic women. *J Reprod Med* 43(11), 959–62.

Gogol, N. V. (1961). *Dead Souls.* Penguin, New York.

Gold, K., & Rabins, P. V. (1989). Isolated visual hallucinations and the Charles Bonnet syndrome: A review of the literature and presentation of six cases. *Compr Psychiatry* 30 (1), 90–8. doi:10.1016/0010-440x(89)90122-3

Golden, E. C., & Josephs, K. A. (2015). Minds on replay: Musical hallucinations and their relationship to neurological disease. *Brain* 138(Pt 12), 3793–802. doi:10.1093/brain/awv286

Goldin, S., & MacDonald, J. E. (1955). The Ganser state. *J Ment Sci* 101(423), 267–80.

Goldwert, M. (1993). Erotic paranoid reaction, the imaginary lover, and the benign conspiracy. *Psychol Rep* 72(1), 258. doi:10.2466/pr0.1993.72.1.258

Golub, D. (1995). Cultural variations in multiple personality disorder. In L. M. Cohen, J. N. Berzoff & M. R. Elin (eds.), *Dissociative Identity Disorder: Theoretical and Treatment Controversies* (pp. 285–326). Jason Aronson, Lanham, MD.

Gonçalves, L. M., & Tosoni, A. (2016). Sudden onset of Côtard's syndrome as a clinical sign of brain tumor. *Arch Clin Psychiatry (São Paulo)* 43(2), 35–6. doi:10.1590/0101-60830000000080.

Gondolf, E. W., & Shestakov, D. (1997). Spousal homicide in Russia versus the United States: Preliminary findings and implications. *J Fam Violence* 12(1), 63–74.

Gönül, M., Kiliç, A., Soylu, S., et al. (2008). Folie à deux, diagnosed by delusional parasitosis. *Eur J Dermatol* 18(1), 95–6. doi:10.1684/ejd.2007.0330

Gordon, K. D. (2016). Prevalence of visual hallucinations in a national low vision client population. *Can J Ophthalmol* 51(1), 3–6. doi:10.1016/j.jcjo.2015.10.006

Graff-Radford, J., Whitwell, J. L., Geda, Y. E., & Josephs, K. A. (2012). Clinical and imaging features of Othello's syndrome. *Eur J Neurol* 19(1), 38–46. doi:10.1111/j.1468-1331.2011.03412.x

Gralnick, A. (1942). Folie a deux: The psychosis of association. *Psychiatric Q* 16(3), 491–520.

Greaves, G. B. (1980). Multiple personality: 165 years after Mary Reynolds. *J Nerv Ment Dis* 168(10), 577–96.

Greaves, G. B. (1993). A history of multiple personality disorder. In R. P. Kluft & C. G. Fine (eds.), *Clinical Perspectives on Multiple Personality Disorder*. American Psychological Association, Washington, DC.

Greenberg, H. P. (1956). Crime and folie à deux: Review and case history. *J Ment Sci* 102(429), 772–9.

Greenberg, J. L., Shaw, A. M., Reuman, L., et al. (2016). Clinical features of olfactory reference syndrome: An internet-based study. *J Psychosom Res* 80, 11–16.

Greyson, B., Fountain, N. B. M. D., & Derr, L. L. M. (2014). Out-of-body experiences associated with seizures. *Front Hum Neurosci* 8, 65. doi:10.3389/fnhum.2014.00065/full

Griesinger, W. (1882). *Mental Pathology and Therapeutics* (p. 69). W. Wood & Company, New York.

Griffiths, T. D. (2000). Musical hallucinosis in acquired deafness: Phenomenology and brain substrate. *Brain* 123(Pt 10), 2065–76. doi:10.1093/brain/123.10.2065

Grossenbacher, P. G., & Lovelace, C. T. (2001). Mechanisms of synesthesia: Cognitive and physiological constraints. *Trends Cogn Sci* 5(1), 36–41.

Gruzelier, J. (1998). A working model of the neurophysiology of hypnosis: A review of evidence. *Contemp Hypnosis* 15(1), 3–21. doi:10.1002/ch.112

Guadagno, R. E., & Sagarin, B. J. (2010). Sex differences in jealousy: An evolutionary perspective on online infidelity. *J Appl Soc Psychol* 40(1), 2636–55. doi:10.1111/j.1559-1816.2010.00674.x

Guisado Macías, J. A., De Miguel Pedrero, J. L., Mesa del Castillo Payá, P. , & Carbonell Masiá, C. (2001). [Clinical perspective in the folie à trois: A case report]. *Acta Esp Psiquiatr* 29(1), 67–9.

Gumus, I. I., Sarifakioglu, E., Uslu, H., & Turhan, N. O. (2008). Vulvodynia: Case report and review of literature. *Gynecol Obstet Invest* 65(3), 155–61.

Gupta, L. C. A., Das, B. R. C., & Panda, M. S. P. (2016). A case of episodic derealisation in focal cortical dysplasia: First looks at the whole elephant. *Neurol Psychiatry & Brain Res* 22(3–4), 135–40.

Hagen, F. W. (1861). *Studien auf dem Gebiete der ärztlichen Seelenheilkunde*. Besold, Erlangen.

Hagen, F. W. (1868). Zur theorie der hallucination. *All Z Psychiatr* 25, 1–107.

Hajnal, L., & Lazary, J. (2019). Côtard-syndrome associated with Hashimoto encephalopathy: A case report. *Neuropharmacol Hung* 21(2), 85–93.

Hammeke, T. A., McQuillen, M. P., & Cohen, B. A. (1983). Musical hallucinations associated with acquired deafness. *J Neurol Neurosurg Psychiatry* 46(6), 570–2. doi:10.1136/jnnp.46.6.570

Hampson, J. P., Reed, B. D., Clauw, D. J., et al. (2013). Augmented central pain processing in vulvodynia. *J Pain* 14(6), 579–89.

Hänggi, J., Beeli, G., Oechslin, M. S., & Jäncke, L. (2008). The multiple synaesthete ES: Neuroanatomical basis of interval-taste and tone-colour synaesthesia. *Neuroimage* 43(2), 192–203.

Hanihara, T., Takahashi, T., Washizuka, S., et al. (2009). Delusion of oral parasitosis and thalamic pain syndrome. *Psychosomatics* 50(5), 534–7. doi:10.1176/appi.psy.50.5.534

Harciarek, M., & Kertesz, A. (2008). The prevalence of misidentification syndromes in neurodegenerative diseases. *Alzheimer Dis Assoc Disord* 22(2), 163–9. doi:10.1097/WAD.0b013e3181641341

Hardeman, W. J. (1970). [Erotic delusions of reference toward the family physician]. *Ned Tijdschr Geneeskd* 114(20), 845–9.

Harlow, B. L., & Stewart, E. G. (2003). A population-based assessment of chronic unexplained vulvar pain: Have we underestimated the prevalence of vulvodynia? *J Am Med Womens Assoc* 58(2), 82–8.

Harlow, B. L., & Stewart, E. G. (2005). Adult-onset vulvodynia in relation to childhood violence victimization. *Am J Epidemiol* 161(9), 871–80.

Harlow, B. L., He, W., & Nguyen, R. H. N. (2009). Allergic reactions and risk of vulvodynia. *Ann Epidemiol* 19(11), 771–7.

Harlow, B. L., Vitonis, A. F., & Stewart, E. G. (2008). Influence of oral contraceptive use on the risk of adult-onset vulvodynia. *J Reprod Med* 53(2), 102–10.

Harlow, B. L., Kunitz, C. G., Nguyen, R. H. N., et al. (2014). Prevalence of symptoms consistent with a diagnosis of vulvodynia: Population-based estimates from 2 geographic regions. *Am J Obstet Gynecol* 210(1), 40.e1–e8.

Harper, R., & Moss, G. (1992). Delusional infestation associated with post-herpetic neuralgia and EEG abnormalities. *Br J Psychiatry* 161, 411–12. doi:10.1192/bjp.161.3.411

Hart, O. V. D., & Bolt, H. (2005). Memory fragmentation in dissociative identity disorder. *J Trauma & Dissoc* 6(1), 55–70. doi:10.1300/J229v06n01_04

Hashmi, F. K., Ogra, S., & Madge, S. (2019) Reversible Charles Bonnet syndrome secondary to upper lid ptosis. *Orbit* 2019, 1–3. doi:10.1080/01676830.2019.1648522

Hedges, T. R. (2007). Charles Bonnet, his life, and his syndrome. *Surv Ophthalmol* 52(1), 111–14. doi:10.1016/j.survophthal.2006.10.007

Heining, M., & Phillips, M. (2006). Role of the insula in smell and disgust. In W Brewer, D Castle, & C Pantelis (eds)., *Olfaction and the Brain*. Cambridge University Press, Cambridge, UK.

Hilti, L. M., & Brugger, P. (2010). Incarnation and animation: Physical versus representational deficits of body integrity. *Exp Brain Res* 204(3), 315–26. doi: 10.1007/s00221-009-2043-7.

Hilti, L. M., Hänggi, J., Vitacco, D. A., et al (2013). The desire for healthy limb amputation: Structural brain correlates and clinical features of xenomelia. *Brain* 136 (Pt 1), 318–29.

Hinkle, N. C. (2010). Ekbom syndrome: The challenge of 'invisible bug' infestations. *Ann Rev Entomol* 55, 77–94.

Hinkle, N. C. (2011). Ekbom syndrome: A delusional condition of 'bugs in the skin'. *Curr Psychiatry Rep* 13(3), 178–86.

Hirjak, D., Huber, M., Kirchler, E., et al. (2017). Cortical features of distinct developmental trajectories in patients with delusional infestation. *Prog Neuropsychopharmacol Biol*

Psychiatry 76, 72–9. doi:10.1016/j.pnpbp.2017.02.018

Hirstein, W., & Ramachandran, V. S. (1997). Capgras syndrome: A novel probe for understanding the neural representation of the identity and familiarity of persons. *Proc Biol Sci* 264(1380), 437–44. doi:10.1098/rspb.1997.0062

Hirstein, W. (2009). *Confabulation.* Oxford University Press, New York.

Hirstein, W. (2010). The misidentification syndromes as mindreading disorders. *Cogn Neuropsychiatry* 15(1), 233–60. doi:10.1080/13546800903414891

Hitomi, K. (2001). A case of autoscopy during glue sniffing. *Acta Med Kinki Univ* 26 (1), 23–5.

Hodgson, R. (1891). A case of double consciousness. *Psychical Res* 7, 221–57.

Hoepner, R., Labudda, K., Hoppe, M., & Schoendienst, M. (2012). Unilateral autoscopic phenomena as a lateralizing sign in focal epilepsy. *Epilepsy Behav* 23(3), 36–363. doi: 10.1016/j.yebeh.2012.01.010.

Hollender, M. H., & Callahan, A. S. (1975). Erotomania or de Clérambault syndrome. *Arch Gen Psychiatry* 32(12), 1574–6.

Hollender, M. H., & Fishbein, J. H. (1979). Recurrent pathological jealousy. *J Nerv Ment Dis* 167(8), 500–1.

Holroyd, S., & Sabeen, S. (2008). Successful treatment of hallucinations associated with sensory impairment using gabapentin. *J Neuropsychiatry Clin Neurosci* 20(3), 364–6. doi:10.1176/jnp.2008.20.3.364

Hougen, H. P., Rogde, S., & Poulsen, K. (2000). Homicide by firearms in two Scandinavian capitals. *Am J Forensic Med Pathol* 21(3), 281–6.

Howard, R., & Levy, R. (1994). Charles Bonnet syndrome plus: Complex visual hallucinations of Charles Bonnet syndrome type in late paraphrenia. *Int J Geriatr Psychiatry* 9(5), 399–404. doi:10.1002/gps.930090509

Howes, C. F., & Sharp, C. (2018). Delusional infestation in the treatment of ADHD with atomoxetine. *BMJ Case Rep* 2018. doi:10.1136/bcr-2018-226020

Huber, C. G., & Agorastos, A. (2012). We are all zombies anyway: Aggression in Côtard's syndrome. *Am Neuropsych Assoc* 24 (3), e21. doi:10.1176/appi.neuropsych.11070155

Huber, M., Karner, M., Kirchler, E., et al. (2008). Striatal lesions in delusional parasitosis revealed by magnetic resonance imaging. *Prog Neuropsychopharmacol Biol Psychiatry* 32(8), 1967–71. doi:10.1016/j.pnpbp.2008.09.014

Huber, M., Kirchler, E., Karner, M., & Pycha, R. (2007). Delusional parasitosis and the dopamine transporter: A new insight of etiology. *Med Hypotheses* 68(6), 1351–8. doi:10.1016/j.mehy.2006.07.061

Huber, M., Wolf, R. C., Lepping, P., et al. (2018). Regional gray matter volume and structural network strength in somatic vs. non-somatic delusional disorders. *Prog Neuropsychopharmacol Biol Psychiatry* 82, 115–22. doi:10.1016/j.pnpbp.2017.11.022

Hudson, A. J., & Grace, G. M. (2000). Misidentification syndromes related to face specific area in the fusiform gyrus, part 1. *J Neurol Neurosurg Psychiatry* 69(5), 645–8.

Hume, D. (1817). *A Treatise of Human Nature.* Oxford University Press, Oxford, UK.

Hunter, E. C. M., Sierra, M., & David, A. S. (2004). The epidemiology of depersonalisation and derealisation. *Soc Psychiatry Psychiatr Epidemiol* 39(1), 9–18. doi: 10.1007/s00127-004-0701-4.

Hunter, R., & Macalpine, I. (1970). *Three Hundred Years of Psychiatry 1535–1860.* Oxford University Press, Oxford, UK.

Huntjens, R. J. C., Postma, A., & Peters, M. L. (2003). Interidentity amnesia for neutral, episodic information in dissociative identity disorder. *J Abnorm Psychol* 112(2), 290–7. doi:10.1.1.1019.1567

Hurley, M., Scallan, E., Johnson, H., & De La Harpe, D. (2000). Adult service refusers in the greater Dublin area. *Ir Med J* 93(7), 208–11.

Husain, F., Levin, J., Scott, J., & Fjeldstad, C. (2014). Recurrent refrains in a patient with multiple sclerosis: Earworms or musical hallucinations. *Mult Scler Relat Disord* 3(2), 276–8. doi:10.1016/j.msard.2013.08.004

Hussain, K., Gkini, M. A., Taylor, R., et al. (2018). A patient with delusional infestation by proxy: Issues for vulnerable adults. *Dermatol Ther* 31(6), e12724. doi:10.1111/dth.12724

Hylwa, S. A., Bury, J. E., Davis, M. D., et al. (2011). Delusional infestation, including delusions of parasitosis: Results of histologic examination of skin biopsy and patient-provided skin specimens. *Arch Dermatol* 147(9), 1041–5. doi:10.1001/archdermatol.2011.114

Iacoboni, M. (2009a). Imitation, empathy, and mirror neurons. *Annu Rev Psychol* 60, 653–70. doi:10.1146/annurev.psych.60.110707.163604

Iacoboni, M. (2009b). Neurobiology of imitation. *Curr Opin Neurobiol* 19(6), 661–5. doi:10.1016/j.conb.2009.09.008

Ibekwe, P. C., & Achor, J. U. (2008). Psychosocial and cultural aspects of pseudocyesis. *Indian J Psychiatry* 50(2), 112–16. doi:10.4103/0019-5545.42398

Iglesias-Rios, L., Harlow, S. D., & Reed, B. D. (2015). Depression and posttraumatic stress disorder among women with vulvodynia: Evidence from the population-based woman to woman health study. *J Women's Health* 24 (7), 557–62. doi:10.1089/jwh.2014.5001

Igreja, V., Dias-Lambranca, B., & Hershey, D. A. (2010). The epidemiology of spirit possession in the aftermath of mass political violence in Mozambique. *Soc Sci Med* 71(3), 592–9.

Iizuka, O., Suzuki, K., Fujii, T., et al. (2005). [Amnesia following left medial frontal subcortical hemorrhage: A case report]. *No To Shinkei* 57(3), 227–31.

Ilzarbe, D., Vigo, L., Ros-Cucurull, E., et al. (2015). A case of folie à trois induced by a child. *J Clin Psychiatry* 76(1), e119. doi:10.4088/JCP.14cr09295

Ionta, S., Gassert, R., & Blanke, O. (2011). Multisensory and sensorimotor foundation of bodily self-consciousness: An interdisciplinary approach. *Front Psychol* 2, 383. doi:10.3389/fpsyg.2011.00383/full

Ionta, S., Heydrich, L., Lenggenhager, B., et al. (2011). Multisensory mechanisms in temporo-parietal cortex support self-location

and first-person perspective. *Neuron* 70(2), 363–74.

Irvine, J. D. C., & Nwachukwu, K. (2014). Recognizing Diogenes syndrome: A case report. *BMC Res Notes* 7(1), 1–4. doi:10.1186/1756-0500-7-276

Ismail, Z., Nguyen, M.-Q., Fischer, C. E., et al. (2012). Neuroimaging of delusions in Alzheimer's disease. *Psychiatry Res* 202(2), 89–95. doi:10.1016/j.pscychresns.2012.01.008

Jackson, G. A. (1997). Diogenes syndrome: How should we manage it? *J Ment Health* 6(2), 113–16.

Jackson, R. S., Naylor, M. W., Shain, B. N., & King, C. A. (1992). Capgras syndrome in adolescence. *J Am Acad Child Adolesc Psychiatry* 31(5), 977–83.

Janet, P. (2018). *The Mental State of Hystericals.* Franklin Classics, London.

Janet, P. (2019). *The Major Symptoms of Hysteria: Fifteen Lectures Given in the Medical School of Harvard University.* Wentworth Press, Sydney, Australia.

Jantos, M. (2008). Vulvodynia: A psychophysiological profile based on electromyographic assessment. *Appl Psychophysiol Biofeedback* 33(1), 29–38. doi:10.1007/s10484-008-9049-y

Jaspers, K. (1997). *General Psychopathology* (vol. 2). Johns Hopkins University Press, Baltimore.

Jáuregui-Renaud, K., & Ramos-Toledo, V. (2008). Symptoms of detachment from the self or from the environment in patients with an acquired deficiency of the special senses. *J Vestib Res* 18 (2–3), 129–37.

Jedidi, H., Daury, N., Capa, R., et al. (2013). Brain metabolic dysfunction in Capgras delusion during Alzheimer's disease: A positron emission tomography study. *Am J Alzheimers Dis Other Demen* 30(7), 699–706. doi:10.1177/1533317513495105

Jegede, O., Virk, I., Cherukupally, K., et al. (2018). Olfactory reference syndrome with suicidal attempt treated with pimozide and fluvoxamine. *Case Rep Psychiatry* 2018, 7876497. doi:10.1155/2018/7876497

Jenkins, S. B., Revita, D. M., & Tousignant, A. (1962). Delusions of childbirth and labor in a bachelor. *Am J Psychiatry* 118, 1048–50. doi:10.1176/ajp.118.11.1048

Jocic, Z., & Staton, R. D. (1993). Reduplication after right middle cerebral artery infarction. *Brain Cogn* 23(2), 222–30. doi:10.1006/brcg.1993.1056

Joe, S., Park, J., Lim, J., & Park, C. (2015). Unilateral musical hallucination after a hybrid cochlear implantation. *Gen Hosp Psychiatry* 37(1), 97.e1–e3. doi:10.1016/j.genhosppsych.2014.09.014

John, S., & Ovsiew, F. (1996). Erotomania in a brain-damaged male. *J Intellect Disabil Res* 40 (Pt 3), 279–83.

Johnson, J. (1969). Organic psychosyndromes due to boxing. *Br J Psychiatry* 115(518), 45–53.

Johnston, J., & Elliott, C. (2002). Healthy limb amputation: Ethical and legal aspects. *Clin Med* 2, 431–5. doi: 10.7861/clinmedicine.3-2-188

Jonas, J., Maillard, L., Frismand, S., & Colnat-Coulbois, S. (2014). Self-face hallucination evoked by electrical stimulation of the human brain. *Neurology* 83(4), 336–8. doi:10.1212/WNL.0000000000000628

Joseph, A. B. (1994). Observations on the epidemiology of the delusional misidentification syndromes in the Boston metropolitan area: April 1983–June 1984. *Psychopathology* 27(3–5), 150–3.

Joseph, A. B., O'Leary, D. H., Kurland, R., & Ellis, H. D. (1999). Bilateral anterior cortical atrophy and subcortical atrophy in reduplicative paramnesia: A case-control study of computed tomography in 10 patients. *Can J Psychiatry* 44(7), 685–9.

Joseph, A. B. (1985a). Bitemporal atrophy in a patient with Fregoli syndrome, syndrome of intermetamorphosis, and reduplicative paramnesia. *Am J Psychiatry* 142(1), 146–7.

Joseph, A. B. (1985b). Focal central nervous system abnormalities in patients with misidentification syndromes. *Bibliotheca Psychiatrica*, 164), 68–79,

Joseph, A. B., & O'Leary, D. H. (1986). Brain atrophy and interhemispheric fissure

enlargement in Côtard's syndrome. *J Clin Psychiatry* 47(10), 518–20.

Joshi, K. G., Frierson, R. L., & Gunter, T. D. (2006). Shared psychotic disorder and criminal responsibility: A review and case report of folie à trois. *J Am Acad Psychiatry Law* 34(4), 511–17.

Kamleiter, M., & Laakmann, G. (2003). [Stalking: Relevance for clinical practice and jurisdiction]. *Psychiatr Prax* 30(3), 152–8. doi:10.1055/s-2003-38609

Kanemura, S., Tanimukai, H., & Tsuneto, S. (2010). Can 'steroid switching' improve steroid-induced musical hallucinations in a patient with terminal cancer. *J Palliat Med* 13(12), 1495–8. doi:10.1089/jpm.2010.9751

Kant, I. (1999). *Critique of Pure Reason*. Cambridge University Press, Cambridge, UK.

Kapur, N., Turner, A., & King, C. (1988). Reduplicative paramnesia: Possible anatomical and neuropsychological mechanisms. *J Neurol Neurosurg Psychiatry* 51(4), 579–81.

Karroum, E., Konofal, E., & Arnulf, I. (2009). Karl-Axel Ekbom (1907–1977). *J Neurol* 256(4), 683–4.

Kas, A., Lavault, S., Habert, M. O., & Arnulf, I. (2014). Feeling unreal: A functional imaging study in patients with Kleine-Levin syndrome. *Brain* 137(7), 2077–87. doi: 10.1093/brain/awu112.

Kasahara, Y., Fujinawa, A., Sekiguchi, H., & Matsumoto, M. (1972). *Fear of Eye-to-Eye Confrontation and Fear of Emitting Bad Odors* (pp. 74–80). Igaku Shoin, Tokyo.

Kashiwase, H., & Kato, M. (1997). Folie à deux in Japan: Analysis of 97 cases in the Japanese literature. *Acta Psychiatr Scand* 96(4), 231–4.

Kassam, A. S., & Cunningham, E. A. (2018). Côtard syndrome resulting from valacyclovir toxicity. *Primary Care Companion for CNS Disord* 20(1), 17102143.

Kawai, N., Honda, M., Nakamura, S., & Samatra, P. (2001). Catecholamines and opioid peptides increase in plasma in humans during possession trances. *NeuroReport* 12(16), 3419–23.

Kawai, N., Honda, M., Nishina, E., et al. (2017). Electroencephalogram characteristics during possession trances in healthy individuals. *NeuroReport* 28(15), 949–55.

Kaya, M. C., & Bulut, M. (2019). Côtard syndrome developed after radioactive iodine treatment. *Klin Psikofarmakol Bul* 1(29), 240.

Kearns, A. (1987). Côtard's syndrome in a mentally handicapped man. *Br J Psychiatry* 150, 112–14. doi: 10.1192/bjp.150.1.112

Kelley, N. J., Eastwick, P. W., & Harmon-Jones, E. (2015). Jealousy increased by induced relative left frontal cortical activity. *Emotion* 15(5), 550–5. doi: 10.1037/emo0000068

Kelly, B. D. (2009). Folie à plusieurs: Forensic cases from nineteenth-century Ireland. *Hist Psychiatry* 20(77 Pt 1), 47–60. doi:10.1177/0957154X08094236

Kelly, D. H. W., & Walter, C. J. S. (1968). The relationship between clinical diagnosis and anxiety, assessed by forearm blood flow and other measurements. *Br J Psychiatry* 114(510), 611–26.

Kendler, K. S., Robinson, G., McGuire, M., & Spellman, M. P. (1986). Late-onset folie simultanée in a pair of monozygotic twins. *Br J Psychiatry* 148, 463–5.

Kennair, L. E. O., Nordeide, J., & Andreassen, S. (2011). Sex differences in jealousy: A study from Norway. *Nordic Psychol* 63(1), 20–34. doi:10.1027/1901-2276/a000025

Kennedy, N., McDonough, M., Kelly, B., & Berrios, G. E. (2002). Erotomania revisited: Clinical course and treatment. *Compr Psychiatry* 43(1), 1–6.

Khalifa, N., & Hardie, T. (2005). Possession and jinn. *J R Soc Med* 98(8), 351–3. doi:10.1177/014107680509800805

Khandker, M., Brady, S. S., Vitonis, A. F., et al. (2011). The influence of depression and anxiety on risk of adult onset vulvodynia. *J Womens Health* 20(10), 1445–51. doi:10.1089/jwh.2010.2661

Khanna, S., & Ramasubbu, R. (1985). A study of depersonalisation neurosis. *Indian J Psychiatry* 27(1), 73–6.

Khanobdee, C., Sukratanachaiyakul, V., & Gay, J. T. (1993). Couvade syndrome in expectant Thai fathers. *Int J Nurs Stud* 30(2), 125–31.

Kianpoor, M., & Rhoades, Jr, G. F. (2006). Djinnati, a possession state in Baloochistan, Iran. *J Trauma Pract* 4(1–2), 147–55. doi:10.1300/J189v04n01_10

Kim, C., Kim, J., Lee, M., & Kang, M. (2003). Delusional parasitosis as 'folie à deux'. *J Korean Med Sci* 18(3), 462–5. doi:10.3346/jkms.2003.18.3.462

Kirov, G., Jones, P., & Lewis, S. W. (1994). Prevalence of delusional misidentification syndromes. *Psychopathology* 27(3–5), 148–9.

Klein, M. (1977). *Envy and Gratitude and Other Works, 1946–1963*. Doubleday, New York.

Kluft, R. P. (1987). The simulation and dissimulation of multiple personality disorder. *Am J Clin Hypnosis* 30(2), 104–18. doi:10.1080/00029157.1987.10404170

Knight, J. A. (1960). False pregnancy in a male. *Psychosom Med* 22, 260–6.

Kohorst, J. J., Bailey, C. H., Andersen, L. K., et al. (2018). Prevalence of delusional infestation: A population-based study. *JAMA Dermatol* 154(5), 615–17. doi:10.1001/jamadermatol.2018.0004

Kok, L. P., Cheang, M., & Chee, K. T. (1994). De Clerambault syndrome and medical practitioners: Medico-legal implications. *Singapore Med J* 35(5), 486–9.

Kopelman, M. D. (1987). Two types of confabulation. *J Neurol Neurosurg Psychiatry* 50(11), 1482–7.

Kopelman, M. D. (2010). Varieties of confabulation and delusion. *Cogn Neuropsychiatry* 15(1), 14–37. doi:10.1080/13546800902732830

Kopelman, M. D. (2015). What does a comparison of the alcoholic Korsakoff syndrome and thalamic infarction tell us about thalamic amnesia? *Neurosci Biobehav Rev* 54, 46–56. doi:10.1016/j.neubiorev.2014.08.014

Kopelman, M. D., Ng, N., & Brouke, O. V. D. (1997). Confabulation extending across episodic, personal, and general semantic memory. *Cogn Neuropsychol* 14(5), 683–712. doi:10.1080/026432997381411

Korsakoff, S. S. (1889/1890). Medizinskoje Obozrenije. *Allegemeine Z Psychiatrie* 46, 475–85.

Korsakoff, S. S. (1955). Psychic disorder in conjunction with multiple neuritis (psychosis polyneuritica cerebropathia psychica toxaemica). *Neurology* 5(6), 396–406. doi:10.1212/WNL.5.6.396

Kraya, N. A., & Patrick, C. (1997). Folie à deux in forensic setting. *Aust NZ J Psychiatry* 31(6), 883–8. doi:10.3109/00048679709065518

Kuhle, B. X., Smedley, K. D., & Schmitt, D. P. (2009). Sex differences in the motivation and mitigation of jealousy-induced interrogations. *Pers Indiv Dif* 46(4), 499–502.

Kumar, S., Sedley, W., Barnes, G. R., et al. (2014). A brain basis for musical hallucinations. *Cortex* 52, 86–97. doi:10.1016/j.cortex.2013.12.002

Kumbier, E., & Kornhuber, M. (2002). [Delusional ectoparasitic infestation in multiple system atrophy]. *Nervenarzt* 73(4), 380–3. doi:10.1007/s00115-002-1273-8

Kuruppuarachchi, K., & Seneviratne, A. N. (2011). Organic causation of morbid jealousy. *Asian J Psychiatry* 4(4), 258–60.

Lader, M. H., & Wing, L. (1966). *Physiological Measures, Sedative Drugs, and Morbid Anxiety* (vol. 14). Oxford University Press, Oxford, UK.

Ladowsky-Brooks, R. L., & Fischer, C. E. (2003). Ganser symptoms in a case of frontal-temporal lobe dementia: Is there a common neural substrate? *J Clin Exp Neuropsychol* 25(6), 761–8. doi:10.1076/jcen.25.6.761.16473

Lai, J., Lu, Q., Xu, Y., & Hu, S. (2016). Severe water intoxication and secondary depressive syndrome in relation to delusional infestation. *Neuropsychiatr Dis Treat* 12, 517–21. doi:10.2147/NDT.S102993

Lai, J., Xu, Z., Xu, Y., & Hu, S. (2018). Reframing delusional infestation: Perspectives on unresolved puzzles. *Psychol Res Behav Manag* 11, 425–32. doi:10.2147/PRBM.S166720

Lambek, M. (1980). Spirits and spouses: Possession as a system of communication among the Malagasy speakers of Mayotte. *Am Ethnol* 7(2), 318–31. doi:10.1525/ae.1980.7.2.02a00060

Lange, E., & Ficker, F. (1976). [Double suicide and symbiontic psychosis (suicide à deux and folie à deux)]. *Psychiatr Clin (Basel)* 9(3–4), 168–82.

Lapid, M. I., Burton, M. C., Chang, M. T., et al. (2013). Clinical phenomenology and mortality in Charles Bonnet syndrome. *J Geriatr Psychiatry Neurol* 26(1), 3–9. doi:10.1177/0891988712473800

Lasegue, C., & Falret, J. P. (1877/1964). La folie à deux (trans. by R. Michaud). *Am J Psychiatry* 121, 2–23.

Lawrence, A. A. (2006). Clinical and theoretical parallels between desire for limb amputation and gender identity disorder. *Arch Sex Behav* 35(3), 263–78. doi:10.1.1.368.6837

Lazarus, A. (1986). Folie a deux in identical twins: interaction of nature and nurture. *The British Journal of Psychiatry, 148*(3), 324–326.

Leandro, J. E., Beato, J., Pedrosa, A. C., et al. (2017). The Charles Bonnet syndrome in patients with neovascular age-related macular degeneration: Association with proton pump inhibitors. *Invest Ophthalmol Vis Sci* 58(10), 4138–42. doi:10.1167/iovs.16-21270

Lee, G. H., & Stewart, J. T. (2018). A case of musical hallucinations related to mirtazapine. *Clin Neuropharmacol* 41(6), 222–23. doi:10.1097/WNF.0000000000000302

Lee, K., Shinbo, M., Kanai, H., & Nagumo, Y. (2011). Reduplicative paramnesia after a right frontal lesion. *Cogn Behav Neurol* 24 (1), 35–9. doi:10.1097/WNN.0b013e31821129b7

Lee, S. M., Lewis, M., Leighton, D., & Harris, B. (2014). Neuropsychological characteristics of people living in squalor. *Int Psychogeriatr* 26 (5), 837–44.

Lemche, E., Anilkumar, A., & Giampietro, V. P. (2008). Cerebral and autonomic responses to emotional facial expressions in depersonalisation disorder. *Br J Psychiatry* 193(3), 222–28. doi: 10.1192/bjp.bp.107.044263

Lenggenhager, B., Hilti, L., & Brugger, P. (2015). Disturbed body integrity and the 'rubber foot illusion'. *Neuropsychology* 29(2), 205–11. doi:10.1037/neu0000143.

Lenggenhager, B., Hilti, L., Palla, A., et al. (2014). Vestibular stimulation does not diminish the desire for amputation. *Cortex* 54, 210–12. doi:10.1016/j.cortex.2014.02.004

Lepping, P., Baker, C., & Freudenmann, R. W. (2010). Delusional infestation in dermatology in the UK: Prevalence, treatment strategies, and feasibility of a randomized, controlled trial. *Clin Exp Dermatol* 35(8), 841–4. doi:10.1111/j.1365-2230.2010.03782.x

Lepping, P., Rishniw, M., & Freudenmann, R. W. (2015). Frequency of delusional infestation by proxy and double delusional infestation in veterinary practice: Observational study. *Br J Psychiatry* 206(2), 160–3. doi:10.1192/bjp.bp.114.144469

Lerner, V., Bergman, J., & Greenberg, D. (1995). Laurence-Moon-Bardet-Biedl syndrome in combination with Côtard's syndrome: Case report. *Israel J Psychiatry Relat Sci* 32(4), 291–4.

Levy, K. N., & Kelly, K. M. (2010.) Sex differences in jealousy: A contribution from attachment theory. *Psychol Sci* 21(2), 168–73. doi:10.1177/0956797609357708

Lewis, D. O., Yeager, C. A., & Swica, Y. (1997). Objective documentation of child abuse and dissociation in 12 murderers with dissociative identity disorder. *Am J Psychiatry* 154(12), 1703–10. doi:10.1176/ajp.154.12.1703

Lewis, I. M. (1989). *Ecstatic Religion*. Routledge, New York.

Lewis, S. W. (1987). Brain imaging in a case of Capgras syndrome. *Br J Psychiatry* 150(1), 117–21.

Lhermwitte, J. (1951) Visual hallucinations of the self. *BMJ* 1(4704), 431–4. doi: 10.1136/bmj.1.4704.431

Lindén, T., & Helldén, A. (2013). Côtard's syndrome as an adverse effect of acyclovir treatment in renal failure. *J Neurol Sci*, 333, s1, E650.

Lipkin, M., & Lamb, G. S. (1982). The couvade syndrome: an epidemiologic study. *Ann Intern Med*, 96(4), 509–511. doi:10.7326/0003-4819-96-4-509

Lochner, C., & Stein, D. J. (2003). Olfactory reference syndrome: diagnostic criteria and differential diagnosis. *Journal of postgraduate medicine*, 49(4), 328.

Lochner, C., & Stein, D. J. (2014). Prevalence of olfactory reference syndrome in obsessive-compulsive disorder and social anxiety disorder. *J Clin Psychiatry* 75(11), 1266.

Locke, J. (1817). *An Essay Concerning Human Understanding: In Two Volumes*. JM Dent, London.

Lodhi, S. (2020). It smells fishy: A case report and discussion of olfactory reference syndrome. *CNS Spectr* 25(2), 310. doi:10.1017/S1092852920000899

López, A. C., Botello, M. C. C., & Romero, V. C. (2016). Côtard syndrome in a young man? *Eur Psychiatry* 33, 5348.

Lopez, C., & Blanke, O. (2010). How body position influences the perception and conscious experience of corporeal and extrapersonal space. *Rev Neuropsychol* 2, 195–202.

Lopez, C., & Elziere, M. (2018). Out-of-body experience in vestibular disorders: A prospective study of 210 patients with dizziness. *Cortex* 104, 193–206. doi: 10.1016/j.cortex.2017.05.026

Lopez, C., Halje, P., & Blanke, O. (2008). Body ownership and embodiment: Vestibular and multisensory mechanisms. *Neurophysiol Clin* 38(3), 149–61. doi: 10.1016/j.neucli.2007.12.006.

Lorente-Rovira, E., Berrios, G., McKenna, P., et al. (2011). Confabulations: I. Concept, classification and neuropathology. *Acta Esp Psiquiatr* 39(4), 251–9.

Lotery, H. E., McClure, N., & Galask, R. P. (2004). Vulvodynia. *Lancet* 363(9414), 1058–60.

Low, W. K., Tham, C. A., D'Souza, V. D., & Teng, S. W. (2013). Musical ear syndrome in adult cochlear implant patients. *J Laryngol Otol* 127(9), 854–8. doi:10.1017/S0022215113001758

Luaute, J. P., Saladini, O., & Luauté, J. (2008). Neuroimaging correlates of chronic delusional jealousy after right cerebral infarction. *J Neuropsychiatry Clin Neurosci* 20(2), 245–7. doi/full/10.1176/jnp.2008.20.2.245

Luke, D., & Terhune, D. B. (2013). The induction of synaesthesia with chemical agents: A systematic review. *Front Psychol.* doi:10.3389/fpsyg.2013.00753

Lukianowicz, N. (1967). 'Body image' disturbances in psychiatric disorders. *Br J Psychiatry* 113(494), 31–47.

Lunn, V. (1970). Autoscopic phenomena. *Acta Psychiatr Scand* 46(Suppl 219), 118–25. doi:10.1111/j.1600-0447.

Lynn, S. J., & Pintar, J. (1997). A social narrative model of dissociative identity disorder. *Aust J Clin Exp Hypn* 25(1), 1–7.

Mackay-Sim, A., & Royet, J. P. (2006). The olfactory system. In W. Brewer, D. Castle & C. Pantelis (eds.), *Olfaction and the Brain.* Cambridge University Press, Cambridge, UK.

Macmillan, D., & Shaw, P. (1966). Senile breakdown in standards of personal and environmental cleanliness. *BMJ* 2(5521), 1032–7. doi:10.1136/bmj.2.5521.1032

Madill, S. A., Lascaratos, G., Arden, G. B., & ffytche, D. H. (2009). Perceived color of hallucinations in the Charles Bonnet syndrome is related to residual color contrast sensitivity. *J Neuroophthalmol* 29(3), 192–6. doi:10.1097/WNO.0b013e3181b1b2bf

Madoz-Gúrpide, A., & Hillers-Rodríguez, R. (2010). [Capgras delusion: A review of aetiological theories]. *Rev Neurol* 50(7), 420–30.

Malaspina, D., Corcoran, C., & Goudsmit, N. (2006). The impact of olfaction on human social functioning. In W. Brewer, D. Castle & C. Pantelis (eds.), *Olfaction and the Brain.* Cambridge University Press, Cambridge, UK.

Malloy, M., Miller, B., & Kane, J. (2015). Apolipoprotein E and neurocognitive function: Reply. *JAMA Neurol* 72(4), 479.

Mann, J., & Foreman, D. M. (1996). Homo-erotomania for a delusional parent: Erotomania with Capgras and Fregoli syndromes in a young male with learning difficulties. *J Intellect Disabil Res* 40(Pt 3), 275–8.

Manzi, D., Greenberg, B., Maier, D., et al. (1995). Bronchogenic carcinoma presenting as a pseudopregnancy. *Chest* 107(2), 567–9. doi:10.1378/chest.107.2.567

Marazziti, D., Poletti, M., Dell'Osso, L., & Baroni, S. (2013). Prefrontal cortex, dopamine, and jealousy endophenotype. *CNS Spectrum* 18(1), 6–14. doi: 10.1017/S1092852912000740

Margariti, M. M., & Kontaxakis, V. P. (2006). Approaching delusional misidentification syndromes as a disorder of the sense of uniqueness. *Psychopathology* 39(6), 261–8. doi:10.1159/000095730

Markos, A. R. (2008). Caffeine-related genital skin pain. *J Low Genit Tract Dis* 12(1), 38–9.

Markos, A. R. (2011). Dysaesthetic penoscrotodynia: Nomenclature, classification, diagnosis and treatment. *Int J STD & AIDS* 22(9), 483–7 doi:10.1258/ijsa.2011.010451

Markos, A. R., & Dinsmore, W. (2013). Persistent genital arousal and restless genitalia: Sexual dysfunction or subtype of vulvodynia. *Int J STD & AIDS* 24(11), 852–8. doi:10.1177/0956462413489276

Marshall, C. L., Williams, V., Ellis, C., Taylor, R. E., & Bewley, A. P. (2017). Delusional infestation may be caused by recreational drug usage in some patients, but they may not disclose their habit. *Clin Exp Dermatol* 42(1), 41–5. doi:10.1111/ced.12999

Martial, C., Larroque, S. K., Cavaliere, C., et al. (2019). Resting-state functional connectivity and cortical thickness characterization of a patient with Charles Bonnet syndrome. *PLoS One* 14(7), e0219656. doi:10.1371/journal.pone.0219656

Martín Juan, A., Madrigal, R., Porta Etessam, J., et al. (2018). Anton-Babinski syndrome: Case report. *Arch Soc Esp Oftalmol* 93(11), 555–7. doi:10.1016/j.oftal.2018.04.004

Martin, K., Fremlin, G. A., Mall, J., & Goulding, J. M. R. (2018). Olfactory reference syndrome: A patient's perspective. *Clin Exp*

Dermatol 43(4), 509–10. doi:10.1111/ced.13421

Martínez-Horta, S., Perez-Perez, J., & Pagonabarraga, J. (2020). Autoscopic phenomena as an atypical psychiatric presentation of Huntington's disease: A case report including longitudinal clinical and neuroimaging data. *Cortex* 125, 299–306. doi: 10.1016/j.cortex.2020.01.024.

Mashayekhi, A., & Ghayoumi, A. (2015). Coexistence of reverse Capgras syndrome, subjective double and Côtard syndrome. *Zahedan J Res Med Sci* 18(1). doi:10.17795/ZJRMS-5878

Masoni, S., Maio, A., Trimarchi, G., et al. (1994). The Couvade syndrome. *J Psychosom Obstet Gynecol* 15(3), 125–31.

Mathew, R. J., Wilson, W. H., Humphreys, D., & Lowe, J. V. (1993). Depersonalization after marijuana smoking. *Biol Psychiatry* 33(6), 431–41. doi: 10.1016/0006-3223(93)90171-9

Maupassant, G. d. (2004). *A Parisian Affair and Other Stories* (trans. Sian Miles). Penguin, New York.

Mayer-Gross, W. (1935). On depersonalization. *Br J Med Psychol* 15, 103–26. doi:10.1111/J.2044-8341.1935.tb01140.x

Mazzoli, M. (1992). Folie à deux and mental retardation. *Can J Psychiatry* 37(4), 278–9.

McConnell, W. B. (1965). The phantom double in pregnancy. *Br J Psychiatry* 111, 67–9. doi: 10.1192/bjp.111.470.67.

McGeoch, P. D., Brang, D., Song, T., & Lee, R. R. (2011). Xenomelia: A new right parietal lobe syndrome. *J Neurol Neurosurg Psychiatry* 82 (12), 1314–19. doi: 10.1136/jnnp-2011-300224

McGuire, M., & Troisi, A. (1998). *Darwinian Psychiatry*. Oxford University Press, Oxford, UK.

McKay, R., & Cipolotti, L. (2007). Attributional style in a case of Côtard delusion. *Consciousness & Cognition* 16(2), 349–59.

McKay, R., & Kinsbourne, M. (2010). Confabulation, delusion, and anosognosia: Motivational factors and false claims. *Cogn Neuropsychiatry* 15(1), 288–318. doi:10.1080/13546800903374871

Meakin, C. J., Renvoize, E. B., & Kent, J. (1987). Folie à deux in Down's syndrome: A case report. *Br J Psychiatry* 151, 258–60.

Meats, P. (1988). Olfactory hallucinations. *BMJ Clin Res* 296, 645.

Medvei, V. C. (1987). The illness and death of Mary Tudor. *J R Soc Med* 80(12), 766–70.

Melzack, R. (1990). Phantom limbs and the concept of a neuromatrix. *Trends Neurosci* 13(3), 88–92.

Melzack, R., Israel, R., & Lacroix, R. (1997). Phantom limbs in people with congenital limb deficiency or amputation in early childhood. *Brain* 120(2), 1603–20. doi: 10.1093/brain/120.9.1603

Mendez, M. F., & Ramírez-Bermúdez, J. (2011). Côtard syndrome in semantic dementia. *Psychosomatics* 52(6), 571–4. doi: 10.1016/j.psym.2011.06.004.

Mendis, S., & Hodgson, R. E. (2012). Ganser syndrome: Examining the aetiological debate through a systematic case report review. *Eur J Psychiatry* 26(2), 96–106. doi.org/10.4321/S0213-61632012000200003

Menninger-Lerchenthal, E. (1935). *Das Truggebilde der eigenen Gestalt*. Karger, Basel.

Menninger-Lerchenthal, E. (1961). Heautoscopy. *Wien Med Wochenschr* 111, 745–56.

Mentis, M. J., Weinstein, E. A., Horwitz, B., et al. (1995). Abnormal brain glucose metabolism in the delusional misidentification syndromes: A positron emission tomography study in Alzheimer disease. *Biol Psychiatry* 38 (7), 438–49.

Merckelbach, H., Peters, M., & Jelicic, M. (2006). Detecting malingering of Ganser-like symptoms with tests: A case study. *Psychiatry Clin Neurosci* 60(5), 636–8. doi:10.1111/J.1440-1819.2006.01571.x

Merleau-Ponty, M. (1966). *Phenomenology of Perception* (trans by Colin Smith). Routledge, London.

Merskey, H. (1995a). Multiple personality disorder and false memory syndrome. *Br J Psychiatry* 166(3), 281–2.

Merskey, H. (1995b). The manufacture of personalities: The production of multiple personality disorder. In L. M. Cohen, J. N. Berzoff & M. R. Elin (eds.), *Dissociative Identity Disorder: Theoretical and Treatment Controversies* (pp. 3–32). Jason Aronson, Lanham, MD.

Merskey, H. (1992). The manufacture of personalities. *Br J Psychiatry* 160(3), 327–40.

Mianji, F., & Semnani, Y. (2015). Zār spirit possession in Iran and African countries: Group distress, culture-bound syndrome or cultural concept of distress. *Iranian J Psychiatry* 10(4), 225–32.

Michael, A., Joseph, A., & Pallen, A. (1994). Delusions of pregnancy. *Br J Psychiatry* 164 (2), 244–46. doi:10.1192/bjp.164.2.244

Middelveen, M. J., Fesler, M. C., & Stricker, R. B. (2018). History of Morgellon's disease: From delusion to definition. *Clin Cosmet Invest Dermatol* 11, 71–90. doi:10.2147/CCID. S152343

Middleton, K. (2000). How Karembola men become mothers. In J. Carsten (ed.), *Cultures of Relatedness: New Approaches to the Study of Kinship* (pp. 104–27). Cambridge University Press, Cambridge, UK.

Miller, L. J., & Forcier, K. (1992). Situational influence on development of delusions of pregnancy in a man. *Am J Psychiatry* 149 (1), 140.

Miller, P., Bramble, D., & Buxton, N. (1997). Case study: Ganser syndrome in children and adolescents. *J Am Acad Child Adolesc Psychiatry* 36(1), 112–15.

Minkowski, E. (1970). *Lived Time*. Northwestern University Press, Evanston, IL.

Mischel, W., & Mischel, F. (1958). Psychological aspects of spirit possession. *Am Anthropol* 60 (2), 249–60. doi:10.1525/ aa.1958.60.2.02a00040

Mitchill, S. L. (1816). A double consciousness, or a duality of person in the same individual. *Med Reposit* 3, 185–6.

Miyaoka, T., Yasukawa, R., Sukegawa, T., et al. (2005). Late-onset persistent visual hallucinations with epileptiform discharge. *Int J Psychiatry Clin Pract* 9(1), 71–4. doi:10.1080/13651500510018220

Mocellin, R., Walterfang, M., & Velakoulis, D. (2006). Neuropsychiatry of complex visual hallucinations. *Aust NZ J Psychiatry* 40(9), 742–51. doi:10.1080/j.1440-1614.2006.01878.x

Modestin, J. (1992). Multiple personality disorder in Switzerland. *Am J Psychiatry* 149(1), 88–92.

Moftah, N. H., Kamel, A. M., Attia, H. M., et al. (2013). Skin diseases in patients with primary psychiatric conditions: A hospital-based study. *J Epidemiol Glob Health* 3, 131–8. doi:10.1016/j.jegh.2013.03.005

Money, J., Jobaris, R., & Furth, G. (1977). Apotemnophilia: Two cases of self-demand amputation as a paraphilia. *J Sex Res* 13(2), 115–25. doi:10.1080/00224497709550967

Moore, D. L. (1966). *Marie and the Duke of H.: The Daydream Love Affair of Marie Bashkirtseff*. Cassell, London.

Mora, J. M. R. D., & Jenner, F. A. (1980). On heautoscopy or the phenomenon of the double: Case presentation and review of the literature. *Br J Med Psychol* 53(1), 75–83. doi:10.1111/j.2044-8341.1980.tb02871.x

Moran, C. (1986). Depersonalization and agoraphobia associated with marijuana use. *Br J Med Psychol* 59(2), 187–96. doi/pdf/ 10.1111/j.2044–8341.1986.tb02684.x

Moroy, A., Bellivier, F., & Fénelon, G. (2012). Olfactory reference syndrome: An unusual delusion in a patient with Parkinson's disease. *J Neuropsychiatry Clin Neurosci* 24(3), E2. doi:10.1176/appi.neuropsych.11070163

Morris, M. (1991). Delusional infestation. *Br J Psychiatry* 159(S14), 83–7.

Morse, J. M., & Mitcham, C. (1997). Compathy: The contagion of physical distress. *J Adv Nurs* 26(4), 649–57.

Morton, J. (2017). Interidentity amnesia in dissociative identity disorder. *Cogn Neuropsychiatry* 22(4), 315–30. doi: 10.1080/ 13546805.2017.1327848

Moseley, P., Alderson-Day, B., Kumar, S., & Fernyhough, C. (2018). Musical hallucinations, musical imagery, and earworms: A new phenomenological survey. *Conscious Cogn* 65, 83–94. doi:10.1016/j. concog.2018.07.009

Moselhy, H., & Oyebode, F. (1997). Delusional misidentification syndromes: A review of the anglophone literature. *Neurol Psychiatry Brain Res.* 5(1), 21–6.

Moser, D. J., Cohen, R. A., Malloy, P. F., et al. (1998). Reduplicative paramnesia: Longitudinal neurobehavioral and neuroimaging analysis. *J Geriatr Psychiatry Neurol* 11(4), 174–80. doi:10.1177/089198879901100402

Mosiołek, A., Jakima, S., Małachowska, E., & Gierus, J. (2016). Persistent genital arousal disorder: The case of a 35-year-old patient. *Seksuolog Polska* 14(1), 46–51.

Moskowitz, J. A. (1972). Capgras symptom in modern dress. *Int J Child Psychother* 1(2), 45–64.

Moyal-Barracco, M., & Lynch, P. J. (2004). 2003 ISSVD terminology and classification of vulvodynia: A historical perspective. *J Reprod Med* 49(10),772–777.

Muggleton, N., Tsakanikos, E., Walsh, V., & Ward, J. (2007). Disruption of synaesthesia following TMS of the right posterior parietal cortex. *Neuropsychologia* 45(7), 1582–5. doi:10.1016/j.neuropsychologia.2006.11.021.

Mullen, P. E., & Martin, J. (1994). Jealousy: A community study. *Br J Psychiatry* 164(1), 35–43.

Mullen, P. E., & Pathé, M. (1994a). The pathological extensions of love. *Br J Psychiatry* 165(5), 614–23.

Mullen, P. E. (1991). Jealousy: The pathology of passion. *Br J Psychiatry* 158, 593–601.

Mullen, P. E., & Pathé, M. (1994b). Stalking and the pathologies of love. *Aust NZ J Psychiatry* 28(3), 469–77. doi:10.3109/00048679409075876

Munro, A. (1994). Delusional disorders are a naturally occurring 'experimental psychosis'. *Psychopathology* 27(3–5), 247–50.

Munro, A. (1978a). Monosymptomatic hypochondriacal psychoses: A diagnostic entity which may respond to pimozide. *Can Psychiatric Assoc J* 23(7), 497–500. doi:10.1177/070674377802300712

Munro, A. (1978b). Monosymptomatic hypochondriacal psychosis manifesting as delusions of parasitosis: A description of four cases successfully treated with pimozide. *Arch Dermatol* 114(6), 940–3.

Murai, T., Toichi, M., Sengoku, A., et al. (1997). Reduplicative paramnesia in patients with focal brain damage. *Neuropsychiatry Neuropsychol Behav Neurol* 10(3), 190–6.

Murata, S., Naritomi, H., & Sawada, T. (1994). Musical auditory hallucinations caused by a brainstem lesion. *Neurology* 44(1), 156–8. doi:10.1212/wnl.44.1.156

Murray, J. L., & Abraham, G. E. (1978). Pseudocyesis: A review. *Obstet Gynecol* 51(5), 627–31.

Musalek, M., & Kutzer, E. (1990). The frequency of shared delusions in delusions of infestation. *Eur Arch Psychiatry Neurol Sci* 239(4), 263–6.

Myers, C. S. (1911). A case of synaesthesia. *Br J Psychol* 4(2), 228–38.

Myers, C. S. (1914). Two cases of synaesthesia. *Br J Psychol* 7(1), 112–17.

Myers, D. H., & Grant, G. (1972). A study of depersonalization in students. *Br J Psychiatry* 121(560), 59–65.

Myles, K. M., Dixon, M. J., Smilek, D., & Merikle, P. M. (2003). Seeing double: The role of meaning in alphanumeric-colour synaesthesia. *Brain & Cognition* 53(2),342–5. doi: 10.1016/s0278-2626(03)00139-8.

Nahum, L., Ptak, R., Leemann, B., et al. (2010). Behaviorally spontaneous confabulation in limbic encephalitis: The roles of reality filtering and strategic monitoring. *J Int Neuropsychol Soc* 16(6), 995–1005. doi:10.1017/S1355617710000780

Nakul, E., & Lopez, C. (2017). Commentary: Out-of-body experience during awake craniotomy. *Front Hum Neurosci.* doi:10.3389/fnhum.2017.00417.

Narang, T., Kumaran, M. S., Dogra, S., et al. (2013). Red scrotum syndrome: idiopathic neurovascular phenomenon or steroid addiction? *Sexual Health* 10(5), 452–455.

Narumoto, J., Ueda, H., Tsuchida, H., et al. (2006). Regional cerebral blood flow changes in a patient with delusional parasitosis before and after successful treatment with risperidone: A case report. *Prog Neuropsychopharmacol Biol Psychiatry* 30(4), 737–40. doi:10.1016/j.pnpbp.2005.11.029

Neary, D., Snowden, J. S., Gustafson, L., et al. (1998). Frontotemporal lobar degeneration: A consensus on clinical diagnostic criteria. *Neurology* 51(6), 1546–54.

Nejad, A. G. (2002). Hydrophobia as a rare presentation of Côtard's syndrome: A case report. *Acta Psychiatr Scand* 106(2), 156–8, doi:10.1034/j.1600-0447.2002.02252.x

Nejad, A. G., Anari, A. M. Z., & Pouya, F. (2013). Effect of cultural themes on forming Côtard's syndrome: Reporting a case of Côtard's syndrome with depersonalization and out of body experience symptoms. *Iran J Psychiatry Behav Sci* 7(2), 91–3.

Nersesjan, V., Bogwardt, H. G., & Kondziella, D. (2020). Mesial bifrontal stroke presenting as isolated spontaneous confabulations. *Pract Neurol* 20(5). doi:10.1136/practneurol-2020-002518

Neuner, F., Pfeiffer, A., & Schauer-Kaiser, E. (2012). Haunted by ghosts: Prevalence, predictors and outcomes of spirit possession experiences among former child soldiers and war-affected civilians in Northern Uganda. *Soc Sci Med* 75(3), 548–54. doi: 10.1016/j.socscimed.2012.03.028.

Newman, W. J., & Harbit, M. A. (2010). Folie à deux and the courts. *J Am Acad Psychiatry Law* 38(3), 369–75.

Niazi, S., Krogh Nielsen, M., Singh, A., et al. (2019). Prevalence of Charles Bonnet syndrome in patients with age-related macular degeneration: Systematic review and meta-analysis. *Acta Ophthalmol* 98(2), 121–31. doi:10.1111/aos.14287

Nielssen, O., Langdon, R., & Large, M. (2013). Folie à deux homicide and the two-factor model of delusions. *Cogn Neuropsychiatry* 18 (5), 390–408. doi:10.1080/13546805.2012.718246

Nijenhuis, E. R. S., Hart, O. V. D., & Steele, K. (2002). The emerging psychobiology of trauma-related dissociation and dissociative disorders. In H. D'Haenen, J. A. den Boer & P. Willner (eds.), *Biological Psychiatry* doi:10.1002/0470854871.chxxi

Nissen, M. J., Ross, J. L., Willingham, D. B., & Mackenzie, T. B. (1988). Memory and awareness in a patient with multiple personality disorder. *Brain & Cognition* 8(1), 117–34. doi: 10.1016/0278-2626(88)90043-7

O'Connor, J. J. M., & Feinberg, D. R. (2012). The influence of facial masculinity and voice pitch on jealousy and perceptions of intrasexual rivalry. *Pers Indiv Dif* 52(3), 369–73.

Oaklander, A. L., Sharma, S., Kessler, K., & Price, B. H. (2020). Persistent genital arousal disorder: A special sense neuropathy. *Pain Rep* 5(1), e801. doi: 10.1097/PR9.0000000000000801.

Oberndorfer, R., Schönauer, C., & Eichbauer, H. (2017). Côtard syndrome in hypoactive delirium: A case report. *Psychiatr Danube* 29(4), 500–2. doi: 10.24869/psyd.2017.500.

Oesterreich, T. K. (2013). *Possession, Demoniacal and Other: Among Primitive Races, in Antiquity, the Middle Ages and Modern*. Routledge, London.

Ogata, H., Shigeto, H., Torii, T., et al. (2011). [A case of Charles Bonnet syndrome following syphilitic optic neuritis]. *Rinsho Shinkeigaku* 51(8), 595–8. doi:10.5692/clinicalneurol.51.595

Ohnuma, T., & Arai, H. (2015). Genetic or psychogenic? A case study of 'folie à quatre' including twins. *Case Rep Psychiatry* 2015, 983212. doi:10.1155/2015/983212

Olojugba, C., de Silva, R., Kartsounis, L. D., et al. (2007). De Clerambault's syndrome (erotomania) as a presenting feature of fronto-temporal dementia and motor neurone disease (FTD-MND). *Behav Neurol* 18(3), 193–5.

Oohashi, T., Kawai, N., Honda, M., & Nakamura, S. (2002). Electroencephalographic measurement of possession trance in the field. *Clin Neurophysiol* 113(3), 435–45. doi: 10.1016/s1388-2457(02)00002-0.

Orne, M. T., Dinges, D. F., & Orne, E. C. (1984). On the differential diagnosis of multiple personality in the forensic context. *Int J Clin Exp Hypn* 32(2), 118–69. doi:10.1080/00207148408416007

Örüm, M. H., & Kalenderoğlu, A. (2018). Côtard and Capgras delusions in a patient with bipolar disorder: 'I'll prove, I'm dead!'.

Psychiatr Clin Psychopharmacol 28(1), 110–12. doi:10.1080/24750573.2017.1371661

Ospina-García, N., Román, G. C., Pascual, B., et al. (2018). Hypothalamic relapse of a cardiac large B-cell lymphoma presenting with memory loss, confabulation, alexia-agraphia, apathy, hypersomnia, appetite disturbances and diabetes insipidus. *BMJ Case Rep* 2018. doi:10.1136/bcr-2016-217700

Ossola, M., Romani, A., Tavazzi, E., et al. (2010). Epileptic mechanisms in Charles Bonnet syndrome. *Epilepsy Behav* 18(1–2), 119–22. doi:10.1016/j.yebeh.2010.03.010

Österholm, M. (2010). Beliefs: A theoretically unnecessary construct. In V. Durand-Guerrier, S. Soury-Lavergne & F. Arzarello (eds.), *Proceedings of the Sixth Congress of the European Society for Research in Mathematics Education (Proc CERME 6)*. Institut National Recherche Pedagogique, Lyon.

Ouj, U. (2009). Pseudocyesis in a rural southeast Nigerian community. *J Obstet Gynaecol Res* 35(4), 660–5. doi:10.1111/j.1447-0756.2008.00997.x

Ouyang, D., Duggal, H. S., & Jacob, N. J. (2003). Neurobiological basis of Ganser syndrome. *Indian J Psychiatry* 45(4), 255–6.

Oyama, H., Mabuchi, T., Niwa, M., et al. (1998). Traumatic Korsakoff syndrome. *J Clin Neurosci* 5(4), 441–4. doi:10.1016/s0967-5868(98)90284-3

Oyebode, F., & Sargeant, R. (1996). Delusional misidentification syndromes: A descriptive study. *Psychopathology* 29(4), 209–14.

Oyebode, F. (2008). The neurology of psychosis. *Med Princ Pract* 17(4), 263–9. doi:10.1159/000129603

Oyebode, F. (2018). *Sims' Symptoms in the Mind: Textbook of Descriptive Psychopathology*. Elsevier Health Sciences, Edinburgh.

Ozkan, N., & Caliyurt, O. (2016). Brain metabolism changes with ^{18}F-fluorodeoxy-glucose-positron emission tomography in a patient with Côtard's syndrome. *Aust NZ J Psychiatry* 50(6), 600–1. doi:10.1177/0004867415622273

Paavonen, J. (1995). Vulvodynia a complex syndrome of vulvar pain. *Acta Obstet Gynecol Scand* 74(4), 243–7. doi:10.3109/00016349509024442

Pagonabarraga, J., Llebaria, G., García-Sánchez, C., et al. (2008). A prospective study of delusional misidentification syndromes in Parkinson's disease with dementia. *Mov Disord* 23(3), 443–8. doi:10.1002/mds.21864

Paillère-Martinot, M. L., Dao-Castellana, M. H., Masure, M. C., et al. (1994). Delusional misidentification: A clinical, neuropsychological and brain imaging case study. *Psychopathology* 27(3–5), 200–10.

Painter, D. R., Dwyer, M. F., Kamke, M. R., & Mattingley, J. B. (2018). Stimulus-driven cortical hyperexcitability in individuals with Charles Bonnet hallucinations. *Curr Biol* 28 (21), 3475–80.e3. doi:10.1016/j.cub.2018.08.058

Papageorgiou, C., Lykouras, L., Alevizos, B., et al. (2005). Psychophysiological differences in schizophrenics with and without delusional misidentification syndromes: A P300 study. *Prog Neuropsychopharmacol Biol Psychiatry* 29(4), 593–601. doi:10.1016/j.pnpbp.2005.01.016

Papageorgiou, C., Lykouras, L., Ventouras, E., et al. (2002). Abnormal P300 in a case of delusional misidentification with coinciding Capgras and Frégoli symptoms. *Prog Neuropsychopharmacol Biol Psychiatry* 26(4), 805–10.

Papageorgiou, C., Ventouras, E., Lykouras, L., et al. (2003). Psychophysiological evidence for altered information processing in delusional misidentification syndromes. *Prog Neuropsychopharmacol Biol Psychiatry* 27(3), 365–72. doi:10.1016/S0278-5846(02)00353-6

Paradowski, B., Kowalczyk, E., Chojdak-Łukasiewicz, J., et al. (2013). Three cases with visual hallucinations following combined ocular and occipital damage. *Case Rep Med* 2013, 450725. doi:10.1155/2013/450725

Park, J. H., Ahn, J. H., Park, J. B., & Joe, S. (2016). Charles Bonnet syndrome following trans-sphenoidal adenomectomy without optic nerve atrophy. *Psychiatry Invest* 13(5), 577–9. doi:10.4306/pi.2016.13.5.577

Parks, N. E., Rigby, H. B., Gubitz, G. J., & Shankar, J. J. (2014). Dysmetropsia and

Côtard's syndrome due to migrainous infarction – or not? *Cephalagia* 34(9), 717–20. doi:10.1177/0333102414520765

Pasquini, F., & Cole, M. G. (1997). Idiopathic musical hallucinations in the elderly. *J Geriatr Psychiatry Neurol* 10(1), 11–14. doi:10.1177/089198879701000103

Pathé, M., & Mullen, P. E. (1993). Medical victims of pathological love: The Hippocratic curse. *Med J Aust* 159(9), 632.

Patterson, M. B., & Mack, J. L. (1985). Neuropsychological analysis of a case of reduplicative paramnesia. *J Clin Exp Neuropsychol* 7(1), 111–21. doi:10.1080/01688638508401245

Pearce, J. M. S. (2007). Synaesthesia. *Eur Neurol* 57(2), 120–4.

Pearson, M. L., Selby, J. V., Katz, K. A., et al. (2012). Clinical, epidemiologic, histopathologic and molecular features of an unexplained dermopathy. *PLoS One* 7(1), e29908. doi:10.1371/journal.pone.0029908

Pechey, R., & Halligan, P. (2012). Prevalence and correlates of anomalous experiences in a large non-clinical sample. *Psychol Psychother Theory* 85(2), 150–62. doi:10.1111/j.2044-8341.2011.02024.x

Penfield, W., & Perot, P. (1963). The brain's record of visual and auditory experience: A final summary. *Brain* 86, 595–696.

Perceval, J. (1840/1962). *Perceval's Narrative: A Patient's Account of His Psychosis, 1830–1832.* Edited by G. Bateson. Hogarth Press, London.

Perez, D. L., Fuchs, B. H., & Epstein, J. (2014). A case of Côtard syndrome in a woman with a right subdural hemorrhage. *J Neuropsychiatry Clin Neurosci* 26(1), E29–30. doi:10.1176/appi.neuropsych.13020021

Phillips, K. A., & Menard, W. (2011). Olfactory reference syndrome: Demographic and clinical features of imagined body odor. *Gen Hosp Psychiatry* 33(4), 398–406. doi:10.1016/j.genhosppsych.2011.04.004

Pick, A. (1903). On reduplicative paramnesia. *Brain* 26, 242–67.

Pignat, J. M., Ptak, R., Leemann, B., et al. (2013). Modulation of environmental reduplicative paramnesia by perceptual experience.

Neurocase 19(5), 445–50. doi:10.1080/13554794.2012.690428

Piper, Jr, A. (1994). Multiple personality disorder. *Br J Psychiatry* 164(5), 600–12.

Piper, A., & Merskey, H. (2004a). The persistence of folly: A critical examination of dissociative identity disorder, part I. The excesses of an improbable concept. *Can J Psychiatry* 49(9), 592–600. doi:10.1177/070674370404900904

Piper, A., & Merskey, H. (2004b). The persistence of folly: Critical examination of dissociative identity disorder, part II. The defence and decline of multiple personality or dissociative identity disorder. *Can J Psychiatry* 49(10), 678–83. doi:10.1177/070674370404901005

Pliskin, N. H., Kiolbasa, T. A., Towle, V. L., et al. (1996). Charles Bonnet syndrome: An early marker for dementia. *J Am Geriatr Soc* 44(9), 1055–61. doi:10.1111/j.1532-5415.1996.tb02937.x

Podoll, K., & Robinson, D. (1999). Out-of-body experiences and related phenomena in migraine art. *Cephalalgia* 19, 886–96. doi:10.1046/j.1468-2982.1999.1910886.x

Poletti, M., Perugi, G., Logi, C., & Romano, A. (2012). Dopamine agonists and delusional jealousy in Parkinson's disease: A cross-sectional prevalence study. *Mov Disord* 27 (13), 1679–82. doi:10.1002/mds.25129

Pollio, H. R., Henley, T., & Thompson, C. B. (1997). *The Phenomenology of Everyday Life.* Cambridge University Press, Cambridge, UK.

Ponson, L., Andersson, F., & El-Hage, W. (2015). Neural correlates of delusional infestation responding to aripiprazole monotherapy: A case report. *Neuropsychiatr Dis Treat* 11, 257–61. doi:10.2147/NDT.S74786

Ponte, M., Klemperer, E., Sahay, A., & Chren, M.-M. (2009). Effects of vulvodynia on quality of life. *J Am Acad Dermatol* 60(1), 70–6.

Potts, C. S. (1891). Two cases of hallucination of smell. *University of Pennsylvania Medical Magazine* 226–7.

Prevost, N., & English, 3rd, J. C. (2007). Red scrotal syndrome: A localized phenotypical expression of erythromelalgia. *J Drugs Dermatol* 6(9), 935–6.

Prince, M. (1906). *The Dissociation of a Personality: A Biographical Study in Abnormal Psychology.* Longmans, Green, and Company, London.

Pryse-Phillips, W. (1971). An olfactory reference syndrome. *Acta Psychiatr Scand* 47(4), 484–509. doi/pdf/10.1111/j.1600-0447.1971.tb03705.x

Putnam, F. W., Guroff, J. J., & Silberman, E. K. (1986). The clinical phenomenology of multiple personality disorder: Review of 100 recent cases. *J Clin Psychiatry* 47(6), 285–93.

Radebaugh, T. S., Hooper, F. J., & Gruenberg, E. M. (1987). The social breakdown syndrome in the elderly population living in the community: The helping study. *Br J Psychiatry* 151(3), 341–6.

Radhakrishnan, R., Satheeshkumar, G., & Chaturvedi, S. K. (1999). Recurrent delusions of pregnancy in a male. *Psychopathology* 32(1), 1–4. doi:10.1159/000029059

Radojević, N., Radnić, B., Petković, S., et al. (2013). Multiple stabbing in sex-related homicides. *J Forens Leg Med* 20(5), 502–7. doi:10.1016/j.jflm.2013.03.005

Rahman, T., Grellner, K. A., Harry, B., et al. (2013). Infanticide in a case of folie à deux. *Am J Psychiatry* 170(10), 1110–12. doi:10.1176/appi.ajp.2013.13010027

Ramachandran, V. S., Blakeslee, S., & Dolan, R. J. (1998). Phantoms in the brain: Probing the mysteries of the human mind. *Nature* 396(6712), 639–40.

Ramachandran, V. S., Brang, D., & McGeoch, P. D. (2009). Sexual and food preference in apotemnophilia and anorexia: Interactions between 'beliefs' and 'needs' regulated by two-way connections between body image. *Perception* 38(5), 775–7. doi:10.1068/p6350

Ramachandran, V. S., & Hubbard, E. M. (2001). Synaesthesia: A window into perception, thought and language. *J Conscious Stud* 8 (12), 3–34.

Ramachandran, V. S., & McGeoch, P. (2007). Can vestibular caloric stimulation be used to treat apotemnophilia. *Med Hypoth* 69(2), 250–2. doi:10.1016/j.mehy.2006.12.013

Ramachandran, V. S. (2001). Psychophysical investigations into the neural basis of synaesthesia. *Proc R Soc B: Biol Sci* 268(1470), 973–83. doi:10.1098/rspb.2000.1576

Ramirez-Bermudez, J. (2010). Côtard syndrome in neurological and psychiatric patients. *J Neuropsychiatry Clin Sci* 22(4), 409–16. doi:10.1176/jnp.2010.22.4.409

Ramirez-Bermudez, J., Espinola-Nadurille, M., & Loza-Taylor, N. (2010). Delusional parasitosis in neurological patients. *Gen Hosp Psychiatry* 32(3), 294–9. doi:10.1016/j.genhosppsych.2009.10.006

Ranjan, S., Chandra, P. S., Gupta, A. K., & Prabhu, S. (2007). Clonal pluralization of self, relatives and others. *Psychopathology* 40(6), 465–7. doi:10.1159/000108126

Rao, K. N. (1992). Internal autoscopy: A case report. *Indian J Psychiatry* 34(3), 280–2.

Rather, L. J. (1965). *Mind and Body in Eighteenth Century Medicine.* University of California Press, Berkeley, CA.

Reed, B. D., Haefner, H. K., & Cantor, L. (2003). Vulvar dysesthesia (vulvodynia): A follow-up study. *Obstet Gynecol Surv* 58 (10), 658–60.

Reed, B. D., Haefner, H. K., Punch, M. R., et al. (2000). Psychosocial and sexual functioning in women with vulvodynia and chronic pelvic pain: A comparative evaluation. *J Reprod Med* 45(8), 624–32.

Reed, B. D., Haefner, H. K., Sen, A., & Gorenflo, D. W. (2008). Vulvodynia incidence and remission rates among adult women: A 2-year follow-up study. *Obstet Gynaecol* 112(2), 231–7.

Reed, B. D., Legocki, L. J., Plegue, M. A., et al. (2014). Factors associated with vulvodynia incidence. *Obstet Gynecol* 123(201), 225–31.

Reed, B. D., Harlow, S. D., Sen, A., & Edwards, R. M. (2012). Relationship between vulvodynia and chronic comorbid pain conditions. *Obstet Gynaecol* 120(1), 145–51. doi: 10.1097/AOG.0b013e31825957cf.

Reed, B. D., Harlow, S. D., Sen, A., & Legocki, L. J. (2012). Prevalence and demographic characteristics of vulvodynia in a population-based sample. *Am J Obstet Gynecol* 206(2), 170. e1–9.

Regis, E. (1881). Unilateral hallucinations: A contribution to the pathogenic study of hallucinations. *Alienist and Neurologist (1880-1920)* 2(3), 346.

Reif, A., Murach, W. M., & Pfuhlmann, B. (2003). Delusional paralysis: An unusual variant of Côtard's syndrome. *Psychopathology* 36, 218–20.

Reik, T. (1974). *Ritual.* International Universities Press, Madison, CT.

Reilly, T. M. (1988). Delusional infestation. *Br J Psychiatry* 153(Suppl 2), 44–6.

Reinders, A. A. T. S., Nijenhuis, E. R. S., Quak, J., & Korf, J. (2006). Psychobiological characteristics of dissociative identity disorder: A symptom provocation study. *Biol Psychiatry* 60(7), 730–40. doi: 10.1016/j.biopsych.2005.12.019.

Remington, G. J. (1997). Erotomanic delusions focused on a child. *J Clin Psychiatry* 58(9), 406.

Restrepo-Bernal, D., Gómez-González, A., & Gaviria, S. L. (2014). [Deliberate burning with acid: New expressions of violence against women in Medellín, Colombia. Series of cases]. *Vertex* 25(115), 179–85.

Restrepo-Martínez, M., & Espinola-Nadurille, M. (2019). FDG-PET in Côtard syndrome before and after treatment: Can functional brain imaging support a two-factor hypothesis of nihilistic delusions? *Cognitive Neuropsychiatry* 24(6), 470–80. doi:10.1080/13546805.2019.1676710

Retterstøl, N., & Opjordsmoen, S. (1991). Erotomania: Erotic self-reference psychosis in old maids. A long-term follow-up. *Psychopathology* 24(6), 388–97. doi:10.1159/000284743

Rival, L. (1998). Androgynous parents and guest children: The Huaorani Couvade. *J R Anthropol Inst* 4(4), 619–42.

Rivera, M. (1991). Multiple personality disorder and the social systems: 185 cases. *Dissociation* 4(2), 79–82.

Rizzolatti, G., & Craighero, L. (2004). The mirror-neuron system. *Annu Rev Neurosci* 27, 169–92. doi:10.1146/annurev.neuro.27.070203.144230

Roane, D. M., Rogers, J. D., Robinson, J. H., & Feinberg, T. E. (1998). Delusional misidentification in association with parkinsonism. *J Neuropsychiatry Clin Neurosci* 10(2), 194–8.

Robaeys, G., De Bie, J., Van Ranst, M., & Buntinx, F. (2007). An extremely rare case of delusional parasitosis in a chronic hepatitis C patient during pegylated interferon alpha-2b and ribavirin treatment. *World J Gastroenterol* 13(16), 2379–80. doi:10.3748/wjg.v13.i16.2379

Roessner, V., & Rössner, V. (2002). A new classification of the delusional misidentification syndromes. *Psychopathology* 35(1), 3–7. doi:56209

Roh, J. H., Lee, B. H., Chin, J., et al. (2012). Graphabulation: A graphic form of confabulation. *Cortex* 48(3), 356–9. doi:10.1016/j.cortex.2011.05.004

Romanov, D. V., Lepping, P., Bewley, A., et al. (2018). Longer duration of untreated psychosis is associated with poorer outcomes for patients with delusional infestation. *Acta Derm Venereol* 98(9), 848–54. doi:10.2340/00015555-2888

Romero Sandoval, K., Festa Neto, C., & Nico, M. M. S. (2018). Delusional infestation caused by pramipexole. *Clin Exp Dermatol* 43(2), 192–3. doi:10.1111/ced.13292

Rosen, B. K. (1981). Suicide pacts: A review. *Psychol Med* 11(3), 525–33.

Ross, C. A. (1989). *Multiple Personality Disorder: Diagnosis, Clinical Features, and Treatment.* John Wiley & Sons, New York.

Ross, C. A. (1991). Epidemiology of multiple personality disorder and dissociation. *Psychiatr Clin North Am* 14(3), 503–17.

Ross, C. A., Anderson, G., & Fleishe, W. P. (1991). The frequency of multiple personality disorder among psychiatric inpatients. *Am J Psychiatry* 148(12), 1717–20.

Ross, C. A., Miller, S. D., & Bjornso, L. (1991). Abuse histories in 102 cases of multiple personality disorder. *Can J Psychiatry* 36(2), 97–101. doi/abs/10.1177/070674379103600204

Ross, C. A., Miller, S. D., Reagor, P., & Bjornson, L. (1990). Structured interview data on 102 cases of multiple personality disorder from four centers. *Am J Psychiatry* 147(5), 596–601. doi: 10.1176/ajp.147.5.596.

Rothen, N., & Meier, B. (2010). Higher prevalence of synaesthesia in art students. *Perception* 39(5), 18–20. doi:10.1068/p6680

Rothen, N., Meier, B., & Ward, J. (2012). Enhanced memory ability: Insights from synaesthesia. *Neurosci Biobehav Rev* 36(8), 1952–63. doi: 10.1016/j. neubiorev.2012.05.004.

Rudden, M., Sweeney, J., & Frances, A. (1990). Diagnosis and clinical course of erotomanic and other delusional patients. *Am J Psychiatry* 147(5), 625–8. doi:10.1176/ ajp.147.5.625

Rūmī, J. A.-D. (2007). *The Masnavi* (trans J. A. D. R. Maulana & J. Mojaddedi). Oxford University Press, Oxford, UK.

Russell, G., & Burns, A. (2014). Charles Bonnet syndrome and cognitive impairment: A systematic review. *Int Psychogeriatr* 26(9), 1431–43. doi:10.1017/S1041610214000763

Russell, G., Harper, R., Allen, H., et al. (2018). Cognitive impairment and Charles Bonnet syndrome: A prospective study. *Int J Geriatr Psychiatry* 33(1), 39–46. doi:10.1002/ gps.4665

Saad, L., Silva, L. F., Banzato, C. E., et al. (2010). Anorexia nervosa and Wernicke-Korsakoff syndrome: A case report. *J Med Case Rep* 4, 217. doi:10.1186/1752-1947-4-217

Sachs, G. T. L. (1812). *Historia naturalis duorum Leucaethiopum, auctoris ipsius et sororis ejus.* Sulzbach, Germany.

Sacks, O. (2013). Hallucinations of musical notation. *Brain* 136(Pt 7), 2318–22. doi:10.1093/brain/awt057

Sadownik, L. A. (2000). Clinical profile of vulvodynia patients: a prospective study of 300 patients. *J Reprod Med* 45, 679–84.

Saetta, G., Hänggi, J., Gandola, M., et al. (2020). Neural correlates of body integrity dysphoria. *Curr Biol* 30(11), 2191–5.e3. doi: 10.1016/j. cub.2020.04.001

Sagarin, B. J., Martin, A. L., Coutinho, S. A., & Edlund, J. E. (2012). Sex differences in jealousy: A meta-analytic examination. *Evol Hum Behav* 33(6), 595–614.

Sahoo, A., & Josephs, K. A. (2018). A neuropsychiatric analysis of the Côtard delusion. *Neuropsychiatry Clin Neurosci* 30 (1), 58–65. doi:10.1176/appi. neuropsych.17010018

Saldarriaga-Cantillo, A., & Rivas Nieto, J. C. (2015). Noah syndrome: A variant of Diogenes syndrome accompanied by animal hoarding practices. *J Elder Abuse Negl* 27(3), 270–5. doi:10.1080/08946566.2014.978518

Salih, M. A. (1981). Suicide pact in a setting of folie à deux. *Br J Psychiatry* 139, 62–7.

Salviati, M., Bersani, F. S., Macrì, F., et al. (2013). Capgras-like syndrome in a patient with an acute urinary tract infection. *Neuropsychiatr Dis Treat* 9, 139–42. doi:10.2147/NDT.S39077

Sang, F. Y. P., Jauregui-Renaud, K., & Green, D. A. (2006). Depersonalisation/ derealisation symptoms in vestibular disease. *J Neurol Neurosurg Psychiatry* 77(6), 760–6.

Santhouse, A. M., Howard, R. J., & Ffytche, D. H. (2000). Visual hallucinatory syndromes and the anatomy of the visual brain. *Brain* 123(Pt 10), 2055–64. doi:10.1093/brain/123.10.2055

Santos-Bueso, E., Sáenz-Francés, F., Serrador-García, M., et al. (2014a). Prevalence and clinical characteristics of Charles Bonnet syndrome in Madrid, Spain. *Eur J Ophthalmol* 24(6), 960–3. doi:10.5301/ ejo.5000483

Santos-Bueso, E., Serrador-García, M., Sáenz-Francés, F., et al. (2014b). [Paradoxical cessation in a case of Charles Bonnet syndrome]. *Arch Soc Esp Oftalmol* 89(10), 418–20. doi:10.1016/j.oftal.2013.01.017

Santos-Bueso, E., Serrador-García, M., Sáenz-Francés, F., et al. (2017). [Charles Bonnet syndrome in a child with congenital glaucoma]. *Arch Soc Esp Oftalmol* 92(8), 398–400. doi:10.1016/j.oftal.2016.11.008

Sapkota, R. P., Gurung, D., Neupane, D., & Shah, S. K. (2014). A village possessed by 'witches': A mixed-methods case. Control study of possession and common mental disorders in rural Nepal. *Culture Med Psychiatry* 38(4), 642–8. doi:10.1007/s11013-014-9393-8

Sar, V., Alioğlu, F., & Akyüz, G. (2014). Experiences of possession and paranormal phenomena among women in the general population: Are they related to traumatic stress and dissociation. *J Trauma Dissoc* 15 (3), 303–18. doi:10.1080/15299732.2013.849321

Sar, V., Unal, S. N., & Ozturk, E. (2007). Frontal and occipital perfusion changes in dissociative identity disorder. *Psychiatry Res Neuroimag* 156(3), 217–27. doi: 10.1016/j.pscychresns.2006.12.017

Şar, V., Yargic, I., & Tutkun, H. (1996). Structured interview data on 35 cases of dissociative identity disorder in Turkey. *Am J Psychiatry* 153(10), 1329–33. doi: 10.1176/ajp.153.10.1329.

Sasaki, J., Wada, K., & Tanno, Y. (2013). Understanding egorrhea from cultural-clinical psychology. *Front Psychol* 4, 894. doi:10.3389/fpsyg.2013.00894

Schacter, D. L., Kihlstrom, J. F., & Kihlstrom L. C. (1989). Autobiographical memory in a case of multiple personality disorder. *J Abnorm Psychol* 98(4), 508–14. doi: 10.1037//0021-843x.98.4.508

Scharfetter, C. (2003). The self-experience of schizophrenics. In T. Kircher & A. David (eds.), *The Self in Neuroscience and Psychiatry*. Cambridge University Press, Cambridge, UK.

Scharfetter, C. (1981). Ego-psychopathology: The concept and its empirical evaluation, part 1. *Psychol Med* 11(2), 273.

Schilder, P. (1914). Die depersonalisation. In *Selbstbewusstsein und Persönlichkeitsbewusstsein. Monographien aus dem Gesamtgebiete der Neurologie und Psychiatrie*, vol 9. Springer, Berlin. doi:10.1007/978-3-642-47702-7_2

Schilder, P. (1953). *Medical Psychology*. International Universities Press, Madison, CT.

Schilder, P. (1936). The image and appearance of the human body: Studies in the constructive energies of the psyche. Psyche monograph no. 4. *J Nerv Ment Dis* 83(2), 227–8.

Schnider, A. (2008). *The Confabulating Mind*. Oxford University Press, Oxford, UK.

Schnider, A., Nahum, L., Pignat, J. M., et al. (2013). Isolated prospective confabulation in Wernicke-Korsakoff syndrome: A case for reality filtering. *Neurocase* 19(1), 90–104. doi:10.1080/13554794.2011.654221

Schodt, C. M. (1989). Parental-fetal attachment and couvade: A study of patterns of human-environment integrality. *Nurs Sci Q* 2, 88–97. doi:0.1.1.922.8682

Schorer, C. E., & Scott, P. D. (1965). The Ganser syndrome. *Br J Criminol* 5(2), 120–6.

Schreber, D. P. (1955). *Memoirs of My Nervous Illness* (trans and ed I. Macalpine & R. A. Hunter). Wm Dawson & Sons, London.

Schwartz, T. L., & Vahgei, L. (1998). Charles Bonnet syndrome in children. *J AAPOS* 2(5), 310–13. doi:10.1016/s1091-8531(98)90091-x

Sedda, A. (2011). Body integrity identity disorder: From a psychological to a neurological syndrome. *Neuropsychol Rev* 21(4), 334–6. doi: 10.1007/s11065-011-9186-6

Sedda, A., & Bottini, G. (2014). Apotemnophilia, body integrity identity disorder or xenomelia? Psychiatric and neurologic etiologies face each other. *Neuropsychiatr Dis Treat* 10, 1255–65.

Sedman, G. (1966). Depersonalization in a group of normal subjects. *Br J Psychiatry* 112(490), 907–12.

Sedman, G. (1970). Theories of depersonalization: A re-appraisal. *Br J Psychiatry* 117(536), 1–14.

Seeman, M. V. (2014). Pseudocyesis, delusional pregnancy, and psychosis: The birth of a delusion. *World J Clin Cases* 2(8), 338–44. doi:10.12998/wjcc.v2.i8.338

Seeman, M. V. (1971). The search for cupid or the phantom-lover syndrome. *Can Psychiatr Assoc J* 16(2), 183–4.

Serino, A., Alsmith, A., Costantini, M., et al. (2013). Bodily ownership and self-location: components of bodily self-consciousness. *Conscious Cogn* 22(4), 1239–52. doi:10.1016/j.concog.2013.08.013

Serra, M., La Corte, V., Migliaccio, R., et al. (2014). Confabulators mistake multiplicity for uniqueness. *Cortex* 58, 239–47. doi:10.1016/j.cortex.2014.06.011

Sethi, S., & Bhargava, S. C. (2009). Mass possession state in a family setting. *Transcult Psychiatry* 46(2), 372–4.

Shaan, F., Rizvi, A., & Sharma, G. (2018). Cotard syndrome in tumefactive multiple sclerosis: A case report. *Asian J Psychiatry* 34, 57–8. doi: 10.1016/j.ajp.2018.04.002.

Shah, R., Taylor, R. E., & Bewley, A. (2017). Exploring the psychological profile of patients with delusional infestation. *Acta Derm Venereol* 97(1), 98–101. doi:10.2340/00015555-2423

Shakespeare, W. (2008). *The Oxford Shakespeare: The Winter's Tale*. Oxford Paperbacks, Oxford, UK.

Shakespeare, W. (2003). *Othello (The New Cambridge Shakespeare)*. Ed. Norman Sanders; Introduction by Christina Lucky. Cambridge University Press, Cambridge, UK.

Shepherd, M. (1961). Morbid jealousy: Some clinical and social aspects of a psychiatric symptom. *J Ment Sci* 107 (449), 687–753.

Shiraishi, Y., Terao, T., Ibi, K., et al. (2004). The rarity of Charles Bonnet syndrome. *J Psychiatr Res* 38(2), 207–13. doi:10.1016/s0022-3956(03)00090-6

Shiwach, R. S., & Sobin, P. B. (1998). Monozygotic twins, folie à deux and heritability: A case report and critical review. *Med Hypoth* 50(5), 369–74.

Shorvon, H. J. (1946). The depersonalization syndrome. *Proc R Soc Med* 39(12), 779–92. doi:0.1177/003591574603901206

Shorvon, H. J. (1947). Prefrontal leucotomy and the depersonalisation syndrome. *Lancet* 2 (6481), 714–18.

Sidoti, V., & Lorusso, L. (2007). Multiple sclerosis and Capgras' syndrome. *Clin Neurol Neurosurg* 109(9), 786–7. doi:10.1016/j.clineuro.2007.05.022

Sierra, M. (2009). *Depersonalization: A New Look at a Neglected Syndrome*. Cambridge University Press, Cambridge, UK.

Sierra, M., & Berrios, G. E. (1998). Depersonalization: Neurobiological perspectives. *Biol Psychiatry* 44(9), 898–908.

Sierra, M., & David, A. S. (2011). Depersonalization: A selective impairment of self-awareness. *Conscious Cogn* 20(1), 99–108. doi: 10.1016/j.concog.2010.10.018

Sierra, M., Nestler, S., Jay, E. L., et al. (2014). A structural MRI study of cortical thickness in depersonalisation disorder. *Psychiatr Res* 224(1), 1–7. doi: 10.1016/j.pscychresns.2014.06.007.

Sierra, M., & Berrios, G. E. (2001). The phenomenological stability of depersonalization: Comparing the old with the new. *J Nerv Ment Dis* 189(9), 629–36.

Signer, S. F. (1991). 'Les psychoses passionnelles' reconsidered: A review of de Clérambault's cases and syndrome with respect to mood disorders. *J Psychiatry Neurosci* 16(2), 81–90.

Signer, S. F., & Cummings, J. L. (1987). De Clerambault's syndrome in organic affective disorder: Two cases. *Br J Psychiatry* 151(3), 404–7.

Silva, J. A., & Leong, G. B. (1992). The Capgras syndrome in paranoid schizophrenia. *Psychopathology* 25(3), 147–53.

Silva, J. A., Leong, G. B., Garza-Treviño, E. S., et al. (1994). A cognitive model of dangerous delusional misidentification syndromes. *J Forens Sci* 39(6), 1455–67.

Silva, J. A., Leong, G. B., & Shaner, A. L. (1990). A classification system for misidentification syndromes. *Psychopathology* 23(1), 27–32.

Silva, J. A., Leong, G. B., & Weinstock, R. (2000). A case of Côtard's syndrome associated with self-starvation. *J Forens Sci* 45(1), 188–90.

Silva, J. A., Leong, G. B., Weinstock, R., & Klein, R. L. (1995). Psychiatric factors associated with dangerous misidentification delusions. *Bull Am Acad Psychiatry Law* 23(1), 53–61.

Silva, J. A., Leong, G. B., Weinstock, R., & Wine, D. B. (1993). Delusional misidentification and dangerousness: A neurobiologic hypothesis. *J Forens Sci* 38(4), 904–13.

Silveira, J. M., & Seeman, M. V. (1995). Shared psychotic disorder: A critical review of the literature. *Can J Psychiatry* 40(7), 389–95.

Simeon, D., Guralnik, O., & Hazlett, E. A. (2000). Feeling unreal: A PET study of depersonalization disorder. *Am J Psychiatry* 157(11), 1782–8. doi:10.1176/appi.ajp.157.11.1782

Simeon, D., Knutelska, M., & Nelson, D. (2003). Feeling unreal: A depersonalization disorder update of 117 cases. *J Clin Psychiatry* 64(19), 990–7. doi: 10.4088/jcp.v64n0903

Simner, J., Glover, L., & Mowat, A. (2006). Linguistic determinants of word colouring in grapheme-colour synaesthesia. *Cortex* 42(2), 281–9. doi: 10.1016/s0010-9452(08)70353-8.

Simner, J., Harrold, J., Creed, H., et al. (2009). Early detection of markers for synaesthesia in childhood populations. *Brain* 132(1), 57–64. doi: 10.1093/brain/awn292.

Simner, J., Mulvenna, C., Sagiv, N., & Tsakanikos, E. (2006). Synaesthesia: The prevalence of atypical cross-modal experiences. *Perception* 35(8), 1024–33. doi:10.1068/p5469

Sims, A., Salmons, P., & Humphreys, P. (1977). Folie à quatre. *Br J Psychiatry* 130, 134–8.

Sims, A. C. P., & White, A. C. (1973). Coexistence of the Capgras and de Clérambault syndromes: A case history. *Br J Psychiatry* 123(577), 635–7.

Singer, I. (2009). *The Nature of Love.* MIT Press, Cambridge, MA.

Singh, A., & Sørensen, T. L. (2012). The prevalence and clinical characteristics of Charles Bonnet syndrome in Danish patients with neovascular age-related macular degeneration. *Acta Ophthalmol* 90(5), 476–80. doi:10.1111/j.1755-3768.2010.02051.x

Singh, G. P. (2006). Is olfactory reference syndrome an OCD. *Indian J Psychiatry* 48(3), 476–80.

Skene, A. J. C. (1889). *Treatise on the Diseases of Women.* D. Appleton & Company, New Tork.

Skimming, K. A., & Miller, C. W. T. (2019). Transdiagnostic approach to olfactory reference syndrome: Neurobiological considerations. *Harv Rev Psychiatry* 27(3), 193–200. doi:10.1097/HRP.0000000000000215

Skott, A. (1978). *Delusions of Infestation: Dermatozoenwahn-Ekbom's Syndrome.* University of Goteborg Press, Goteborg.

Slater, E., & Roth, M. (1970). *Clinical Psychiatry.* Bailliere, Tindall and Cassell, London.

Sluhovsky, M. (1996). A divine apparition or demonic possession? Female agency and church authority in demonic possession in sixteenth-century France. *Sixteenth Century Journal* 27(4),1039–55.

Smilek, D., Callejas, A., Dixon, M. J., & Merikle, P. M. (2007). Ovals of time: Time-space associations in synaesthesia. *Conscious Cogn* 16(2),507–19. doi: 10.1016/j.concog.2006.06.013.

Smilek, D., Dixon, M. J., Cudahy, C., & Merikle, P. M. (2001). Synaesthetic photisms influence visual perception. *J Cogn Neurosci* 13(7), 930–6. doi:0.1.1.383.8926

Smulevich, A. B., Lvov, A. N., & Romanov, D. V. (2016). Hypochondriasis circumscripta: A neglected concept with important implications in psychodermatology. *Acta Derm Venereol* 96(217), 64–8. doi:10.2340/00015555-2371

Sno, H. N. (1994). A continuum of misidentification symptoms. *Psychopathology* 27(3–5), 144–7.

Snyder, S. L., & Buchsbaum, M. S. (1998). Unusual visual symptoms and Ganser-like state due to cerebral injury: A case study using ^{18}F-deoxyglucose positron emission tomography. *Behav Neurol* 11, 51–4. doi: 10.1155/1998/907914

Sofko, C., Tremont, G., Tan, J. E., et al. (2020). Olfactory and neuropsychological functioning in olfactory reference syndrome. *Psychosomatics* 61(3), 261–7. doi:10.1016/j.psym.2019.12.009

Solimine, S., Chan, S., & Morihara, S. K. (2016). Côtard syndrome: 'I'm dead, so why do I need to eat?'. *Primary Care Companion CNS Disorders* 18(2). doi:10.4088/PCC.15l01862

Solla, P., Cannas, A., Orofino, G., & Marrosu, F. (2015). Fluctuating Côtard syndrome in a patient with advanced Parkinson disease. *Neurologist* 19(3), 70–2. doi: 10.1097/NRL.0000000000000010

Song, C. I., & Jung, Y. E. (2019). Musical hallucination caused by ceftazidime in a woman with a hearing impairment. *Clin Psychopharmacol Neurosci* 17(2), 326–8. doi:10.9758/cpn.2019.17.2.326

Sonnenblick, M., Nesher, R., Rozenman, Y., & Nesher, G. (1995). Charles Bonnet syndrome in temporal arteritis. *J Rheumatol* 22(8), 1596–7.

Sottile, F., Bonanno, L., Finzi, G., & Ascenti, G. (2015). Côtard and Capgras syndrome after ischemic stroke. *J Stroke Cerebrovasc Dis* 24 (4), e103–4. doi: 10.1016/j. jstrokecerebrovasdis.2015.01.001.

Soultanian, C., Perisse, D., & Révah-Levy, A. (2005). Côtard's syndrome in adolescents and young adults: A possible onset of bipolar disorder requiring a mood stabilizer? *J Child Adolesc Psychopharmacol* 15(4), 706–11. doi:10.1089/cap.2005.15.706

Spanos, N. P. (1994). Multiple identity enactments and multiple personality disorder: A sociocognitive perspective. *Psychol Bull* 116(1), 143–65. doi: 10.1037/ 0033-2909.116.1.143

Spitzer, D., White, S. J., Mandy, W., & Burgess, P. W. (2017). Confabulation in children with autism. *Cortex* 87, 80–95. doi:10.1016/j.cortex.2016.10.004

Stanton, B. R., David, A. S., Cleare, A. J., & Sierra, M. (2001). Basal activity of the hypothalamic–pituitary–adrenal axis in patients with depersonalization disorder. *Psychiatr Res* 104(1), 85–9. doi: 10.1016/ s0165-1781(01)00291-8

Staton, R. D., Brumback, R. A., & Wilson, H. (1982). Reduplicative paramnesia: A disconnection syndrome of memory. *Cortex* 18(1), 23–35.

Stein, D. J., Le Roux, L., Bouwer, C., & Van Heerden, B. (1998). Is olfactory reference syndrome an obsessive-compulsive spectrum disorder? Two cases and a discussion. *J Neuropsychiatry Clin Neurosci* 10(1), 96–9. doi/pdfplus/10.1176/jnp.10.1.96

Steinert, T., & Studemund, H. (2006). Acute delusional parasitosis under treatment with ciprofloxacin. *Pharmacopsychiatry* 39(4), 159–60. doi:10.1055/s-2006-947183

Sternberg, R. J. (1986). A triangular theory of love. *Psychol Rev* 93(2), 119–35.

Sternberg, R. J. (1988). Triangulating love. In R. J. Sternberg & M. L. Barnes (eds.), *The Psychology of Love* (pp. 119–38). Yale University Press, New Haven, CT.

Stevens, A., & Price, J. (2015). *Evolutionary Psychiatry*. Routledge, London.

Stewart, L., von Kriegstein, K., Warren, J. D., & Griffiths, T. D. (2006). Music and the brain: Disorders of musical listening. *Brain* 129(Pt 10), 2533–53. doi:10.1093/ brain/awl171

Stickley, T., & Nickeas, R. (2006). Becoming one person: Living with dissociative identity disorder. *J Psychiatric Ment Health* 13(2), 180–7. doi/abs/10.1111/ j.1365–2850.2006.00939.x

Strawhun, J., Adams, N., & Huss, M. T. (2013). The assessment of cyberstalking: An expanded examination including social networking, attachment, jealousy, and anger in relation to violence and abuse. *Violence Vict* 28(4), 715–30.

Stricker, R. B., & Winger, E. E. (2003). Musical hallucinations in patients with Lyme disease: Case report. *South Med J* 96(7), 711–16.

Strickland, O. L. (1987). The occurrence of symptoms in expectant fathers. *Nurs Res* 36 (3), 184–9.

Suárez-Richards, M., & Fournes, O. (2002). Erotomania preceding an aneurysmal subarachnid hemorrhage: Is there an association. *J Affect Disord* 70(3), 333–6.

Sutton, R. L. (1919). Bromidrosiphobia. *JAMA* 72(18), 1267–8.

Suzuki, K., Takei, N., Iwata, Y., et al. (2004). Do olfactory reference syndrome and jiko-shu-kyofu (a subtype of taijin-kyofu) share a common entity? *Acta Psychiatr Scand* 109(2), 150–5. doi:10.1046/j.1600-0447.2003.00195.x

Tagler, M. J. (2010). Sex differences in jealousy: Comparing the influence of previous infidelity among college students and adults. *Soc Psychol Person Sci* 1(4), 353–60. doi:10.1177/1948550610374367

Takahashi, Y. (1990). Is multiple personality disorder really rare in Japan. *Dissociation* 3 (2), 57–9.

Tamam, L., Karatas, G., Zeren, T., & Ozpoyraz, N. (2003). The prevalence of Capgras syndrome in a university hospital setting. *Acta Neuropsychiatry* 15(5), 290–5. doi:10.1034/j.1601-5215.2003.00039.x

Tan, C. S., & Au Eong, K. G. (2007). Charles Bonnet syndrome associated with first attack of MS. *Jpn J Ophthalmol* 51 (1),82; author reply 82–3. doi:10.1007/s10384-006-0401-6

Taylor, F. K. (1966). *Psychopathology.* Butterworths, London.

Taylor, F. K. (1981). On pseudo-hallucinations. *Psychol Med* 11(2), 265–71.

Teixeira, B. , & Araújo, A. F. (2015). Côtard's syndrome: Two cases of self-starvation. *Psilogos Revista* 13(1), 124–33. doi:10.25752/PSI.6296

Teja, J. S., & Khanna, B. S. (1970). 'Possession states' in Indian patients. *Indian J Psychiatry* 12, 71–87.

Tényi, T., Herold, R., Fekete, S., et al. (2001). Coexistence of delusions of pregnancy and infestation in a male. *Psychopathology* 34(4), 215–16. doi:10.1159/000049310

Tényi, T., Trixler, M., & Jádi, F. (1996). Psychotic couvade: 2 case reports. *Psychopathology* 29(4), 252–4. doi:10.1159/000285002

Terao, T. (1995). Tricyclic-induced musical hallucinations and states of relative sensory deprivation. *Biol Psychiatry* 38(3), 192–3.

Teunisse, R. J., & Rikkert, M. G. M. O. (2012). Prevalence of musical hallucinations in patients referred for audiometric testing. *Am J Geriatr Psychiatry* 20(12), 1075–7.

Teunisse, R. J., Zitman, F. G., & Raes, D. C. (1994). Clinical evaluation of 14 patients with the Charles Bonnet syndrome (isolated visual hallucinations). *Compr Psychiatry* 35(1), 70–5. doi:10.1016/0010-440x(94)90172-4

Teunisse, R. J., Cruysberg, J. R., Hoefnagels, W. H., et al. (1999). Social and psychological characteristics of elderly visually handicapped patients with the Charles Bonnet Syndrome. *Compr Psychiatry* 40(4), 315–19. doi:10.1016/s0010-440x(99)90133-5

Teunisse, R. J., Cruysberg, J. R., Verbeek, A., & Zitman, F. G. (1995). The Charles Bonnet syndrome: A large prospective study in the Netherlands. A study of the prevalence of the Charles Bonnet syndrome and associated factors in 500 patients attending the University Department of Ophthalmology at Nijmegen. *Br J Psychiatry* 166(2), 254–7. doi:10.1192/bjp.166.2.254

Thaipisuttikul, P., Lobach, I., Zweig, Y., et al. (2013). Capgras syndrome in dementia with Lewy bodies. *Int Psychogeriatr* 25(5), 843–9. doi:10.1017/S1041610212002189

Thiel, C. M., Studte, S., Hildebrandt, H., et al. (2014). When a loved one feels unfamiliar: A case study on the neural basis of Capgras delusion. *Cortex* 52, 75–85. doi:10.1016/j.cortex.2013.11.011

Thompson, A. E., & Swan, M. (1993). Capgras' syndrome presenting with violence following heavy drinking. *Br J Psychiatry* 162, 692–4.

Thorpe, J. G. (1961). Sensory deprivation. *J Ment Sci* 107(451), 1047–59.

Tilley, H. (1895). Three cases of parosmia: Causes, treatment. *Lancet* 146(3763), 907–8.

Todd, J., Dewhurst, K., & Wallis, G. (1981). The syndrome of Capgras. *Br J Psychiatry* 139, 319–27.

Todd, J., & Dewhurst, K. (1955). The Othello syndrome: A study in the psychopathology of sexual jealousy. *J Nerv Ment Dis* 122(4), 367–74.

Tolstoy, G. L. (1985). *The Kreutzer Sonata and Other Stories.* Penguin Books Ltd, London.

Toone, B. K. (1978). Psychomotor seizures, arterio-venous malformation and the olfactory reference syndrome: A case report. *Acta Psychiatr Scand* 58(1), 61–6. doi:10.1111/j.1600-0447.1978.tb06921.x

Trabert, W. (1995). 100 years of delusional parasitosis: Meta-analysis of 1,223 case reports. *Psychopathology* 28(5), 238–46. doi:10.1159/000284934

Trangkasombat, U., & Su-Umpan, U. (1998). Risk factors for spirit possession among school girls in southern Thailand. *J Med Assoc Thai* 81(7), 541–6.

Traver, J. (1951). Unusual scalp dermatitis in humans caused by the mite Dermatophagoides (Acarina, Epidermoptidae). *Proc Entomol Soc Washington* 53(1), 1–25.

Trethowan, W. H., & Conlon, M. F. (1965). The couvade syndrome. *Br J Psychiatry* 111, 57–66.

Trevisani, M., Smart, D., Gunthorpe, M. J., et al. (2002). Ethanol elicits and potentiates nociceptor responses via the vanilloid receptor-1. *Nat Neurosci* 5, 546–51.

Tsoi, W. F. (1973). The Ganser syndrome in Singapore: A report on ten cases. *Br J Psychiatry* 123(576), 567–72). doi: 10.1192/bjp.123.5.567.

Turner, M. L., & Marinoff, S. C. (1988). Association of human papillomavirus with vulvodynia and the vulvar vestibulitis syndrome. *J Reprod Med* 33(6), 533–7.

Tympanidis, P., Terenghi, G., & Dowd, P. (2003). Increased innervation of the vulval vestibule in patients with vulvodynia. *Br J Dermatol* 148(5), 1021–7. doi:10.1046/j.1365-2133.2003.05308.x

Tympanidis, P., Casula, M. A., Yiangou, Y., et al. (2004). Increased vanilloid receptor VR1 innervation in vulvodynia. *Eur J Pain* 8 (2), 129–33. doi:10.1016/S1090-3801(03) 00085-5

Tyndel, M. (1956). Some aspects of the Ganser state. *J Ment Sci* 102(427), 324–9.

Uguru, C., Umeanuka, O., Uguru, N. P., et al. (2011). The delusion of halitosis: Experience at an Eastern Nigerian tertiary hospital. *Niger J Med* 20(2), 236–40.

Ukai, S., Yamamoto, M., Tanaka, M., et al. (2007). Donepezil in the treatment of musical hallucinations. *Psychiatry Clin Neurosci* 61 (2), 190–2. doi:10.1111/j.1440-1819.2007.01636.x

Ulzen, T. P., & Carpentier, R. (1997). The delusional parent: Family and multisystemic issues. *Can J Psychiatry* 42(6), 617–22. doi:10.1177/070674379704200608

Vaitl, D., Birbaumer, N., & Gruzelier, J. (2005). Psychobiology of altered states of consciousness. *Psychol Bull* 131(1), 98–127. doi: 10.1037/0033-2909.131.1.98

Varma, S. L., & Katsenos, S. (1999). Delusion of pregnancy. *Aust NZ J Psychiatry* 33(1), 118.

Veale, D., & Matsunaga, H. (2014). Body dysmorphic disorder and olfactory reference disorder: Proposals for ICD-11. *Brazil J Psychiatry* 36, 14–20.

Venkataramaiah, V., & Mallikarjunaiah, M. (1981). Possession syndrome: An epidemiological study in West Karnataka. *Indian J Psychiatry* 23(3), 213–18.

Vermetten, E., Schmahl, C., & Lindner, S. (2006). Hippocampal and amygdalar volumes in dissociative identity disorder. *Am J Psychiatry* 163(4), 630–6. doi:10.1176/ajp.2006.163.4.630

Victor, M., Adams, R. D., & Collins, G. H. (1971). The Wernicke-Korsakoff syndrome: A clinical and pathological study of 245 patients, 82 with post-mortem examinations. *Contemp Neurol Ser* 7, 1–203.

Victor, M., & Yakovlev, P. I. (1955). SS Korsakoff's psychic disorder in conjunction with peripheral neuritis: A translation of Korsakoff's original article with brief comments on the author and his contribution to clinical medicine. *Neurology* 5(6), 394. doi.org/10.1212/WNL.5.6.394

Vieira-Baptista, P., Lima-Silva, J., Cavaco-Gomes, J., & Beires, J. (2014). Prevalence of vulvodynia and risk factors for the condition in Portugal. *Int J Gynecol Obstet* 127(3), 283–7. doi:10.1016/j.ijgo.2014.05.020

Vogel, B. F. (1974). The Capgras syndrome and its psychopathology. *Am J Psychiatry* 131(8), 922–4.

Vukicevic, M., & Fitzmaurice, K. (2008). Butterflies and black lacy patterns: The prevalence and characteristics of Charles Bonnet hallucinations in an Australian population. *Clin Exp Ophthalmol* 36(7), 659–65. doi:10.1111/j.1442-9071.2008.01814.x

Wainwright, W. H. (1966). Fatherhood as a precipitant of mental illness. *Am J Psychiatry* 123(1), 40–4.

Waldinger, M. D., Venema, P. L., van Gils, A. P. G., et al. (2011). Stronger evidence for small fiber sensory neuropathy in restless genital syndrome: Two case reports in males. *J Sex Med* 8(1), 325–30. doi:10.1111/j.1743-6109.2010.02079.x

Waldinger, M. D., Venema, P. L., Van Gils, A. P. G., & Schweitzer, D. H. (2009). New insights into restless genital syndrome: Static mechanical hyperesthesia and neuropathy of the nervus dorsalis clitoridis. *J Sex Med* 6(10), 2778–87. doi:10.1111/j.1743-6109.2009.01435.x

Walker, J. D., & Keys, M. A. (2008). Dementia with Lewy bodies and Charles Bonnet syndrome. *Retin Cases Brief Rep* 2(1), 27–30. doi:10.1097/01.iae.0000243039.22011.5f

Walloch, J. E., Klauwer, C., Lanczik, M., et al. (2007). Delusional denial of pregnancy as a special form of Côtard's syndrome. *Psychopathology* 40(1), 61–4. doi: 10.1159/000096685.

Walther, S., Federspiel, A., Horn, H., et al. (2010a). Performance during face processing differentiates schizophrenia patients with delusional misidentifications. *Psychopathology* 43(2), 127–36. doi:10.1159/000277002

Wang, T., Parish, W. L., & Laumann, E. O. (2009). Partner violence and sexual jealousy in China: A population-based survey. *Violence Against Women* 15(7), 774–88. doi:10.1177/1077801209334271

Ward, J. (2009). *The Frog Who Croaked Blue: Synesthesia and the Mixing of the Senses.* Routledge, London.

Ward, J., Simner, J., & Auyeung, V. (2005). A comparison of lexical-gustatory and grapheme-colour synaesthesia. *Cognit Neuropsychol* 22(1), 28–41. doi: 10.1080/02643290442000022

.Ward, J., Thompson-Lake, D. , & Ely, R. (2008). Synaesthesia, creativity and art: What is the link. *Br J Psychol* 99(1), 127–41. doi:10.1348/000712607X204164

Ward, J., Li, R., Salih, S., & Sagiv, N. (2007). Varieties of grapheme-colour synaesthesia: A new theory of phenomenological and behavioural differences. *Conscious Cognit* 16(4), 913–31.

Wardener, H. E. D., & Lennox, B. (1947). Cerebral beriberi (Wernicke's encephalopathy): Review of 52 cases in a Singapore prisoner-of-war hospital. *Lancet* 1(6436), 11–17.

Weinstein, E. A. (1994). The classification of delusional misidentification syndromes. *Psychopathology* 27(3–5), 130–5.

Weiss, C., Santander, J., & Torres, R. (2013). Catatonia, neuroleptic malignant syndrome, and Côtard syndrome in a 22-year-old woman: A case report. *Case Rep Psychiatry* 2013:452646. doi: 10.1155/2013/452646.

Wertham, F. (1949). *The Shadow of Violence.* Gollancz, London.

Westermeyer, J., Lyfoung, T., Wahmanholm, K., & Westermeyer, M. (1989). Delusions of fatal contagion among refugee patients. *Psychosomatics* 30(4), 374–82.

White, G. L., & Mullen, P. E. (1992). *Jealousy.* Guilford Press, New York.

White, T. G. (1995). Folie simultanée in monozygotic twins. *Can J Psychiatry* 40(7), 418–20.

Whitlock, F. A. (1967). The Ganser syndrome. *Br J Psychiatry* 113(494), 19–29. doi: 10.1192/bjp.113.494.19

Wilkins, L. K., Girard, T. A., & Cheyne, J. A. (2011). Ketamine as a primary predictor of out-of-body experiences associated with multiple substance use. *Conscious Cognit* 20(3), 943–50. doi: 10.1016/j.concog.2011.01.005

Wilkins, L. K., Girard, T. A., & Cheyne, J. A. (2012). Anomalous bodily-self experiences among recreational ketamine users. *Cognit Neuropsychiatry* 17(5),415–30. doi:10.1080/13546805.2012.663162

Wilson, E. O. (2000). *Sociobiology.* Harvard University Press, Cambridge, MA.

Wilson, J. W., & Miller, H. E. (1946). Delusion of parasitosis (acarophobia). *Arch Dermatol Syphilol* 54(1), 39–56.

Wilson, L. G. (1977). The couvade syndrome. *Am Fam Phys* 15(5), 157–60.

Wilson, M., & Daly, M. (1993). Spousal homicide risk and estrangement. *Violence Vict* 8, 3–16.

Wilson, M., Daly, M., & Daniele, A. (1995). Familicide: The killing of spouse and children. *Aggressive Behavior* 21(4), 275–91.

Wilson, M. E., Pointdujour-Lim, R., Lally, S., et al. (2016). Acute Charles Bonnet syndrome following Hughes procedure. *Orbit* 35(5), 292–4. doi:10.1080/01676830.2016.1176218

Wilson, P. J. (1967). Status ambiguity and spirit possession. *Man* 2(3), 366–78.

Witztum, E., & Grisaru, N. (1996). The 'Zar'possession syndrome among Ethiopian immigrants to Israel: Cultural and clinical aspects. *Br J Med Psychol* 69(3), 207–25. doi:10.1111/j.2044-8341.1996.tb01865.x

Wodarz, N., Becker, T., & Deckert, J. (1995). Musical hallucinations associated with post-thyroidectomy hypoparathyroidism and symmetric basal ganglia calcifications. *J Neurol Neurosurg Psychiatry* 58(6), 763–4. doi:10.1136/jnnp.58.6.763

Wolf, R. C., Huber, M., Depping, M. S., et al. (2013). Abnormal gray and white matter volume in delusional infestation. *Prog Neuropsychopharmacol Biol Psychiatry* 46, 19–24. doi:10.1016/j.pnpbp.2013.06.004

Wolf, R. C., Huber, M., Lepping, P., et al. (2014). Source-based morphometry reveals distinct patterns of aberrant brain volume in delusional infestation. *Prog Neuropsychopharmacol Biol Psychiatry* 48, 112–16. doi:10.1016/j.pnpbp.2013.09.019

Wollina, U. (2011). Red scrotum syndrome. *J Dermatol Case Rep* 5(3), 38–41.

Woo, P. Y., Leung, L. N., Cheng, S. T., & Chan, K. Y. (2014). Monoaural musical hallucinations caused by a thalamocortical auditory radiation infarct: A case report. *J Med Case Rep* 8, 400. doi:10.1186/1752-1947-8-400

Wood, W. (2000). Attitude change: Persuasion and social influence. *Ann Rev Psychol* 51(1), 539–70.

Woodruff, P. W., Higgins, E. M., du Vivier, A. W., & Wessely, S. (1997). Psychiatric illness in patients referred to a dermatology-psychiatry clinic. *Gen Hosp Psychiatry* 19(1), 29–35. doi:10.1016/s0163-8343(97)00155-2

Woytassek, L. E., & Atwal, S. S. (1985). Capgras syndrome in court. *Nebr Med J* 70(11), 392–4.

Wright, S., & Young, A. W. (1993). Sequential cotard and capgras delusions. *Br J Clin Psychol* 32(3), 345–9. doi:10.1111/j.2044-8260.1993.tb01065.x

Wylie, K., Hallam-Jones, R., & Harrington, C. (2004). Psychological difficulties within a group of patients with vulvodynia. *J Psychosom Obstet Gynecol* 25(3–4), 257–65.

Yalin, Ş. , Varol Taş, F., & Gunevir, T. (2008). The coexistence of Capgras, Fregoli and Côtard's syndromes in an adolescent case. *Arch Neuropsychiatry* 45, 149–51.

Yang, E. J., Beck, K. M., & Koo, J. (2019). Folie à famille: A systematic review of shared delusional infestation. *J Am Acad Dermatol* 81(5), 1211–15. doi:10.1016/j.jaad.2019.04.023

Yap, P. M. (1960). The possession syndrome: A comparison of Hong Kong and French findings. *J Ment Sci* 106, 114–37. doi:10.1192/bjp.106.442.114.

Yarnada, K., Katsuragi, S., & Fujii, I. (1999). A case study of Côtard's syndrome: Stages and diagnosis. *Acta Psychiatr Scand* 100(5), 396–8. doi:10.1111/j.1600-0447.1999.tb10884.x

Yorston, G., Miesch, M., Pleasance, S., & Rubbert, S. (2003). The pre-senile delusion of infestation. *Hist Psychiatry* 14, 229–56.

Young, A. (1975). Why Amhara get kureynya: Sickness and possession in an Ethiopian zar cult. *Am Ethnologist* 2(3), 567–84. doi:10.1525/ae.1975.2.3.02a00130

Young, A. W., Leafhead, K. M., & Szulecka, K. (1994). The Capgras and Côtard delusions. *Psychopathology* 27(3), 226–31. doi: 10.1159/000284874.

Young, A. W., Robertson, I. H., & Hellawell, D. J. (1992). Côtard delusion after brain injury. *Psychol Med* 22(3), 799–804.

Young, L. J. (2009). Being human: Love. Neuroscience reveals all. *Nature* 457 (7226), 148.

Zamboni, G., Budriesi, C., & Nichelli, P. (2005). 'Seeing oneself': A case of autoscopy. *Neurocase* 11(3), 212–15. doi:10.1080/13554790590944799

Zarrouk, E. T. (1991). The co-existence of erotomania and Capgras' syndrome. *Br J Psychiatry* 159, 717–19. doi:10.1192/bjp.159.5.717

Zhang, J., Waisbren, E., Hashemi, N., & Lee, A. G. (2013). Visual hallucinations (Charles Bonnet syndrome) associated with neurosarcoidosis. *Middle East Afr J Ophthalmol* 20(4), 369–71. doi:10.4103/0974-9233.119997

Zhang, Z., Zolnoun, D. A., Francisco, E. M., et al. (2011). Altered central sensitization in subgroups of women with vulvodynia. *Clin J Pain* 27(9), 755.

Zhou, Y., Fox, D., Anand, A., et al. (2015). Artery of percheron infarction as an unusual cause of Korsakoff's syndrome. *Case Rep Neurol Med* 2015, 927809. doi:10.1155/2015/927809

Zhu, T. H., Werchan, I. A., Escamilla, K. V., et al. (2018). Association between delusions of infestation and prescribed narcotic and stimulant use. *J Psychiatr Pract* 24(6), 428–31. doi:10.1097/PRA.0000000000000338

Zilles, D., Zerr, I., & Wedekind, D. (2012). Successful treatment of musical hallucinations with the acetylcholinesterase inhibitor donepezil. *J Clin Psychopharmacol* 32(3), 422–4. doi:10.1097/JCP.0b013e318253a086

Zivković, V., & Nikolić, S. (2014). Philemon and Baucis, Diogenes and syllogomania, Wischnewski and hypothermia: Gastric mucosal lesions in partially mummified bodies. *Med Sci Law* 54(3), 177–80. doi:10.1177/0025802413502331

Index